Handbook of
CLINICAL TRIALS IN OPHTHALMOLOGY

Handbook of
CLINICAL TRIALS IN OPHTHALMOLOGY

Second Edition

Editors

Vinod Kumar MS
Associate Professor
Dr Rajendra Prasad Center for Ophthalmic Sciences
All India Institute of Medical Sciences
New Delhi, India

Neha Goel MS
Co-founder, Director and Senior Consultant
Tetravue Superspecialty Eye Center
New Delhi, India

Pooja Shah MD DNB FICO FAICO
Assistant Professor and Associate Consultant
Bombay Hospital and Medical Research Center
Mumbai, Maharashtra, India

AK Gupta MS
Director Academics
ICARE Eye Hospital and Postgraduate Institute
Noida, Uttar Pradesh
Shroff Eye Center, Kailash Colony
New Delhi, India

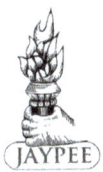

JAYPEE BROTHERS MEDICAL PUBLISHERS
The Health Sciences Publisher
New Delhi | London

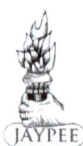 **Jaypee Brothers Medical Publishers (P) Ltd**

Headquarters
Jaypee Brothers Medical Publishers (P) Ltd
EMCA House, 23/23-B
Ansari Road, Daryaganj
New Delhi 110 002, India
Landline: +91-11-23272143, +91-11-23272703
+91-11-23282021, +91-11-23245672
Email: jaypee@jaypeebrothers.com

Corporate Office
Jaypee Brothers Medical Publishers (P) Ltd
4838/24, Ansari Road, Daryaganj
New Delhi 110 002, India
Phone: +91-11-43574357
Fax: +91-11-43574314
Email: jaypee@jaypeebrothers.com

Overseas Office
J.P. Medical Ltd
83 Victoria Street, London
SW1H 0HW (UK)
Phone: +44 20 3170 8910
Fax: +44 (0)20 3008 6180
Email: info@jpmedpub.com

Website: www.jaypeebrothers.com
Website: www.jaypeedigital.com

© 2022, Jaypee Brothers Medical Publishers

The views and opinions expressed in this book are solely those of the original contributor(s)/author(s) and do not necessarily represent those of editor(s) of the book.

All rights reserved. No part of this publication may be reproduced, stored or transmitted in any form or by any means, electronic, mechanical, photocopying, recording or otherwise, without the prior permission in writing of the publishers.

All brand names and product names used in this book are trade names, service marks, trademarks or registered trademarks of their respective owners. The publisher is not associated with any product or vendor mentioned in this book.

Medical knowledge and practice change constantly. This book is designed to provide accurate, authoritative information about the subject matter in question. However, readers are advised to check the most current information available on procedures included and check information from the manufacturer of each product to be administered, to verify the recommended dose, formula, method and duration of administration, adverse effects and contraindications. It is the responsibility of the practitioner to take all appropriate safety precautions. Neither the publisher nor the author(s)/editor(s) assume any liability for any injury and/or damage to persons or property arising from or related to use of material in this book.

This book is sold on the understanding that the publisher is not engaged in providing professional medical services. If such advice or services are required, the services of a competent medical professional should be sought.

Every effort has been made where necessary to contact holders of copyright to obtain permission to reproduce copyright material. If any have been inadvertently overlooked, the publisher will be pleased to make the necessary arrangements at the first opportunity. The **CD/DVD-ROM** (if any) provided in the sealed envelope with this book is complimentary and free of cost. **Not meant for sale.**

Inquiries for bulk sales may be solicited at: jaypee@jaypeebrothers.com

Handbook of Clinical Trials in Ophthalmology

First Edition: 2014

Second Edition: 2022

ISBN: 978-93-90595-07-5

Dedicated to

The participants and investigators of clinical trials

Contributors

AK Gupta MS
Director Academics
ICARE Eye Hospital and
Postgraduate Institute
Noida, Uttar Pradesh
Shroff Eye Center, Kailash Colony
New Delhi, India

Anju Bhari MD
Senior Resident
Strabismus, Neuro-ophthalmology
and Oculoplasty
Dr Rajendra Prasad Center for
Ophthalmic Sciences
All India Institute of Medical
Sciences
New Delhi, India

Archita Singh MD FICO FAICO
Senior Resident
Cornea and Refractive Surgery
Dr Rajendra Prasad Center for
Ophthalmic Sciences
All India Institute of Medical
Sciences
New Delhi, India

Arpit Sharma MD
Fellow
Vitreo-retina
Arvind Eye Institute
Madurai, Tamil Nadu, India

Brijesh Takkar MD
Consultant
Retina Services
LV Prasad Eye Institute
Hyderabad, Telangana, India

Mohammad Sabir MBBS
Junior Resident
Dr Rajendra Prasad Center for
Ophthalmic Sciences
All India Institute of Medical
Sciences
New Delhi, India

Neha Goel MS
Co-founder, Director and Senior
Consultant
Tetravue Superspeciality Eye Center
New Delhi, India

Noopur Gupta MD
Associate Professor
Cornea and Refractive Surgery
Dr Rajendra Prasad Center for
Ophthalmic Sciences
All India Institute of Medical
Sciences
New Delhi, India

Pooja Shah MD DNB FICO FAICO
Assistant Professor and Associate
Consultant
Bombay Hospital and Medical
Research Center
Mumbai, Maharashtra, India

Priyanka Ramesh MD
Senior Resident
Glaucoma Services
Dr Rajendra Prasad Center for
Ophthalmic Sciences
All India Institute of Medical
Sciences
New Delhi, India

Rohan Chawla MD FRCS
Associate Professor
Retina Services
Dr Rajendra Prasad Center for
Ophthalmic Sciences
All India Institute of Medical
Sciences
New Delhi, India

Saurabh Verma MD
Senior Resident
Retina Services
Dr Rajendra Prasad Center for
Ophthalmic Sciences
All India Institute of Medical
Sciences
New Delhi, India

Shikha Gupta MD
Assistant Professor
Glaucoma Services
Dr Rajendra Prasad Center for
Ophthalmic Sciences
All India Institute of Medical
Sciences
New Delhi, India

Shorya Azad MD
Assistant Professor
Retina Services
Dr Rajendra Prasad Center for
Ophthalmic Sciences
All India Institute of Medical
Sciences
New Delhi, India

Sonali Gupta MS
Specialist
ESIC Model Hospital
Noida, Uttar Pradesh, India

Sumit Monga MS DNB FRCS
Senior Consultant
Pediatric Ophthalmology
Centre for Sight
New Delhi, India

Swati Phuljhele MD
Associate Professor
Squint and Neuro-ophthalmology
Dr Rajendra Prasad Center for
Ophthalmic Sciences
All India Institute of Medical
Sciences
New Delhi, India

Vinod Kumar MS
Associate Professor
Dr Rajendra Prasad Center for
Ophthalmic Sciences
All India Institute of Medical
Sciences
New Delhi, India

Preface to the Second Edition

The impact of clinical trials on the practice of medicine cannot be underestimated. Anyone involved in healthcare today must know the basics of running and interpreting clinical trial data. In order to form opinions and make judgments, clinicians require access to reliable sources of evidence. Ideally, this data should be easily accessible to the practitioners in order to implement the latest findings in their respective field. Also for students in this area of specialization, this data is an invaluable resource of information on previously conducted research. Not only does this add to their clinical acumen, but this knowledge is also frequently tested in all examinations and reviews.

Although the clinical trials in the field of ophthalmology are numerous, yet one would need to spend considerable time and effort to locate each relevant one and learn from it. This book offers every clinical ophthalmologist complete guidance as it compiles the results of the latest multicenter clinical trials in the practice of ophthalmology with relevant references. The trials have been organized into chapters, covering all ophthalmic sub-specialties. Each pertinent trial is described under similar subject headings/styles and has been formatted accordingly for easy reading and recall. A summary at the end of each chapter has been provided for easy reference. All the major and latest clinical trials have been recorded but it must be understood that the list is not exhaustive.

Such significant consolidated information can be uniquely valuable to a wide audience. The first edition of the book was in fact a recommended read by the prestigious International Council of Ophthalmology. In the second edition, the individual chapters have been authored by respective experts in the field. Over 70 different trials have been added to make the knowledge of the reader contemporary.

Knowledge of these trials in clinical practice can lead to significant improvements in patient care and patient outcome in ophthalmology. General ophthalmologists will have the current standard of patient care across the spectrum of ophthalmology at their fingertips, in an easily digestible format. Residents reviewing the major subspecialties for board examinations, comprehensive ophthalmologists keeping abreast of all areas of ophthalmology, and subspecialists interested in future direction of their area of focus, will all find the second edition of this book a good reference.

Vinod Kumar
Neha Goel
Pooja Shah
AK Gupta

Preface to the First Edition

The impact of clinical trials on the practice of medicine cannot be underestimated. Anyone involved in healthcare today must know the basics of running and interpreting clinical trial data. In order to form opinions and make judgments, clinicians require access to reliable sources of evidence. Ideally, this data should be easily accessible to the practitioners in order to implement the latest findings in their respective field. Also, for students in this area of specialization, this data is an invaluable resource of information on previously conducted research. Not only does this add to their clinical acumen, this knowledge is frequently tested in all examinations and reviews.

Although the clinical trials in the field of ophthalmology are numerous, yet one would need to spend considerable time and effort to locate each relevant one and learn from it. This book offers every clinical ophthalmologist complete guidance as it compiles the results of the latest multicenter clinical trials in the practice of ophthalmology with relevant references. The trials have been organized into chapters, covering all ophthalmic subspecialties. Each pertinent trial is described under similar subject headings/styles and has been formatted accordingly for easy reading and recall. A summary at the end of each chapter has been provided for easy reference. All the trials have been listed alphabetically and indexed at the end.

Such significant consolidated information can be uniquely valuable to a wide audience. The individual studies can be traced for details as the book provides all the relevant references. This handbook is not distorting any facts or adding any other perspective, suggestions or implications. It is an effort to provide a convenient and quick reference for the vast data available. All the major and latest clinical trials have been recorded but it must be understood that the list is not exhaustive.

Knowledge of these trials in clinical practice can lead to significant improvements in patient care and patient outcome in ophthalmology. General ophthalmologists will have the current standard of patient care across the spectrum of ophthalmology at their fingertips, in an easily digestible format. Residents reviewing the major subspecialties for board examinations, comprehensive ophthalmologists keeping abreast of all areas of ophthalmology, and subspecialists interested in future direction of their area of focus, will all find this book a good reference.

AK Gupta
Vinod Kumar Aggarwal
Neha Goel

Contents

1. Clinical Trials in Cornea 1
Archita Singh, Noopur Gupta

Herpetic Eye Disease Study (HEDS) I   *1*
Herpetic Eye Disease Study (HEDS) II   *3*
Mycotic Ulcer Treatment Trial (MUTT) I   *5*
Mycotic Ulcer Treatment Trial (MUTT) II   *7*
Steroid in Corneal Ulcers Trial (SCUT)   *8*
Collaborative Longitudinal Evaluation of
Keratoconus (CLEK) Study   *9*
Collaborative Corneal Transplantation Studies (CCTS)   *11*
Cornea Donor Study   *13*
Dream Study (Dry Eye Assessment and Management)   *15*
Prospective Evaluation of Radial Keratotomy (PERK) Study   *16*
Pioneer Study—Prospective Intraoperative and Perioperative
Ophthalmic ImagiNg with Optical CoherEncE TomogRaphy   *17*

2. Clinical Trials in Glaucoma 27
Priyanka Ramesh, Shikha Gupta

Early Manifest Glaucoma Trial (EMGT)   *27*
Collaborative Initial Glaucoma Treatment Study (CIGTS)   *29*
Ocular Hypertension Treatment Study (OHTS)   *30*
European Glaucoma Prevention Study   *32*
Collaborative Normal Tension Glaucoma Study (CNTGS)   *34*
Advanced Glaucoma Intervention Study (AGIS)   *36*
Glaucoma Laser Trial Follow-up Study (GLTFS)   *38*
Fluorouracil Filtering Surgery Study (FFSS)   *40*
Tube Versus Trabeculectomy Study (TVT)   *42*
Trabeculectomy Versus Canaloplasty (TVC Study) in the
Treatment of Patients with Open Angle Glaucoma: A Prospective
Randomized Clinical Trial   *43*
Effectiveness of Early Lens Extraction for the Treatment of
Primary Angle Closure Glaucoma (EAGLE): A Randomized
Control Trial   *45*
Early Lens Extraction with Intraocular Lens Implantation for the
Treatment of Primary Angle Closure Glaucoma: An Economic
Evaluation Based on Data from the EAGLE Trial   *47*
The Ahmed Versus Baerveldt Study (AVB Study). 5-Year
Treatment Outcomes   *49*

A Randomized, Controlled Comparison of Latanoprostene Bunod and Latanoprost 0.005% in the Treatment of Ocular Hypertension and Open Angle Glaucoma: The VOYAGER Study *52*
A Prospective, Randomized, Placebo Controlled, Double-Masked, Three-Armed, Multicenter Phase II/III Trial for the Study of a Topical Treatment of Ischemic Central Retinal Vein Occlusion to Prevent Neovascular Glaucoma—the STRONG Study: Study Protocol for A Randomized Controlled Trial *54*
Glaucoma Epidemiological Studies in India *57*
Other Recent Trails *66*

3. Clinical Trials in Diabetic Retinopathy-I 78
Neha Goel, Vinod Kumar

Wisconsin Epidemiological Study of Diabetic Retinopathy (WESDR) *78*
Diabetes Control and Complications Trial (DCCT) *80*
Epidemiology of Diabetes Interventions and Complications (EDIC) *82*
United Kingdom Prospective Diabetes Study (UKPDS) *83*
Appropriate Blood Pressure Control in NIDDM (ABCD) *85*

4. Clinical Trials in Diabetic Retinopathy-II 90
Neha Goel, Vinod Kumar

Diabetic Retinopathy Study (DRS) *90*
Early Treatment Diabetic Retinopathy Study (ETDRS) *93*
Diabetic Retinopathy Vitrectomy Study (DRVS) *98*

5. Clinical Trials in Diabetic Retinopathy-III 103
Neha Goel, Brijesh Takkar, Pooja Shah

Diabetic Retinopathy Clinical Research Network (DRCR.net) *103*
Other Important Conclusions of Various DRCR.net Studies *122*

6. Clinical Trials in Diabetic Retinopathy-IV..................... 131
Neha Goel, Saurabh Verma, Shorya Azad

Ranibizumab for Edema of the Macula in Diabetes: A Phase 2 Study (READ-2) *132*
A Study of Ranibizumab Injection in Subjects with Clinically Significant Macular Edema with Center Involvement Secondary to Diabetes Mellitus (RISE and RIDE) *134*
Safety and Efficacy of Ranibizumab in Diabetic Macular Edema with Center Involvement (RESOLVE) *136*
Ranibizumab Monotherapy or Combined with Laser Versus Laser Monotherapy for Diabetic Macular Edema (RESTORE) *137*

A Prospective Randomized Trial of Intravitreal Bevacizumab or Laser Therapy in the Management of Diabetic Macular Edema (BOLT)   *139*
DME and VEGF TRAP-EYE: Investigation of Clinical Impact (DA VINCI)   *140*
VEGF Trap-Eye in Vision Impairment due to DME (Vista DME)   *142*
Fluocinolone Acetonide in Diabetic Macular Edema (FAME)   *143*
Three-Year, Randomized, Sham-Controlled Trial of Dexamethasone Intravitreal Implant in Patients with Diabetic Macular Edema (MEAD study)   *144*
A Randomized Clinical Trial of Intravitreal Bevacizumab Versus Intravitreal Dexamethasone for Diabetic Macular Edema: The Bevordex Study   *146*
Dexamethasone Implant for Diabetic Macular Edema in Naive Compared with Refractory Eyes: The International Retina Group Real-Life 24-Month Multicenter Study. The IRGREL-DEX Study   *147*

7. Clinical Trials in Retinal Vascular Occlusions 153
Neha Goel, Pooja Shah, Vinod Kumar

Branch Vein Occlusion Study (BVOS)   *153*
Central Vein Occlusion Study (CVOS)   *156*
Standard Care Versus Corticosteroid for Retinal Vein Occlusion (SCORE) Study   *161*
Ranibizumab for the Treatment of Macular Edema Following Branch Retinal Vein Occlusion: Evaluation of Efficacy and Safety (BRAVO)   *165*
Central Retinal Vein Occlusion Study: Evaluation of Efficacy and Safety (CRUISE)   *167*
Global Evaluation of Implantable Dexamethasone in Retinal Vein Occlusion with Macular Edema (GENEVA)   *168*
Controlled Phase 3 Evaluation of Repeated Intravitreal Administration of VEGF Trap-Eye in Central Retinal Vein Occlusion: Utility and Safety (COPERNICUS)   *171*
General Assessment Limiting Infiltration of Exudates in Central Retinal Vein Occlusion with VEGF Trap-Eye (GALILEO)   *173*
Study of Comparative Treatments for Retinal Vein Occlusion 2 (SCORE 2)   *174*
Study to Assess the Clinical Efficacy and Safety of Intravitreal Aflibercept Injection in Patients with Branch Retinal Vein Occlusion (VIBRANT)   *175*
Head-To-Head Comparison of Ranibizumab PRN Versus Single-Dose Dexamethasone for Branch Retinal Vein Occlusion (COMRADE-B)   *177*
Clinical Efficacy and Safety of Ranibizumab Versus Dexamethasone for Central Retinal Vein Occlusion (COMRADE-C): A European Label Study   *178*

Comparison of Ranibizumab Versus Dexamethasone for Macular Edema Following Retinal Vein Occlusion: 1-year Results of the COMRADE Extension Study *179*

8. Clinical Trials in Age-related Macular Degeneration-I .. 186
Neha Goel, Vinod Kumar

Laser Photocoagulation *186*
Verteporfin Photodynamic Therapy *190*

9. Clinical Trials in Age-related Macular Degeneration-II 207
Neha Goel, Arpit Sharma, Rohan Chawla

Pegaptanib Sodium (Macugen) *208*
Ranibizumab (Lucentis) *210*
Bevacizumab (Avastin) *227*
Ranibizumab Versus Bevacizumab *230*
VEGF Trap-Eye (Aflibercept, Eylea) *238*
Brolucizumab *243*

10. Clinical Trials in Age-related Macular Degeneration-III 253
Pooja Shah, Vinod Kumar

RhuFab V2 Ocular Treatment Combining the Use of Visudyne to Evaluate Safety (FOCUS) *253*
Protect Study *255*
Torpedo Trial *255*
Summit Trials *257*
Radical (Reduced Fluence Visudyne-Anti-VEGF-Dexamethasone in Combination for AMD Lesions) *262*
Cabernet (The Choroidal neovascularization Secondary to AMD Treated with Beta Radiation Epiretinal Therapy) *264*
Initial Versus Delayed Photodynamic Therapy in Combination with Ranibizumab for Treatment of Polypoidal Choroidal Vasculopathy: The Fujisan Study *266*
Aflibercept in Polypoidal Choroidal Vasculopathy (PLANET) Study *267*

11. Clinical Trials in Age-related Macular Degeneration-IV 273
Pooja Shah, Arpit Sharma, Neha Goel

Age-related Eye Disease Study (AREDS) *273*
Age-related Eye Disease Study 2 *276*
Complications of Age-related Macular Degeneration Prevention Trial (CAPT) *278*

12. Clinical Trials in Retinal Detachment 284
Vinod Kumar, Neha Goel

Silicone Oil Study   284
Scleral Buckling Versus Primary Vitrectomy in Rhegmatogenous
Retinal Detachments (SPR) Study   287
Pneumatic Retinopexy versus Vitrectomy for the Management of
Primary Rhegmatogenous Retinal Detachment Outcomes
Randomized Trial (PIVOT)   290

13. Miscellaneous Clinical Trials: Endophthalmitis Vitrectomy Study 295
Vinod Kumar, Neha Goel

Endophthalmitis Vitrectomy Study (EVS)   295
Limitations   299

14. Clinical Trials in Retinopathy of Prematurity 301
Pooja Shah, Neha Goel

Cryotherapy for Retinopathy of Prematurity (CRYO-ROP)   301
Early Treatment for Retinopathy of Prematurity Study (ETROP)   304
Bevacizumab Eliminates the Angiogenic Threat of Retinopathy
of Prematurity (BEAT-ROP)   309
Supplemental Therapeutic Oxygen for Prethreshold Retinopathy of
Prematurity (STOP-ROP)   312
High Oxygen Percentage in Retinopathy of Prematurity Study
(HOPE-ROP)   314
Effects of Light Reduction on Retinopathy of Prematurity
(LIGHT-ROP)   315
Photographic Screening for Retinopathy of Prematurity Study
(PHOTO-ROP)   316
Ranibizumab Versus Laser Therapy for the Treatment of Very Low
Birth Weight Infants with Retinopathy of Prematurity (RAINBOW):
An Open-Label Randomized Controlled Trial   319

15. Miscellaneous Clinical Trials: Infant Aphakia Treatment Study 324
Neha Goel, Sonali Gupta

Infant Aphakia Treatment Study (IATS)   324

16. Clinical Trials in Amblyopia: Pediatric Eye Disease Investigator Group (PEDIG) Studies 328
Sumit Monga, Neha Goel

Amblyopia Treatment Study (ATS)–1   328
Amblyopia Treatment Study (ATS)–2A, 2B, 2C   331
Amblyopia Treatment Study–3   335

Amblyopia Treatment Study–4 338
Amblyopia Treatment Study–5(1) 339
Amblyopia Treatment Study–5(2) 340
Amblyopia Treatment Study–6 342
Amblyopia Treatment Study–7 343
Amblyopia Treatment Study–8 344
Amblyopia Treatment Study–9(1) 345
Amblyopia Treatment Study–9(2) 346
Amblyopia Treatment Study–10 347
Amblyopia Treatment Study–11 349
Amblyopia Treatment Study–12 349
Amblyopia Treatment Study–13 350
Amblyopia Treatment Study–14 352
Amblyopia Treatment Study–15 353
Amblyopia Treatment Study–16 354
Amblyopia Treatment Study–17 355
Amblyopia Treatment Study–18 357
Amblyopia Treatment Study–18 358
Amblyopia Treatment Study–19 359
Amblyopia Treatment Study–20 360

17. Clinical Trials in Neuro-ophthalmology 372
Anju Bhari, Swati Phuljhele

Optic Neuritis and Multiple Sclerosis 372
Clinically Isolated Syndrome (CIS) and Related Clinical Trials 375
Traumatic Optic Neuropathy 385
Leber's Hereditary Optic Neuropathy (LHON) 390

18. Miscellaneous Clinical Trials: Collaborative Ocular Melanoma Study 396
Neha Goel, Vinod Kumar

Collaborative Ocular Melanoma Study (COMS) 396

19. Clinical Trials in Ocular Complications of AIDS 402
Neha Goel, Vinod Kumar

Longitudinal Study of the Ocular Complications of AIDS (LSOCA) 402
Foscarnet–Ganciclovir Cytomegalovirus Retinitis Trial (FGCRT) 409

Index 415

Clinical Trials in Cornea

Archita Singh, Noopur Gupta

■ HERPETIC EYE DISEASE STUDY (HEDS) I[1-3]

Purpose
- To evaluate the efficacy of topical corticosteroids in treating herpes simplex stromal keratitis in conjunction with topical trifluridine.
- To evaluate the efficacy of oral acyclovir in treating herpes simplex stromal keratitis in patients receiving concomitant topical corticosteroids and trifluridine.
- To evaluate the efficacy of oral acyclovir in treating herpes simplex iridocyclitis in conjunction with treatment with topical corticosteroids and trifluridine.

Background
Despite the availability of antiviral agents that are effective in treating herpes simplex epithelial keratitis, inflammation in the corneal tissue and iris can lead to corneal scarring and visual impairment in many patients. Prior to the HEDS-I trials, the role of topical corticosteroids in the management of herpes simplex virus (HSV) stromal keratitis was uncertain. The value of adding an oral antiviral agent to topical corticosteroids and topical antiviral agents was also unknown.

Description
Herpetic Eye Disease Study-I consisted of three randomized, placebo-controlled trials (1992–1996). All patients received the topical antiviral trifluridine as prophylaxis against recurrences of HSV epithelial ulceration. Patients were evaluated weekly for 10 weeks, every other week through week 16, and again at 6 months.

Herpes Stromal Keratitis, Not on Steroid Trial (HEDS-SKN): Patients with active HSV stromal keratitis who had not used a topical corticosteroid in the preceding 10 days were randomized to treatment with topical 1% prednisolone phosphate drops (8 times a day for 7 days, progressively decreased over 10 weeks to once a day) or topical placebo drops (same schedule was followed).

Herpes Stromal Keratitis, on Steroid Treatment (HEDS-SKS): Patients with active HSV stromal keratitis who already were being treated with a topical corticosteroid were randomized either to oral treatment with acyclovir (400 mg five times daily) for 10 weeks or to the identical dose of placebo capsules. Patients also received topical prednisolone phosphate in the dosage schedule described above for the SKN trial.

Herpes Simplex Virus Iridocyclitis, Receiving Topical Steroids (HEDS-IRT): Patients with active HSV iridocyclitis were randomized either to oral treatment with acyclovir (400 mg five times daily) for 10 weeks or to the identical dose of placebo capsules. Patients also received topical prednisolone phosphate in the dosage schedule described above for the SKN trial.

Inclusion Criteria

Patients ≥12 years, no active HSV epithelial keratitis, no prior keratoplasty of the involved eye, and not pregnant.

Study Measures

The primary outcome was the time to development of preset criteria for treatment failure during the 16-week period of examination.

Results

HEDS-SKN: 106 patients were enrolled. Compared with the patients in the placebo group, the patients who received prednisolone phosphate drops had faster resolution of the stromal keratitis and fewer treatment failures. However, delaying the initiation of corticosteroid treatment did not affect the eventual outcome of the disease.

HEDS-SKS: 104 patients were enrolled. Over the 16-week follow-up period, there was no difference in the rate of treatment failure between the two groups. Thus there was no apparent benefit in the addition of oral acyclovir to the treatment regimen of a topical corticosteroid and a topical antiviral.

HEDS-IRT: 50 patients were enrolled during a 4-year recruitment period. Although the number of patients enrolled in this trial was too small to achieve statistically conclusive results, the trend in the results suggested a benefit in adding oral acyclovir to the treatment of HSV iridocyclitis in patients receiving topical corticosteroids and trifluridine prophylaxis.

HERPETIC EYE DISEASE STUDY (HEDS) II[4-6]

Purpose

- To determine whether early treatment (with oral acyclovir) of HSV ulcerations of the corneal epithelium prevents progression to the blinding complications of stromal keratitis and iridocyclitis.
- To determine the efficacy of low-dose oral acyclovir in preventing recurrent HSV eye infection in patients with previous episodes of herpetic eye disease.
- To determine the role of external factors (such as ultraviolet light or corneal trauma) and behavioral factors (such as life stress) on the induction of ocular recurrences of HSV eye infections and disease.

Background

Ocular HSV infection can lead to corneal scarring and neovascularization, permanent endothelial dysfunction and corneal edema, secondary glaucoma, and cataract. Despite the availability of topical antiviral agents that are highly active against HSV keratitis, there is still no known effective method for reducing the frequency of recurrence or severity of stromal keratitis and iridocyclitis. In addition, the prognosis is poor for recovery of good vision following penetrating keratoplasty (PK) for actively inflamed or highly vascularized herpetic corneas.

Description

Herpetic Eye Disease Study-II consisted of two randomized, placebo-controlled trials that assessed the role of oral acyclovir in the management of herpetic eye disease (1992–1996) and one epidemiologic study that investigated risk factors, including stress, for the development of ocular recurrences of the disease.

Herpes Simplex Virus Epithelial Keratitis Trial (HEDS-EKT): Evaluated the benefit of oral acyclovir (400 mg five times a day for 21 days) given during treatment of an acute HSV keratitis (dendritic or geographic keratitis) in preventing the occurrence of later blinding complications.

Study Measures

The primary outcome was the time to the first occurrence of stromal keratitis or iridocyclitis in the study eye (eye with epithelial keratitis at time of study entry).

Acyclovir Prevention Trial (HEDS-APT): Evaluated the benefit of long-term acyclovir treatment (400 mg twice a day for 1 year) in patients with a recent history of HSV eye disease but no current active disease. Episodes of recurrent

HSV eye disease during the trial were treated with topical corticosteroids and antivirals as indicated, but patients continued to receive the oral acyclovir or placebo for the entire 365-day period.

Inclusion Criteria

To be eligible, a patient must have experienced any kind of ocular herpes simplex infection (blepharitis, conjunctivitis, keratitis, or iridocyclitis) in the preceding year. The infection must have been inactive and untreated for at least the previous 30 days.

Study Measures

The primary outcome was the time to the first recurrence of any type of HSV eye disease in either eye.

Ocular HSV Recurrence Factor Study (HEDS-RFS): Evaluated the effect of psychological, environmental, and biological factors on recurrence episodes of herpetic eye disease. Patients recruited into the HEDS-APT trial were eligible to participate in HEDS-RFS if they are 18 years or older. At entry, all subjects filled out a questionnaire to estimate the negative affectivity trait measure. Subjects also filled out a short questionnaire every week for 52 weeks to track acute and chronic stressors (e.g., illnesses, injuries, menstrual periods, sun exposure, and emotional and financial stress). The investigators ensured patient privacy by the patients' mailing of the weekly logs directly to the HEDS National Coordinating Center.

Results

HEDS-EKT: Patient recruitment was stopped after enrolment of 287 of the originally planned 502 patients because of a lack of any suggested efficacy of the treatment protocol. In the treatment of acute HSV epithelial keratitis, there was no benefit on addition of oral acyclovir to treatment with topical trifluridine in preventing the development of stromal keratitis or iritis. Importantly, the study found that the risk of stromal keratitis or iridocyclitis was quite low (much lower than the published risk in the literature) in the year following an episode of epithelial keratitis treated with topical trifluridine alone.

HEDS-APT: Of the 703 patients enrolled, 357 were randomly assigned to the acyclovir group, and 346 to the placebo group. Only 4% of patients in the acyclovir group and 5% in the placebo group stopped treatment because of side effects. One-half of these side effects were due to gastrointestinal upset; some patients may have had intolerance to the lactose contained in the study capsules (treatment medication that does not contain lactose is now available). The study concluded that prophylactic oral acyclovir reduced the probability of recurrence of any form of ocular HSV by 41%. Importantly, researchers noted a 50% reduction in the rate of return of the more severe form of the disease—stromal keratitis—among patients who had this infection during the past year.

In addition to the main findings, it was also noted that during the 12 months of treatment:
- Oral acyclovir reduced the incidence of epithelial keratitis from 11% to 9%, and the incidence of stromal keratitis from 13% to 8%.
- 4% of patients in the acyclovir group and 9% in the placebo group had more than one recurrence.

HEDS-RFS: Psychological stress does not appear to be a trigger of recurrences of ocular HSV disease. If not accounted for, recall bias can substantially overestimate the importance of factors that do not have a causal association with HSV infection.

> **CLINICAL IMPLICATION**
> - Topical steroids help in faster resolution of viral stromal keratitis.
> - Oral acyclovir was helpful in treatment of viral iridocyclitis as an adjunct to topical antivirals and steroids.
> - Oral acyclovir prevents recurrent episodes of viral keratitis.

■ MYCOTIC ULCER TREATMENT TRIAL (MUTT) I[7]

Purpose
To evaluate outcomes of topical natamycin vs. voriconazole in cases of fungal corneal ulcers.

Background
Infectious keratitis is a leading cause of monocular vision loss worldwide. Fungal keratitis is endemic in tropical regions, accounting for as many as half of all corneal ulcers. Mycotic ulcer tends to have guarded visual prognosis contributing significantly to ocular morbidity. Fungal corneal ulcers can be more difficult to treat than bacterial corneal ulcers, with worse outcomes. Prior to the onset of this study natamycin was the only FDA approved topical antifungal agent in ophthalmology; though the use of topical voriconazole had been documented in few reports. The role of topical voriconazole in treatment of mycotic corneal ulcer and its comparison with topical natamycin was not studied in a randomized controlled trial.

Description
Mycotic Ulcer Treatment Trial I (2013) was a National Eye Institute-supported, randomized, double-masked, active comparator-controlled

multicentric interventional trial. The enrolled participants were randomized into two groups based upon the therapy they received into topical natamycin 5% and topical voriconazole 1%. The patients were advised to use the topical medication one drop every hour while awake for the first week followed by every 2 hourly till 3 weeks.

Inclusion Criteria

Patients above 16 years of age that presented with smear positive filamentous fungal keratitis (KOH wet mount, Giemsa or Gram stain) with a visual acuity in between 20/40 and 20/400 in the affected eye were included. Patients presenting with an impending perforation, bilateral corneal ulcers, visual acuity worse than 20/200 in nonaffected eye or those with mixed infections such as viral, bacterial, or acanthamoeba keratitis were excluded.

Study Measures

- The primary outcome measure was the best spectacle corrected visual acuity (BSCVA) at 3 months in terms of log MAR.
- The secondary outcome measures were BSCVA at 3 weeks, time to re-epithelialization, size of infiltrate or the scar at 3 weeks and 3 months, microbiological cure at 6 days, corneal perforation and/or the need full-thickness therapeutic keratoplasty.

Results

The trial suspended recruitment after 323 patients as per recommendations of Data Safety and Monitoring Committee based on higher perforations/therapeutic keratoplasty occurring in voriconazole group ($n = 34$) compared to natamycin group ($n = 18$) ($p = 0.02$).
- The most commonly identified organism was the *Fusarium* species (40% cases) followed by *Aspergillus* species (17% cases).
- The median duration of follow-up was 31 days in natamycin group and 39 days in voriconazole group.
- At 3 months visual acuity was worse by 1.8 lines in voriconazole group as compared to natamycin group. The mean BSCVA for *Fusarium* species was 4.1 lines better in natamycin prescribed group as compared to the voriconazole group.
- The mean BSCVA was 0.49 log MAR in natamycin treated group and 0.60 log MAR in voriconazole treated group at 3 weeks follow-up.
- 48% patients in the voriconazole group had culture positive at 6 days in contrast to 15% in natamycin treatment arm. Subgroup analysis revealed higher percentage in the *Fusarium* group.
- Re-epithelialization was faster in *Fusarium* group when treated with natamycin. Otherwise no significant difference was seen in overall epithelialization rate.

- The scars were smaller in *Fusarium* only group in the natamycin treated arm at 3 months follow-up, but no such difference was noted in the *non-Fusarium* group.
- Perforation of ulcer with or without therapeutic keratoplasty was seen in 34 patients in voriconazole group and only 18 in natamycin treatment group.

■ MYCOTIC ULCER TREATMENT TRIAL (MUTT) II[8]

Purpose
To assess the role of oral voriconazole therapy as compared to placebo as an adjunct to topical antifungal agents in filamentous fungal keratitis.

Background
Mycotic Ulcer Treatment Trial I demonstrated better response of filamentous mycotic ulcers to topical natamycin 5% than topical voriconazole 1%. This result was attributed to subtherapeutic drug levels achieved in the tissue after intermittent topical drug use by the authors. Oral voriconazole has good ocular penetration and may provide consistent tissue drug levels especially in deep mycotic infections. Thus MUTT II investigated the role of adjuvant oral voriconazole therapy.

Description
Mycotic Ulcer Treatment Trial II (2016) was a National Eye Institute-funded, placebo-controlled, double-masked, randomized clinical trial where in effect of oral voriconazole vs. placebo was studied in severe fungal corneal ulcer. The enrolled participants initially received topical 1% voriconazole, but after the results of MUTT I topical natamycin 5% was added in both arms. One group received oral voriconazole and second group received placebo drug.

Inclusion Criteria
Smear positive filamentous fungal keratitis patients with a vision of 20/400 or worse were enrolled for the study. Patients excluded were those with bilateral ulcers, coinfection, vision <20/200 in fellow eye, impending perforation, pregnancy, weight <40 kg or younger than 16 years.

Study Measures
The primary outcome was to measure the rate of ulcer perforation and/or therapeutic keratoplasty within 3 months of inclusion. Secondary outcomes were measure of BSCVA at 3 weeks and 3 months, infiltrates and/or scarring at 3 weeks and 3 months, time to re-epithelialize, microbiological cure at 6 days and complications.

Results

- A total of 240 patients from India and Nepal were enrolled, out of which follow-up (3 months) data for only 207 patients was available.
- Of the 119 patients (49.6%) in the oral voriconazole treatment group, 65 were male (54.6%), and the median age was 54 years (interquartile range, 42–62 years).
- 46.2% perforations occurred in the placebo arm and 53.8% in the oral voriconazole group. There was no statistically significant difference in both groups in the rate of perforation and need for therapeutic PK [hazard ratio: 0.82; 95% confidence interval (CI): 0.57–1.18; $p = 0.29$].
- The mean BSCVA and size of infiltrate and/or scar was comparable at 3 weeks and 3 months.
- No significant difference was noted in microbiological cure (culture positivity at 6 day) amongst both groups.
- The adverse events were more in oral voriconazole group (48.7%) vs. placebo group (23.1%).
- There was a significant increase in the voriconazole-associated adverse effects such as elevated liver enzymes and visual hallucinations.

CLINICAL IMPRESSION
- Topical natamycin is beneficial for treatment of mycotic keratitis over topical voriconazole.
- Oral voriconazole had no added benefits in Fusarium keratitis.

STEROID IN CORNEAL ULCERS TRIAL (SCUT)[9]

Purpose
To determine the effect of topical corticosteroids as adjunctive therapy in bacterial keratitis to improve long-term clinical outcomes.

Background
The use of topical steroids in cases of bacterial keratitis is potentially controversial with different studies suggesting variable outcomes. While anti-inflammatory action of steroids may decrease scarring and improve visual outcomes of bacterial keratitis there exist a potential risk of exacerbation of the pre-existing infection and secondary complications. There is lack of substantial evidence to support their use in cases of bacterial keratitis for long-term clinical improvements.

Description
Steroid in Corneal Ulcers Trial (2012) is a National Eye Institute-funded, double-masked, placebo controlled, randomized multicentric clinical trial comparing placebo vs. topical corticosteroids in patients receiving treatment for bacterial keratitis. A total of 500 culture positive patients of bacterial keratitis after receiving 48 hours of topical moxifloxacin 0.5% were randomized to receive either topical prednisolone phosphate 1% or placebo.

The steroids were administered as 1 drop 4 times per day for 1 week, then twice a day for 1 week, and then once per day for 1 week.

Inclusion Criteria

Culture-proven patients of bacterial keratitis were recruited. All eyes with perforated corneal ulcer, impending perforation, evidence of fungal, and viral or acanthamoeba keratitis were excluded. Patients with previous PK, use of steroids during the course of present ulcer, or fellow eye vision lower than 6/60 were not included in the study.

Study Measures

The primary outcome was BSCVA at 3 months. Other measures were the size of the scar at 12 months.

Results

- At 12 months follow-up a total of 399 patients were assessed.
- There was no significant difference in clinical outcomes in steroid vs. placebo group at 3 months.
- No significant difference was seen in BSCVA at 3–12 months.
- Further analysis in non-*Nocardia* ulcer group demonstrated one-line difference (improvement) in BSCVA in steroid group vs. placebo arm at 12 months. No such difference was seen in *Nocardia* ulcers.
- Steroids were also associated with a larger scar size in Nocardia ulcer group.
- There was no significant difference in the rate of healing between treatment arms among patients whose re-epithelialization occurred within 21 days from enrolment. However, among patients with an epithelial defect at 21 days or later from enrolment, a higher proportion had received corticosteroids.

CLINICAL IMPRESSION

- Topical steroids have no significant benefit in cases of bacterial keratitis.
- Cautious use of topical steroids may be considered after microbiological testing in ulcers not caused by Nocardia.

COLLABORATIVE LONGITUDINAL EVALUATION OF KERATOCONUS (CLEK) STUDY[10,11]

Purpose

- To describe the clinical course of keratoconus and to describe its visual and physiological manifestations, including high- and low-contrast visual acuity, corneal curvature, slit lamp biomicroscopic findings, corneal scarring, and quality of life.
- To identify risk factors and protective factors that influence the severity and progression of keratoconus.

Background
Previous large-scale studies of keratoconus focused on incidence and prevalence, etiology, or clinical management of keratoconus. Few studies have characterized the course of the disease and risk factors for its progression in large number of keratoconus patients. The incidence of vision-threatening corneal scarring in keratoconus is unknown.

Description
Prospective, multicenteric, natural history cohort study of 1,209 patients with mild-to-moderate keratoconus followed up for 8 years (1995–2004).

Inclusion Criteria
Patients with keratoconus ≥12 years; Vogt's striae, Fleischer's ring, or corneal scarring characteristic of keratoconus in at least one eye.

Study Measures
Patients were examined annually for visual acuity, patient-reported quality of life, manifest refraction, keratometry, photo documentation of cornea (to identify central corneal scarring), photo documentation of the flattest contact lens that just clears the cornea, slit lamp biomicroscopy, and corneal topography. In rigid contact lens wearers, the fluorescein pattern of the patient's habitual contact lens was documented.

Results
- Keratoconus patients are generally rigid gas permeable contact lens wearers with moderately steep corneas.
- Advanced keratoconus (steeper average keratometric reading) was associated with a greater likelihood of Vogt's striae, Fleischer's ring, and/or corneal scarring.
- The study group had asymmetric keratoconus. More the severity of disease, more the asymmetric disease status. Patient-reported unilateral eye rubbing, unilateral eye trauma was associated with steeper cornea. Asymmetric refractive spherical equivalent predisposes them to functional difficulties owing to reduced stereopsis.
- Central corneal scarring is associated with decreased vision, and increased glare. Contact lens wear increased the risk of incident scarring in keratoconus more than twofold. It is implied that corneal scarring might be reduced by modifying the contact lens fit.
- Over 8 years of follow-up, CLEK subjects exhibited a slow but clear increase in corneal curvature. Younger age and poorer high-contrast manifest refraction visual acuity at baseline predicted the rate of change in corneal curvature.

- Over 7 years of follow-up, CLEK subjects exhibited a slow but clear decrease in their best-corrected visual acuity (vision under low-contrast conditions decreasing more rapidly than vision under high-contrast viewing conditions). Better best-corrected visual acuity, steeper corneal curvature, and fundus abnormalities were predictive of greater acuity loss with time.
- Progression of disease as measured by changes in visual acuity and corneal curvature resulted in continued decline in vision-related quality of life albeit this effect on vision-specific quality of life is worse than expected based on the condition's relatively low prevalence and clinical severity.
- There was no difference in self-reported contact lens comfort between patients fitted with apical touch vs. apical clearance. No association was found between disease severity and contact lens discomfort.
- After controlling for disease severity in the form of corneal curvature, a keratoconic eye fitted with a rigid contact lens resulting in an apical touch fluorescein pattern did not have an increased risk of being scarred centrally at baseline. This "natural history" sample cannot determine causal proof that one method of fitting lenses is safer than another. To achieve this, a randomized clinical trial is needed.
- Increased likelihood of PK was associated with corneal scarring, steeper keratometry values, poorer visual acuity, and poorer contact lens comfort. CLEK study for the first time reported an increased risk of PK associated with younger age, worse vision-related quality of life, and flatter contact lens fits.

> **CLINICAL IMPRESSION**
> - CLEK reported average measures of disease severity and visual function in patients with keratoconus over 8 years.
> - Clinicians should be cognizant of the documented impact on quality of life when correlating the disease burden with clinical findings.

COLLABORATIVE CORNEAL TRANSPLANTATION STUDIES (CCTS)[12-14]

Purpose
To determine the effect of histocompatibility matching and crossmatching of corneal transplant donors and recipients on the survival of corneal graft in high-risk patients.

Background
Histocompatibility antigen matching and/or cross matching may have offered these patients an improved chance for successful outcome.

Description

Two multicenter double-masked, controlled, clinical trials (1986-1989) consisting of 400 patients each with a follow-up of 3 years.
1. The Cross Match Study was a randomized study assessing the effectiveness of cross matching in preventing graft rejection among high-risk patients with lymphocytotoxic antibodies.
2. The Antigen Matching Study was a prospective, observational study to assess the effectiveness of human leukocyte antigen (HLA)-A, B, and donor-recipient (D-R) matching in high-risk patients who had no lymphocytotoxic antibodies.

Blood samples from each enrolled patient were sent to the local CCTS tissue typing laboratory for HLA typing, and serum samples were sent to the Central Laboratory to be screened for preformed lymphocytotoxic antibodies. Depending on the results of the testing, patients were entered into the Crossmatch Study or the Antigen Matching Study. Patients in the Crossmatch Study received a cornea from either a positively cross matched donor or a negatively cross matched donor. Patients in the Antigen Matching Study received a cornea with 0 to 6 matched antigens.

Transplant patients were followed intensively during the first month after surgery. The number of clinic visits was tapered to 2 during the third and final year of follow-up, resulting in a total of 17 postoperative visits. Standard postoperative treatment regime, recognition and treatment of immunologic allograft reactions were developed and used.

Inclusion Criteria

Males and females aged 10 years or older with two to four quadrants of corneal stromal vascularization or a history of allograft rejection in the eye considered for surgery were eligible for both studies in the CCTS. Patients with conditions that would increase the risk of nonrejection graft failure, such as xerophthalmia or severe exposure keratopathy and patients with systemic diseases or with medication usage that might alter their immune response were excluded.

Study Measures

Irreversible failure of the corneal allograft due to all causes was the primary outcome variable in both studies. Allograft reaction episodes, irreversible failure due to rejection, and visual acuity were secondary outcome variables.

Results

- Donor-recipient tissue typing had no significant long-term effect on the success of corneal transplantation.
- Data from the CCTS indicate that matching patient and donor blood types combined with treating patients with high-dose topical steroids after

surgery may be potentially more effective in improving high-risk corneal transplantation. These two inexpensive strategies are considerably more economical than the more expensive donor-recipient tissue typing.

> **CLINICAL IMPRESSION**
> - CCTS helped to describe a high-risk graft.
> - Tissue typing did not change the outcomes in those at high risk of rejection.

CORNEA DONOR STUDY[15-26]

Purpose
- To determine long-term graft failure rate following keratoplasty when utilizing corneas from donors over 65 years of age in comparison to younger donors.
- To assess the relation between donor/recipient ABO compatibility and graft rejection.
- To assess if the corneal endothelial cell density (ECD) is an indicator of corneal health [in an optional Specular Microscopy Ancillary Study (SMAS)].

Background
Whether donor age should be used to determine suitability of a cornea for transplantation has been controversial. Before the onset of this study there existed a surgeon bias toward preference for younger tissues for keratoplasties in view of better outcomes. This study was designed to assess the role of donor age in long-term corneal graft survival. The SMAS was developed to evaluate the effect of donor age on endothelial cell loss (ECL) during the 5 years after PK in the Cornea Donor Study (CDS) population.

Description
It was a prospective, multicentric, intervention cohort study with triple masking (participant, investigator, assessor of outcomes). The study enrolled 1,101 patients (11 excluded due to ineligible diagnosis) between 2000 and 2002 and included 105 surgeons at 80 sites. 43 participating eye banks provided corneas with donor age range of 12–65 years and 65–75 years of age with endothelial cell densities of 2,300 to 3,300 cells/mm^2. The results were assessed at 5-year and 10-year follow-up.

Inclusion Criteria
Any patient in the age group of 40–80 years with significant corneal disease (endothelial dysfunction, such as pseudophakic corneal edema, Fuchs' dystrophy, posterior polymorphous dystrophy, endothelial failure from another cause, interstitial keratitis—nonherpetic type, or perforating corneal injury).

Study Measures
- Primary outcome was incidence of graft failure.
- Secondary outcome measure was to measure ECD.

Results

5-year Results
- Graft failure was not affected by type of retrieval, tissue processing, time between death and retrieval or between retrieval and utilization, donor characteristics (including age), and characteristics of donor cornea.
- Graft failure was higher (fourfold) in eyes undergoing keratoplasty for postcataract surgery decompensation/bullous keratoplasty (irrespective of lens status) and previous history of glaucoma surgery.
- Preoperative ECD did not affect graft failure occurring secondary to endothelial decompensation. Lower 6-month ECD correlated with graft failure. Irrespective of donor age, ECL was substantial over the first 5 years even after successful transplant.
- Higher ECD at 5 years was seen in those cases with larger grafts, female donors, and younger donor age.
- ABO blood group incompatibility was not associated with risk of graft failure.
- Donor age did not affect the graft survival. The 5-year survival rate for corneas 12–65 years and >65 years was comparable (86%).
- Dual-grading and adjudication procedures produce reliable and reproducible assessments of ECD.

10-year Results
- Graft failure rates were 12% ± 4% among eyes with no rejection in the first 5 years, 17% ± 12% in eyes with at least one probable rejection episode, and 22% ± 20% in eyes with at least one confirmed rejection episode.
- Preoperative history of glaucoma, particularly previous glaucoma surgery and use of antiglaucoma medications at the time of transplant were associated with risk of graft rejection.
- 10-year graft failure was higher in eyes with pseudophakic/aphakic decompensation, previous history of glaucoma or glaucoma surgery, older recipient age, history of smoking, and African American race.
- Rate of ECL at 10 years was slightly higher with age of graft as compared to lower age donors.

> **CLINICAL IMPRESSION**
> - Graft failure was independent of the donor characteristics.
> - Preoperative history of glaucoma or glaucoma surgery was a high risk for post-transplant rejection and graft failure.
> - Grafts with lower ECD at 6 months, 1 year, and 5 years were at higher risk of failure.

DREAM STUDY (DRY EYE ASSESSMENT AND MANAGEMENT)[27]

Purpose
To evaluate the role of oral omega-3-fatty acid supplements in patients with dry eye disease (DED).

Background
Dry eye disease is a multifactorial disease of the tear film and ocular surface characterized by alteration of the tear film homeostasis. The omega-3-fatty acids are believed to have potential anti-inflammatory action which help break the cycle of chronic inflammation. This trial was designed for evaluating the efficacy and safety of long-term oral omega-3-fatty acids supplementation in DED.

Description
It was a prospective, multicentric, randomized, double-masked "real world" clinical trial (2018). A total of 535 subjects were randomized in a ratio of 2:1 to omega 3 or placebo arm of the trial. A year long course of treatment was given. Participants were instructed to take five capsules per day. Each active capsule contained 400 mg EPA (eicosapentaenoic acid) and 200 mg DHA (docosahexaenoic acid), providing a daily dose of 3,000 mg omega 3 (2,000 mg EPA + 1000 mg DHA) while placebo arm received 5,000 mg olive oil. The patients were examined at 3, 6, and 12 months.

Inclusion Criteria
Patients ≥18 years of age with dry eye for at least 6 months and Ocular Surface Disease Index (OSDI) ≥25 were recruited.

Study Measures
Primary outcome was change in the dry eye symptoms based upon the OSDI score.

Results
- The mean OSDI scores were not significantly different between the omega 3 and placebo group.
- There was no significant change in cornea staining, conjunctival staining, and Schirmer's score between the two groups.
- No significant difference in clinical outcomes were noted in both groups.

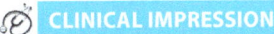
CLINICAL IMPRESSION

Oral supplementation with omega-3-fatty acids did not improve clinical outcomes in patients with DED.

■ PROSPECTIVE EVALUATION OF RADIAL KERATOTOMY (PERK) STUDY[28-30]

Purpose

- To determine whether radial keratotomy (RK) is effective in reducing myopia.
- To detect complications of the surgery.
- To discover patient characteristics and surgical factors affecting the results.
- To determine the long-term safety and efficacy of the procedure.

Description

The study, involving 435 patients recruited 1981–1983, was a clinical trial designed to evaluate the short- and long-term safety and efficacy of one technique of RK. The surgical technique was standardized, consisting of eight centrifugal radial incisions made manually with a diamond micrometer knife. The diameter of the central, uncut, clear zone was determined by the preoperative spherical equivalent cycloplegic refraction (−2.00 to −3.12 D = 4.0 mm; −3.25 to −4.3 D = 3.5 mm; −4.50 to −8.00 D = 3.0 mm). The blade length, which determined the depth of the incision, was set at 100% of the thinnest of four intraoperative ultrasonic corneal thickness readings taken paracentrally at the 3-, 6-, 9-, and 12-o'clock meridians just outside the mark delineating the clear zone. The incisions were made from the edge of the trephine mark to the limbal vascular arcade and were spaced equidistantly around the cornea.

Patients were examined preoperatively and after surgery at 2 weeks, 3 months, 6 months, annually for 5 years, and at 10 years. Examinations in the morning and evening of the same day were done at 3 months, 1 year, 3 years, and 11 years in a subset of the patients to test for diurnal fluctuation of vision and refraction.

Inclusion Criteria

All participants were ≥21 years, had 2–8 diopters (D) of simple myopia correctable to 20/20 or better with glasses or contact lenses and stability of their myopia documented by previous records. Each patient agreed to have surgery on one eye and to wait 1 year for surgery on the other eye. Patients with systemic diseases that might affect corneal wound healing and patients with high corneal astigmatism were excluded from the study.

Study Measures

The primary outcome variables measured at each visit was the uncorrected and spectacle-corrected visual acuity and the refractive error with the pupil dilated and undilated. The corneal shape was measured with central keratometry and photokeratoscopy. Endothelial function was evaluated using specular microscopy. A slit-lamp microscope examination was made to check for complications from the incisions. Contrast sensitivity was tested in a subset of patients. Patient motivation and satisfaction were studied with psychometric questionnaires at baseline, 1 year, 5-6 years, and 10 years.

Results

- The 10-year follow-up PERK study results confirmed that RK reduced myopia but that the effectiveness of the outcome varied among patients.
- These 10-year examinations indicated that the refractive error had not been stable in these eyes during the postoperative interval. There was a mean change in a hyperopic direction of +0.87 D between 6 months and 10 years after surgery. The average rate of change was 0.21 D per year between 6 months and 2 years, and +0.06 D per year between 2 and 10 years after surgery. Between 6 months and 10 years, the refractive error of 43% eyes changed in the hyperopic direction by 1.00 D or more. The hyperopic shift was statistically associated with incision length, with smaller clear zone diameters, and larger overall cornea diameters being associated with a greater change in refraction.
- Few patients lost spectacle-corrected visual acuity, indicating RK is reasonably safe; and that patients' acceptance is extremely high, with the majority stating they would have the surgery again.
- The study demonstrated that for patients to be free of distance optical correction, a refraction within 0.50 D of emmetropia or a visual acuity of 20/20 in at least one eye was necessary.

> **CLINICAL IMPRESSION**
> - High patient satisfaction was correlated with freedom from wearing distance spectacles or contact lenses and a visual acuity of 20/20 or better in at least one eye.
> - Post-RK hyperopic shift was associated with degree of myopia, length of incisions, and residual central clear area.

PIONEER STUDY—PROSPECTIVE INTRAOPERATIVE AND PERIOPERATIVE OPHTHALMIC IMAGING WITH OPTICAL COHERENCE TOMOGRAPHY[31]

Purpose

To assess feasibility, safety, and utility of intraoperative optical coherence tomography (iOCT) in patients undergoing ophthalmic surgeries.

Background

Optical coherence tomography allows high-resolution imaging of ocular tissues in 2 and 3 dimensions providing valuable cross-sectional anatomic information which has revolutionized clinical management of ophthalmic diseases. Integration of OCT in surgical environment can have profound implications in surgical management of ophthalmic diseases.

Description

This was a prospective, single-center, multisurgeon, consecutive, case series (2014). Intraoperative OCT was done using Bioptigen SDOIS portable spectral domain OCT (probe stabilized with microscope mount system or with handheld scanning). Procedure-specific imaging protocol was used for anterior and posterior segment surgeries. Surgeon feedback form was recorded immediately after surgery to assess utility of iOCT. 531 eyes were enrolled (275 anterior segment cases and 256 posterior segment surgical cases) over 24 months.

Inclusion Criteria

Patients over 18 years requiring ophthalmic surgery. Exclusion criteria included any media opacity that precluded OCT scanning of the area of interest and inability to provide written informed consent.

Study Measures

Impact of iOCT on surgical decision-making, time implications of iOCT, and adverse events specifically related to iOCT were recorded.

Results

- Successful imaging was obtained in 98% at some point during the surgical procedure with variable image quality.
- In the anterior segment group, 275 eyes were enrolled, and common surgical procedures performed were DSAEK, phacoemulsification, femtosecond-assisted phacoemulsification, and DALK.
- Role of iOCT in anterior segment surgical decision-making:
  - *DSAEK*:
    - Graft apposition monitoring until optimal fluid removal was achieved.
    - Graft dislocation rate on postoperative day 1 was 3%.
  - *DALK*: Provided depth-related information regarding extent of trephination and residual bed information
  - Phacoemulsification: Allowed assessment of location of intraocular lens and wound architecture
  - *INTACS*: Assessment of location of implant
- 256 eyes were included in posterior segment group, with nearly all eyes requiring vitrectomy and 15 eyes requiring scleral buckling with vitrectomy.
- Common surgical procedures were epiretinal membrane (ERM) removal, full thickness macular hole (FTMH), rhegmatogenous retinal detachment (RRD), proliferative diabetic retinopathy, and vitreous hemorrhage.
- Role of iOCT in posterior segment surgical decision-making:
  - *ERM removal*: To assess completeness of membrane removal, alterations in the outer retinal architecture were noted with

observation of the expansion between the ellipsoid zone and the retinal pigment epithelium (RPE) after peeling.
- *FTMH*: To identify changes in hole architecture, residual ILM, expansion between the ellipsoid zone and RPE after peeling.
- *RRD*: To identify residual subretinal fluid.
- Surgery to relieve vitreomacular traction—confirmation of release of traction and identification of newly formed FTMH.

- Overall, the median number of scan sessions per case was 2 (range: 1-5 sessions) with 6 median total scans (range: 1-24 scans). The overall median time to obtain the first image after pausing surgery was 1.7 minutes (range: 0.3-12.4).
- Overall median time surgery was paused to perform intraoperative OCT imaging was 4.9 minutes (range: 0.4-26.7) with a median duration surgery paused per scanning session of 2.8 minutes.
- No adverse events were reported.

CLINICAL IMPRESSION
- Intraoperative OCT is feasible for anterior and posterior segment surgeries.
- Intraoperative OCT provided useful information which had an impact on surgical decision-making.

Table 1: Summary of clinical trials in cornea.

Title	Purpose	No of patients	Inclusion criteria	Follow-up	Results/conclusion
HEDS-1 SKN 1992-96	Efficacy of topical steroids in herpes simplex stromal keratitis	106	Patients ≥ 12 years, no active HSV epithelial keratitis, active HSV stromal keratitis	16 weeks	Prednisolone drops lead to faster resolution and fewer treatment failures
HEDS-1 SKS	Efficacy of oral acyclovir in herpes simplex stromal keratitis	104	Patients ≥ 12 years, no active HSV epithelial keratitis, active HSV stromal keratitis, already on topical corticosteroid	16 weeks	No apparent benefit of the addition of oral acyclovir
HEDS-1 IRT	Efficacy of oral acyclovir in treating herpes simplex iridocyclitis	50	Patients ≥ 12 years, no active HSV epithelial keratitis, with active HSV iridocyclitis	16 weeks	Benefit in adding oral acyclovir to the treatment of HSV iridocyclitis
HEDS-2 EKT	Does oral acyclovir in HSV epithelium ulcerations prevent progression	287	Eyes with herpes simplex epithelial keratitis within one week of onset	One year	There was no benefit from the addition of oral acyclovir to treatment
HEDS-2 APT	Long-term acyclovir in patients with a recent history of HSV eye disease but no current active disease	703	Any kind of ocular herpes simplex infection in the preceding year. The infection must have been inactive for at least the previous 30 days	One year	Oral acyclovir reduced the probability that any form of herpes of the eye would return in patients

Contd...

Contd...

Title	Purpose	No of patients	Inclusion criteria	Follow-up	Results/conclusion
HEDS-2 RFS	Effect of psychological, environmental, and biological factors on recurrences of herpetic eye disease	–	Same as HEDS – EKT provided the patients were more than 18 years old	One year	Psychological stress does not appear to be a trigger of recurrences of ocular HSV disease
MUTT I 2010-2011	To evaluate outcomes of topical natamycin versus voriconazole in cases of fungal corneal ulcers in terms of visual acuity	323	Patients > 15 years of age that presented with a corneal ulcer which smear positive for fungal filaments, with a visual acuity between 20/40 and 20/400 in affected eye	3 months	Natamycin group was better at 3 months in terms of BSCVA as compared to voriconazole group. The benefits were more pronounced in *Fusarium* species in terms of faster epithelialization, less scarring and more chances of being culture negative at 6 days
MUTT II 2010-2015	To evaluate clinical outcomes of oral voriconazole as an adjunct to topical antifungals in severe fungal keratitis	240	Smear positive filamentous, with vision worse than 20/400 were enrolled	3 months	Voriconazole did not have any additional benefits as an adjunct to topical anti-fungal agents

Contd...

Contd...

Title	Purpose	No of patients	Inclusion criteria	Follow-up	Results/conclusion
SCUT 2006–2010	To determine the effect of topical corticosteroids as adjunctive therapy in bacterial keratitis to improve long-term clinical outcomes	500 (399)	Culture proven bacterial keratitis which received 48 hours of topical antibiotic treatment	12 months	Steroids show some benefit in cases of non-nocardia bacterial keratitis. Clinicians should always be cautious while using steroids depending on the case of keratitis
CLEK 1995–2004	• To describe the clinical course of keratoconus and to describe the relationships among its visual and physiological manifestations, including high- and low-contrast visual acuity, corneal curvature, slit lamp biomicroscopic findings, corneal scarring and quality of life • To identify risk factors and protective factors those influence the severity and progression of keratoconus	1209	Diagnosed Keratoconus, Age > 12 yrs, irregular cornea in at least one eye; Vogt's striae, Fleischer's ring or corneal scarring characteristic of keratoconus in at least one eye	3 years	

Contd...

Contd...

Title	Purpose	No of patients	Inclusion criteria	Follow-up	Results/conclusion
CCTS 1986-1989	To determine whether histocompatibility matching of corneal transplant donors and recipients can reduce the incidence of graft rejection in high-risk patients	400	Males/Female ≥ 10 yrs, with 204 quadrants of deep stromal vessels or a history of graft rejection	3 years	Donor-recipient tissue typing had no significant long-term effect on the success of corneal transplantation
CDS	To assess the effect of donor age on graft survival	1101	Patients with endothelial dysfunction requiring penetrating keratoplasty	10 years	• Graft failure was not affected by donor factors • Higher endothelial cell density was seen in younger grafts at both 5 and 10 years postoperative • ABO incompatibility was not affected by risk of graft failure
DREAM study	To assess the role of oral omega supplements in dry eye	535	≥ 18 years, with dry eye disease (OSDI ≥ 25)	1 year	No significant clinical improvement was seen with long-term supplementation in patients with dry eye disease

Contd...

Contd...

Title	Purpose	No of patients	Inclusion criteria	Follow-up	Results/conclusion
PIONEER study	To assess feasibility of iOCT in clinical practice	18 (in anterior segment arm)	>18 years, willing for ophthalmic surgery when indicated	Observational (Intraoperative) study	iOCT is a useful intraoperative tool for eyes undergoing anterior lamellar surgeries
PERK 1981-83	Determine efficacy, complications and factors affecting the results of RK in myopia. Determine the long-term safety and efficacy of the procedure	435 + 99	Patients with age ≥ 21 years with 2 to 8 diopters of simple myopia correctable to 20/20 or better Stable refraction	10 years	• RK reduced myopia but that the outcome varied • In 43% of patients there is hyperopic shift of 1 D by 10 years • RK is reasonably safe and patient acceptance is high. Residual myopia of -0.50 to -1.00 D is an advantage after RK

REFERENCES

1. Wilhelmus KR, Gee L, Hauck WW; Herpetic Eye Disease Study. A controlled trial of topical corticosteroids for herpes simplex stromal keratitis. Ophthalmology. 1994;101:1883-96.
2. Barron BA, Gee L, Hauck WW; Herpetic Eye Disease Study. A controlled trial of oral acyclovir for herpes simplex stromal keratitis. Ophthalmology. 1994;101:1871-82.
3. Herpetic Eye Disease Study Group. A controlled trial of oral acyclovir for iridocyclitis caused by herpes simplex virus. Arch Ophthalmol. 1996;114:1065-72.
4. Herpetic Eye Disease Study Group. A controlled trial of oral acyclovir for the prevention of stromal keratitis or iritis in patients with herpes simplex virus epithelial keratitis. Arch Ophthalmol. 1997;115:703-12.
5. The Herpetic Eye Disease Study Group. Acyclovir for the prevention of recurrent herpes simplex virus eye disease. N Engl J Med. 1998;339:300-6.
6. Herpetic Eye Disease Study Group. Psychological stress and other potential triggers for recurrences of herpes simplex virus eye infections. Arch Ophthalmol. 2000;118:1617-25.
7. Prajna NV, Krishnan T, Mascarenhas J, Rajaraman R, Prajna L, Srinivasan M, et al.; Mycotic Ulcer Treatment Trial Group. The mycotic ulcer treatment trial: a randomized trial comparing natamycin vs voriconazole. JAMA Ophthalmol. 2013;131(4):422-9.
8. Prajna NV, Krishnan T, Rajaraman R, Patel S, Srinivasan M, Das M, et al. Effect of Oral Voriconazole on Fungal Keratitis in the Mycotic Ulcer Treatment Trial II (MUTT II): A Randomized Clinical Trial. JAMA Ophthalmol. 2016;134(12):1365-72.
9. Srinivasan M, Mascarenhas J, Rajaraman R, Ravindran M, Lalitha P, Glidden DV, et al.; for the Steroids for Corneal Ulcers Trial Group. The Steroids for Corneal Ulcers Trial. Arch Ophthalmol. 2012;130(2):143-50.
10. Szczotka LB, Barr JT, Zadnik K; the CLEK Study Group. A summary of the findings from the Collaborative Longitudinal Evaluation of Keratoconus (CLEK) Study. Optometry. 2001;72:574-87.
11. Barr JT, Zadnik K, Wilson BS, Edrington TB, Everett DF, Fink BA, et al.; the CLEK Study Group. Factors associated with corneal scarring in the Collaborative Longitudinal Evaluation of Keratoconus (CLEK) Study. Cornea. 2000;19(4):501-7.
12. Hahn AB, Foulks GN, Enger C, Fink N, Stark WJ, Hopkins KA, et al. The association of lymphocytotoxic antibodies with corneal allograft rejection in high risk patients. The Collaborative Corneal Transplantation Studies Research Group. Transplantation. 1995; 59(1):21-7.
13. Fink N, Stark WJ, Maguire MG, Stulting D, Meyer R, Foulks G, et al. Effectiveness of histocompatibility matching in high-risk corneal transplantation: A summary of results from the Collaborative Corneal Transplantation Studies. Cesk Oftalmol. 1994;50(1):3-12.
14. Maguire MG, Stark WJ, Gottsch JD, Stulting RD, Sugar A, Fink NE, et al. Risk factors for corneal graft failure and rejection in the Collaborative Corneal Transplantation Studies. Collaborative Corneal Transplantation Studies Research Group. Ophthalmology. 1994;101(9):1536-47.
15. Lass JH, Beck RW, Benetz BA, Dontchev M, Gal RL, Holland EJ, et al. Cornea Donor Study Investigator Group. Baseline factors related to endothelial cell loss following penetrating keratoplasty. Arch Ophthalmol. 2011;129(9):1149-54.
16. Lass JH, Sugar A, Benetz BA, Beck RW, Dontchev M, Gal RL, et al.; for the Cornea Donor Study Investigator Group. Endothelial cell density to predict endothelial graft failure after penetrating keratoplasty. Arch Ophthalmol. 2010;128:63-9.
17. Sugar J, Montoya M, Dontchev M, Tanner JP, Beck R, Gal R, et al. Group Cornea Donor Study Investigator Group. Donor risk factors for graft failure in the cornea donor study. Cornea. 2009;28(9):981-5.

18. Powe A, Gal RL, Beck RW, Mannis MJ, Holland EJ; on behalf of the Cornea Donor Study Investigator Group. The Cornea Donor Study. Vision Pan-America. 2009;8:134-7.
19. Sugar A, Tanner JP, Dontchev M, Tennant B, Schultze RL, Dunn SP, et al.; for the Cornea Donor Study Investigator Group. Recipient risk factors for graft failure in the Cornea Donor Study. Ophthalmology. 2009;116:1023-28.
20. Dunn SP, Stark WJ, Stulting RD, Lass JH, Sugar A, Pavilack MA, et al.; on behalf of the Cornea Donor Study Investigator Group. The effect of ABO blood incompatibility on corneal transplant failure in conditions with low risk of graft rejection. Am J Ophthalmol. 2009;147:432-8.
21. Cornea Donor Study Investigator Group. Donor age and corneal endothelial cell loss five years after successful corneal transplantation: specular microscopy ancillary study results. Ophthalmology. 2008;115:627-32.
22. Cornea Donor Study Investigator Group. The effect of donor age on corneal transplantation outcome: results of the cornea donor study. Ophthalmology. 2008;115:620-6.
23. Dunn SP, Gal RL, Kollman C, Raghinaru D, Dontchev M, Blanton CL, et al.; for the Cornea Donor Study Investigator Group. Corneal Graft Rejection Ten Years after Penetrating Keratoplasty in the Cornea Donor Study. Cornea. 2014;33:1003-9.
24. Lass JH, Benetz BA, Gal RL, Kollman C, Raghinaru D, Dontchev M, et al.; for the Cornea Donor Study Investigator Group. Donor age and factors related to endothelial cell loss ten years after penetrating keratoplasty: Specular Microscopy Ancillary Study. Ophthalmology. 2013;120:2428-35.
25. Mannis MJ, Holland EJ, Gal RL, Dontchev M, Kollman C, Raghinaru D, et al.; for the Cornea Donor Study Investigator Group. The Effect of Donor Age on Penetrating Keratoplasty for Endothelial Disease: Graft Survival after 10 Years in the Cornea Donor Study. Ophthalmology. 2013;120:2419-27.
26. Sugar A, Gal RL, Kollman C, Raghinaru D, Dontchev M, Croasdale CR, et al.; for the Cornea Donor Study Investigator Group. Factors Predictive of Corneal Graft Survival in the Cornea Donor Study. JAMA Ophthalmol. 2015;133(3):246-54.
27. Asbell PA, Maguire MG, Peskin E, Bunya VY, Kuklinski EJ. Dry Eye Assessment and Management (DREAM©) Study Research Group. Dry Eye Assessment and Management (DREAM©) Study: Study design and baseline characteristics. Contemp Clin Trials. 2018;71:70-9.
28. Waring GO, Lynn MJ, McDonnell PJ. Results of the Prospective Evaluation of Radial Keratotomy (PERK) Study 10 years after surgery. Arch Ophthalmol. 1994;112:1298-308.
29. Nizam A, Waring GO, Lynn MJ. Stability of refraction during 11 years in eyes with simple myopia. Invest Ophthalmol Vis Sci. 1996;37:S1004.
30. Rowsey JJ, Waring GO, Monlux RD, Balyeat HD, Stevens SX, Culbertson W, et al. Corneal topography as a predictor of refractive change in the Prospective Evaluation of Radial Keratotomy (PERK) study. Ophthalmic Surgery. 1991;22(7):370-80.
31. Ehlers JP, Dupps WJ, Kaiser PK, Goshe J, Singh RP, Petkovsek D, et al. The Prospective Intraoperative and Perioperative Ophthalmic ImagiNg with Optical CoherEncE TomogRaphy (PIONEER) Study: 2-year results. Am J Ophthalmol. 2014;158(5):999-1007.

Clinical Trials in Glaucoma

Priyanka Ramesh, Shikha Gupta

■ EARLY MANIFEST GLAUCOMA TRIAL (EMGT)[1,2]

Purpose
- Primary purpose—to compare the effect of immediate therapy to lower the intraocular pressure (IOP) versus late or no treatment on the progression of newly detected open-angle glaucoma (OAG), as measured by increasing visual field loss and/or optic disc changes.
- Secondary purposes—to determine the extent of IOP reduction attained by treatment, to explore factors that may influence glaucoma progression, and to describe the natural history of newly detected glaucoma.

Description
Controlled, randomized clinical trial consisting of 255 patients identified by an extensive, population-based screening of successive age cohorts as well as by clinical referral (1992 1997). The diagnosis was confirmed through Humphrey perimetry at two post-screening visits. Eligible patients were randomized to treatment with the beta blocker Betaxolol and argon laser trabeculoplasty (ALT) (treated group) or to no initial treatment (control group).

Patients were followed for a minimum of 4 years to assess the development of glaucoma progression. They were seen every 3 months to collect visual field, IOP, and other data. Disc photographs were taken every 6 months. Technicians and disc photograph graders were masked regarding treatment assignment. Patients in the treated group received Xalatan whenever IOP exceeds 25 mm Hg at more than one visit; patients in the control group received Xalatan whenever IOP reaches 35 mm Hg or higher during the trial. If IOP remained high, individualized treatment was given.

Inclusion Criteria
Men and women between ages 50 and 80 years who have newly detected and untreated chronic OAG with repeatable visual field defects by Humphrey perimetry.

Exclusion Criteria

Advanced visual field loss (MD <16 dB) or threat to fixation; mean IOP >30 mm Hg or any IOP >35 mm Hg in at least one eye; visual acuity <0.5 in either eye; or any conditions precluding reliable fields or photos, use of study treatment, or 4 year follow-up.

Study Measures

The study outcome was glaucoma progression, which was based on specific criteria derived from analyses of Humphrey visual fields and masked evaluations of disc photographs.
- The perimetric outcome was defined as statistically significant deterioration (p <0.05) of the same three or more test points in Pattern Deviation Change Probability Maps in three consecutive 30-2 Humphrey fields.
- Optic disc progression was determined by the following:
  - The presence of definite change (detected by comparison of follow-up photographs with baseline) by flicker chronoscopy in two follow-up photographs from the same visit, with independent confirmation by side-by-side gradings.
  - Final confirmation of change towards progression, by flicker chronoscopy and by side-by-side gradings, at a different follow-up visit.

Results

- The EMGT was the first adequately powered randomized trial with an untreated control arm to evaluate the effects of IOP reduction in patients with OAG who have elevated and normal IOP. Its intent-to-treat analysis showed considerable beneficial effects of treatment that significantly delayed progression. On average, treatment reduced the IOP by 5.1 mm Hg or 25%, a reduction maintained throughout follow-up. Progression was less frequent in the treatment group (45%) than in controls (62%) and occurred significantly later in treated patients. Whereas progression varied across patient categories, treatment effects were present in both older and younger patients, high- and normal-tension glaucoma (NTG), and eyes with less and greater visual field loss.
- Progression was more common in—patients with higher IOP, older patients, patients with more advanced baseline damage, exfoliation glaucoma.
- Treatment was associated with progression of nuclear lens opacities.

COLLABORATIVE INITIAL GLAUCOMA TREATMENT STUDY (CIGTS)[3-5]

Purpose

To compare the long-term effect of treating newly diagnosed OAG with standard medical treatment versus filtration surgery.

Description

A randomized, controlled clinical trial in which eligible patients were randomized to receive either a stepped medication treatment regimen or filtration surgery to control their OAG. Patients, rather than eyes, were randomized to the two treatment arms; if both eyes were eligible for treatment, the treatment course for both eyes were the same. Sample size requirements indicated that 300 patients were needed for each treatment approach; a total of 607 patients were ultimately recruited for the CIGTS (1993–1997).

Patients randomized to the medication treatment arm received a stepped regimen of topical medications, beginning with a single agent (typically a beta blocker), with additional medications added upon documented lack of IOP control or evidence of progressive visual field loss. If medications failed to control the patient's OAG, a series of treatment steps began with ALT and concluded with trabeculectomy.

In the surgical treatment arm, patients underwent immediate trabeculectomy and, with documented failure, proceeded to ALT, then concluded with medications.

All patients were seen for standardized follow-up examinations at 3 and 6 months after treatment and every 6 months thereafter; in addition, patients randomized to the surgical arm received, at a minimum, post-surgical follow-up at 1 day, 1 week, and 1 month. At the visits, examination of the eye(s) included evaluation of visual acuity, visual field, and IOP. The results of these tests determined whether treatment should be changed. In addition, before and at regular intervals after treatment, patients were interviewed by telephone to assess their health-related quality of life. A questionnaire that included the Sickness Impact Profile, Visual Activities Questionnaire, and other components was used.

Inclusion criteria

Patients ranged in age from 25 to 75 with an IOP of 20 mm Hg or greater and evidence of optic nerve damage and/or visual field loss in one or both eyes. The ocular findings must exclude causes of glaucoma other than primary OAG, pigmentary glaucoma, or pseudoexfoliation glaucoma.

Results

Interim results including follow-up as long as 5 years were reported in November, 2001.

- Both treatment groups had substantial and sustained reduction in IOP from baseline with the surgical group running IOPs about 2-3 points lower than the medical group.
- The surgical group had more visual field loss and more visual acuity loss in the first 3 years of the study, but these differences largely disappeared in years 4 and 5 of follow-up.
- The surgery group had more cataract extractions than the medical group.
- Quality of life results indicated that both groups were satisfied with their treatment. While the surgery group reported more local eye symptoms such as feeling something in the eye, most such symptoms were not sustained beyond the first 2-3 years of follow-up. The medical group reported a variety of systemic symptoms that were not consistent over time but were clearly different from the symptoms reported by the surgical group.
- Surgery prevents or delays glaucomatous progression as measured by optic disc criteria in patients with early OAG. Reversal of cupping occurs more frequently in the surgical group than in the medical treatment group. Reversal is associated with lower IOP but is not associated with improved visual function.

Based on these interim follow-up data, the investigators do not recommend changes to current approaches to managing newly diagnosed OAG patients. Longer follow-up is needed before specific treatment recommendations can be made in a chronic disease like glaucoma.

■ OCULAR HYPERTENSION TREATMENT STUDY (OHTS)[6,7]

Purpose

- To determine whether medical reduction of IOP prevents or delays the onset of glaucomatous visual field loss and/or optic disc damage in ocular hypertensive subjects judged to be at moderate risk for developing OAG.
- To produce natural history data to assist in identifying patients at most risk for developing OAG and those most likely to benefit from early medical treatment.
- To quantify risk factors for developing OAG among ocular hypertensive subjects.

Description

A long-term, randomized, controlled multicenter clinical trial (1994-2009). Ocular hypertensive subjects judged to be at moderate risk of developing primary OAG were randomly assigned to either close observation only or a stepped medical regimen. Medical treatment consisted of all commercially available topical antiglaucoma agents. The goal of treatment was a 20% reduction in IOP or IOP <24 mm Hg.

After completion of baseline measures (IOP, visual fields, and disc photos) and randomization, the subjects were followed for a minimum of 5 years with automated threshold central static perimetry (Humphrey program 30-2) twice yearly and stereoscopic optic disc photographs once yearly. Study end points were reproducible visual field loss and/or progressive optic disc damage in either eye of a patient. All visual fields and optic disc photographs were read in a masked fashion in Reading Centers.

In the 1991 Baltimore Eye Survey, African Americans were shown to have a prevalence of OAG four to five times higher than whites. Given this high prevalence of OAG in the African American population, it is important to recruit and follow an adequate sample of African American subjects in the trial (approximately 25% of the total patient sample). Thus 1,637 patients were enrolled, including 409 African Americans.

Inclusion criteria

Men and nonpregnant women between the ages of 40 and 80 with IOP ≥24 mm Hg but ≤32 mm Hg in at least one eye and IOP ≥21 but ≤32 mm Hg in the fellow eye, as well as normal visual fields and optic discs.

Patients presenting with best-corrected visual acuity (BCVA) worse than 20/40 in either eye, previous intraocular surgery, a life-threatening or debilitating disease, secondary causes of elevated IOP, angle-closure glaucoma or anatomically narrow angles, other diseases that can cause visual field loss, background diabetic retinopathy, optic disc abnormalities that can produce visual field loss or obscure the interpretation of the optic disc, or unwillingness to undergo random assignment were excluded from the trial.

Results

- Baseline factors that predicted the development of primary open-angle glaucoma (POAG): *In univariate analyses*—older age, race (African American), sex (male), larger vertical cup-disc ratio, larger horizontal cup-disc ratio, higher IOP, greater Humphrey visual field pattern standard deviation (SD), heart disease, and thinner central corneal measurement. *In multivariate analyses*—older age, larger vertical or horizontal cup-disc ratio, higher IOP, greater pattern SD, and thinner central corneal measurement.
- During the course of the study, the mean ± SD reduction in IOP in the medication group was 22.5 ± 9.9%. The IOP declined by 4.0 ± 11.6% in the observation group. At 60 months, the cumulative probability of developing POAG was 4.4% in the medication group and 9.5% in the

observation group. Thus, a decrease in the IOP by 23% led to a decrease in the incidence of POAG by 60%. The risk of developing POAG at 5 years is 1% per year with treatment, 2% per year on observation and 3-5% per year in the presence of risk factors. There was little evidence of increased systemic or ocular risk associated with ocular hypotensive medication.
- The final goal of the study is to redefine early damage in OAG. The OHTS includes ancillary studies on scanning laser ophthalmoscopy (SLO) of optic nerve and blue on yellow perimetry—whether they can detect changes earlier compared to standard stereoscopic photos and standard white-on-white perimetry.

Thus, topical ocular hypotensive medication was effective in delaying or preventing onset of primary OAG in individuals with elevated IOP. Although this does not imply that all patients with borderline or elevated IOP should receive medication, clinicians should consider initiating treatment for individuals with ocular hypertension (OHT) who are at moderate-or high-risk for developing primary OAG.

EUROPEAN GLAUCOMA PREVENTION STUDY[8]

Purpose
- To evaluate the efficacy of IOP reduction by dorzolamide in preventing or delaying POAG in patients with OHT.
- To obtain information about the natural history of OHT and the risk factors in the onset of POAG.

Description
It was a multicenter, randomized, double masked, placebo-controlled trial. The patients were recruited between 1997 and 1999 and randomized into one group receiving active therapy (dorzolamide 2%) and another group receiving placebo. Both groups were administered eye drops three times a day. Patients were followed up at 6 monthly intervals for 5 years. Baseline and follow-up assessments included refraction, visual acuity testing, Goldmann applanation tonometry, complete ophthalmological examination, Humphrey or Octopus visual field of central 30 degrees using threshold double-crossing strategy and color stereophotography of the optic disc.

Inclusion Criteria
- Age between 30 and 80 years.
- Intraocular pressure between 22 and 29 mm Hg in at least 1 eye without therapy or after a wash out period of at least 3 weeks.
- Open angles on gonioscopy, 2 normal and reliable visual field tests per eye and normal optic discs.

Exclusion Criteria
- Visual acuity worse than 20/40 in either eye.
- Previous intraocular surgery, any sign of diabetic retinopathy or other diseases capable of deterioration of visual fields or optic disc.

Study Measures
The study measured the number of patients who progressed to POAG termed as efficacy end point and the number of patients with uncontrolled high IOP termed as safety end point in both the active treatment and control group.

European Glaucoma Prevention Study (EGPS) criteria for the onset of POAG:
- Occurrence of worsening of visual field.
- Progressive change in the optic disc appearance.
- Both.

Worsening of the visual field occurred when at least one of the following criteria was met and repeatable in 3 visual field tests performed within 3 months.
- Three or more horizontally or vertically adjacent points that differ 5 dB or more from baseline.
- Two or more horizontally or vertically adjacent points that differ 10 dB or more from the baseline.
- A difference of 10 dB or more across the nasal horizontal meridian at 2 or more adjacent points.

Optic disc worsening was defined as a visually recognizable localized or diffuse narrowing of the neuroretinal rim on stereophotographs.

Safety end point: An increase in IOP of ≥35 mm Hg in the same eye on two separate occasions within 1 week.

Results
- A total of 1,081 patients were enrolled. 1,077 patients were included in the final analysis.
- Mean baseline IOP between the two groups was not significantly different. Average IOP across follow ups was 19.3 mm Hg in the dorzolamide group and 20.4 mm Hg in the placebo group and the difference was statistically significant.
- Mean percentage reduction in IOP was 14.5% in the dorzolamide group at 6 months and 22.1% at 5 years and it was statistically significant. The mean percentage reduction of IOP in the placebo group was 9.3% at 6 months and 18.7% at 5 years and it was statistically significant.
- 345 patients in the dorzolamide group completed the study. 46 reached the efficacy end point and 1 reached the safety end point. 407 patients in the placebo group completed the study, out of which 60 patients reached

the efficacy end point and 12 reached the safety end point. Totally 106 patients developed visual field and optic disc changes due to POAG.
- Probability of developing an efficacy end point was 13.4% in the dorzolamide group and 14.1% in the placebo group and the difference was not statistically significant.
- Probability of developing any end point either, efficacy or safety was 13.7% in dorzolamide group and 16.4% in the placebo group and again the difference was not statistically significant.

Conclusion

European Glaucoma Prevention Study failed to detect a protective effect of medical therapy as compared to placebo in the development of POAG in OHT patients at moderate risk over a period of 5 years.

COLLABORATIVE NORMAL TENSION GLAUCOMA STUDY (CNTGS)[9-11]

Purpose

To ascertain the influence of IOP on the course of NTG (whether IOP was or was not involved in NTG, and therefore whether aggressive efforts to lower IOP in patients with NTG are warranted).

Description

Prospective, multicenter study in which 230 patients were enrolled (1988). One eye of patients with NTG was randomized:
- To be followed without treatment until there was evidence of slight deterioration. The other eye could be treated at the discretion of the treating physician, except that systemic carbonic anhydrase inhibitors could not be used.
- To be placed on treatment with medication, laser trabeculoplasty, filtration surgery, or any combination, as required to lower the IOP by 30%.

In both arms, neither eye could receive beta-adrenergic blockers or adrenergic agonists, because they might have systemic cardiovascular effects that could conceivably alter the course of the treated or untreated disease, confounding the analysis of data.

Some patients were randomized immediately, if the field defect threatened the point of fixation or there was previously documented progression of the disease. Other patients were randomized later if there was visual field progression, progression of optic nerve head cupping, or a new disc hemorrhage. By the end of the study, 145 eyes had been randomized:

66 to receive treatment and 79 eyes to serve as untreated controls. Of the 66 assigned to treatment, 5 withdrew before achieving the IOP-lowering goal.

The course of eyes in the control group was followed up from baseline at the time of randomization; the course of treated eyes was followed up from a new baseline established as soon as 30% IOP reduction was stable (usually by filtering surgery). Follow-up examinations were scheduled at a minimal frequency of every 3 months for the first year and every 6 months thereafter, until a visual field change was documented, a change in the optic nerve head appearance was confirmed, or a disc hemorrhage was noted. When an end point was reached by virtue of disc progression or visual field loss, the patient's treatment was according to the clinician, that is, the patient was released from the protocol.

Inclusion Criteria

Unilateral or bilateral NTG evidenced by glaucomatous cupping of the disc and a defined type and severity of field loss with a median IOP of 20 mm Hg or less in 10 baseline measurements with no reading above 24 mm Hg and no more than one reading of 23 or 24 mm Hg.

Results

- There was 80% progression-free survival in the treated group versus 40% in the control arm at the end of 5 years follow-up. The visual field progression was 18% in the treated group versus 30% in the untreated group. 35% of the control eyes and 12% of the treated eyes reached end points (specifically defined criteria of glaucomatous optic disc progression or visual field loss).
- When comparison of control subjects with treated patients is made from the time of their randomization (as opposed to the time of stabilization of decrease in IOP), the intervention is beneficial to those whose IOP were lowered if the visual effects of cataract are excluded from consideration. This suggests that if IOP has been successfully lowered 30% from the baseline with treatment; the rate of progressive visual field loss will be slower.
- Because not all untreated patients progressed (half of the enrolled subjects who did not receive treatment showed no progression within their visual fields within 5 years), the natural history of NTG must be considered before treatment which lowers IOP and increases cataract, unless NTG threatens serious visual loss.
- Risk factors involved in the pathogenesis or that can act as prognostic indicators for the untreated disease are migraine, female sex, a disc hemorrhage at diagnosis, and perhaps racial or genetic heritage.

■ ADVANCED GLAUCOMA INTERVENTION STUDY (AGIS)[12-18]

Purpose
To assess the long-range outcomes of sequences of interventions involving trabeculectomy and ALT in eyes those have failed initial medical treatment for glaucoma.

Background
Sometimes, the first intervention chosen succeeds in controlling IOP for many years; at other times, the success lasts only a few weeks or months. Because success is limited, some patients, over time, need to undergo a sequence of surgical interventions. Little is known about which sequence gives the best long-range outcome.

Description
A total of 591 patients (789 eyes) with advanced glaucoma were enrolled (1988–1992). Eligible eyes were randomly assigned to one of two intervention sequences:
1. Trabeculectomy, followed by ALT should trabeculectomy fail, followed by a second trabeculectomy should ALT fail. *(TAT)*
2. Argon laser trabeculoplasty followed by trabeculectomy should ALT fail; followed by another trabeculectomy should the first trabeculectomy fail. *(ATT)*

Antifibrotic agents may be used as an adjunct to trabeculectomy, but only in eyes with a previous history of invasive surgery. Eyes that failed the entire assigned sequence of interventions were managed at the discretion of the AGIS physician in collaboration with the patient. Interventions were supplemented with medical treatment as needed.

After the initial intervention, follow-up examinations were scheduled at 1 week, 4 weeks, 3 months, 6 months, and every 6 months thereafter. After second and third interventions, follow-up examinations were scheduled at 1 and 4 weeks. Additional visits were scheduled as necessary for the management of the disease. All patients were being followed under a standardized protocol for a minimum of 5 years.

Inclusion Criteria
Men and women between the ages of 35 and 80 with OAG that was not successfully controlled by medication.

Study Measures
The primary outcome variable in AGIS was average percent of eyes with decrease of vision, where decrease of vision is a substantial decline of

either visual field or visual acuity attributable to the effect of glaucoma. Secondary outcome variables included sustained decrease of vision, failure of interventions, number of prescribed glaucoma medications, time to treatment failure and level of IOP. An ancillary study assessed filtering bleb encapsulation.

Results

- After 7 years of follow-up, results revealed that blacks and whites differed in the way they benefited from the two treatment programs. The vision in eyes of black patients with advanced glaucoma tended to be better preserved in the program that started with the laser surgery. From initial treatment through 7 years of follow-up, the average percent of eyes in black patients with decrease of vision was 28% in the program starting with laser surgery, as compared with 37% in the program starting with trabeculectomy.

  Through the first 4 years, the vision in eyes of white patients with advanced glaucoma tended to be better preserved in the program starting with laser surgery. Thereafter, however, the reverse was true; 7 years after the initial treatment, the average percent of eyes in white patients with decrease of vision was 31% in the program starting with a trabeculectomy, as compared with 35% in the program starting with laser surgery.

  Based on the study results, it is recommended that black patients with advanced glaucoma begin a treatment program that starts with laser surgery, which is consistent with current medical practice. In contrast, white patients with advanced glaucoma who have no life-threatening health problems should begin a treatment program that starts with trabeculectomy. This recommendation is inconsistent with current medical practice.

- Lower IOP was associated with a reduced progression of visual field damage. Subjects with IOP <18 mm Hg (target IOP) at 100% of visits had no change in visual field whereas, subjects with IOP <18 mm Hg at <50% of visits had a worsening of visual field by 0.63 units.
- Male gender and previous ALT were found to be a risk factor for bleb encapsulation.[13]
- In the eyes of AGIS patients, after adjustment for age and diabetes, trabeculectomy increased the risk of cataract formation by 78%. Marked postoperative inflammation and flat anterior chamber were the complications associated with the highest risk of cataract.[14]
- Assessment of the optic disc in AGIS was performed by clinical description of stereoscopic slit lamp biomicroscopy. Standardized optic disc photography was not performed in AGIS because of cost issues. The optic disc was noted to have no notching, partial optic disc notching (not to the edge of the disc), or disc notching to the edge of the disc. An analysis of clinical descriptions of the optic disc in AGIS revealed that optic nerves

with partial notching of the neural rim had a lower risk of subsequent visual field loss than eyes with no notching.[15]
- Argon laser trabeculoplasty failure was associated with younger age and higher pre-intervention IOP. Trabeculectomy failure was associated with younger age, higher pre-intervention IOP, diabetes, and one or more postoperative complications, particularly elevated IOP and marked inflammation.[16]
- For sustained decrease of visual field (SDVF), risk factors were better baseline visual field in both treatment sequences, male gender, and worse baseline visual acuity in the ATT sequence, and diabetes in the TAT sequence. For SDVA, risk factors in both treatment sequences were better baseline visual acuity, older age, and less formal education.[17]
- Because glaucoma is a life-long disease, long-term information is important. The AGIS patients were continued to be followed for 10 years and the results are as follows. In black patients the average percent of eyes with visual field loss was less in the ATT sequence than in the TAT sequence, a difference that is not statistically significant at any visit. In white patients, conversely, after 18 months the average percent of eyes with visual field loss was less in the TAT sequence, a difference that increases and is statistically significant in 8–10 years. In both black and white patients, the average percent of eyes with visual acuity loss was less in the ATT sequence; this difference is statistically significant throughout 10 follow-up years in black patients and is statistically significant only for the first year in white patients. In both black and white patients, average IOP reductions were greater in the TAT sequence, though the TAT-ATT difference was substantially greater in white patients. In both black and white patients, first-intervention failure rates were substantially lower for trabeculectomy than for ALT.

Thus, although IOP was lowered in both sequences in black and white patients with medically uncontrolled glaucoma, long-term visual function outcomes were better for the ATT sequence in black patients and better for the TAT sequence in white patients.[18]

GLAUCOMA LASER TRIAL FOLLOW-UP STUDY (GLTFS) [19,20]

Purpose
To compare the safety and long-term efficacy of argon laser treatment of the trabecular meshwork with standard medical treatment for primary OAG.

Background
During the last decade, ALT has often been used instead of surgery as the treatment of choice in cases of OAG that could not be controlled by drugs. ALT treatment consists of tiny laser burns evenly spaced around the trabecular

meshwork. It sometimes has been found to be effective in controlling glaucoma, although many eyes still require some medical treatment.

Description

The Glaucoma Laser Trial (GLT), a randomized, controlled clinical trial, was conducted to determine whether ALT is effective in patients with newly diagnosed, primary OAG (1984–1987). Each of the 271 patients in the trial received argon laser treatment in one eye and standard topical medication in the other eye. The eye to be started on medicine and the eye that would get the laser treatment were randomly selected. The GLTFS was a follow-up study of 203 of the 271 patients who enrolled in GLT. By the close of the GLTFS, median duration of follow-up since diagnosis of primary OAG was 7 years (maximum, 9 years).

The argon laser treatment was done in two sessions 1 month apart, with one-half of the trabecular meshwork treated with 45–55 laser burns in each session. Patients were seen for a follow-up visit 3 months after the first laser treatment and every 3 months thereafter for a period of at least 2 years. At each visit, examination of the eyes included a check of IOP and visual acuity. Visual field examinations were performed 3, 6, and 12 months after randomization and annually thereafter. Disc stereophotographs were taken 6 and 12 months after randomization and annually thereafter.

The results of these examinations determined whether treatment should be changed. If the IOP in either eye had not been reduced to the desired level, the physician changed the medication in the eye treated with drops or started the use of drops in the laser-treated eye according to a standardized procedure being used in the trial. If IOP was still not successfully reduced, surgery or further laser treatment may have been required.

Inclusion Criteria

At the time of recruitment, patients had to be at least 35 years old with an IOP of at least 22 mm Hg or greater in each eye and evidence of optic nerve damage in at least one eye.

Results

Over the course of the GLT and GLTFS, the eyes treated initially with ALT had lower IOP and better visual field and optic disk status than their fellow eyes treated initially with topical medication. As compared with eyes initially treated with medication, eyes initially treated with ALT had a 1.2 mm Hg greater reduction in IOP ($p < 0.001$) and 0.6 dB greater improvement in the visual field ($p < 0.001$) from entry into the GLT. The overall difference between eyes with regard to change in ratio of optic cup area to optic disk area from entry into the GLT was -0.01 ($p = 0.005$), which indicated slightly more deterioration for eyes initially treated with medication.

Thus, initial treatment with ALT was at least as efficacious as initial treatment with topical medication.

■ FLUOROURACIL FILTERING SURGERY STUDY (FFSS)[21,22]

Purpose

- To determine whether postoperative subconjunctival injections of 5-fluorouracil (5-FU) increase the success rate of filtering surgery in patients at high risk for failure after standard glaucoma filtering surgery.
- To compare the success rate of standard glaucoma filtering surgery to the success rate of standard surgery with adjunctive 5-FU treatment.
- To evaluate the frequency and severity of possible adverse effects related to 5-FU injections.

Background

Filtering surgery adequately lowers IOP in most glaucoma patients. However, the prognosis is less favorable for aphakic patients with glaucoma or glaucoma in phakic eyes following unsuccessful filtering operations. Failure of filtering surgery is usually attributed to the proliferation of fibroblasts at the filtering site. The use of 5-FU, an antimetabolite, has been shown to inhibit the proliferation of fibroblasts in tissue culture, and in preliminary studies it has increased the success of filtering surgery in a nonhuman primate model.

Description

A randomized, controlled clinical trial (1985–1988). There were 213 patients recruited into the study, 162 with previous cataract extraction and 51 with previous filtering surgery.

Detailed preoperative and postoperative examinations of the cornea, lens, and retina were performed. Systemic toxicity was assessed by preoperative and postoperative hematologic studies.

After the investigators performed the filtering surgery and determined that the new outlet channel was working, patients were randomized to receive either 5-FU injections or standard postsurgical care without 5-FU. The patients treated with 5-FU received subconjunctival injections of 5 mg of 5-FU twice daily on postoperative days 1 through 7 and once daily on postoperative days 8 through 14.

All patients were examined at 1 month, 3 months, 6 months, 1 year, 18 months, and 2 years postoperatively and at yearly intervals thereafter until 5 years postoperatively. Possible concomitant risks of 5-FU treatment, such as toxic effects to the cornea, lens, or retina, were monitored.

Inclusion Criteria

Men and women with uncontrolled IOP greater than 21 mm Hg in one or both eyes despite maximal tolerated therapy and who were aphakic or had undergone previous filtering surgery.

Study Measures

Success was defined as no reoperation for IOP control and no IOP over 21 mm Hg at or after the 1-year visit.

Results

- The data demonstrate improved surgical control of glaucoma using 5-FU in patients at high risk for trabeculectomy failure. At 1 year the cumulative success rates as calculated by survival analysis were 80% for the 5-FU group and 60% for the standard surgery group; at 3 years the success rates were 56% for the 5-FU group and 28% for the standard group; at 5 years the success rates were 48% in the 5-FU group and 21% in the standard.
- Visual acuity results [logarithm of the minimal angle of resolution (logMAR scale)] in the 5-FU group were worse than results in the standard therapy group at 1 month; however, the visual acuity change from the qualifying visit was better in the 5-FU group at 1, 2, and 3 years. The difference was not statistically significant at 4 or 5 years. This study showed that, regardless of treatment group, patients with controlled IOP had less visual acuity loss than patients whose IOP was not controlled. No difference between treatment groups was found in change in visual field sensitivity. Patients who underwent reoperation showed more visual field loss than those who did not undergo reoperation; the results also suggest that visual field loss is associated with high IOP. Both treatment groups lost visual acuity and visual field throughout the 5 years of the study.
- Risk factors other than treatment that clearly affect success are preoperative IOP, the number of previous ocular procedures with a conjunctival incision, and the time interval between the last ocular surgery and the study filtering surgery.
- The development of a late-onset leak in the filtering bleb was more likely to occur in the 5-FU group (9%) than in the standard therapy group (2%). No other long-term adverse effects were significantly different between the two groups. Two cases of endophthalmitis developed in the 5-FU group versus one case in the standard group.
- The risk of a suprachoroidal hemorrhage was not related to 5-FU. However, an important finding concerning suprachoroidal hemorrhage after filtering surgery is that the risk of hemorrhage was strongly associated with the preoperative IOP.

The association between high preoperative IOP and acute postoperative hypotony was not suspected as a risk factor for the development of suprachoroidal hemorrhage prior to this study. This observation has contributed to a change in ophthalmic surgical practice. Patients with very high preoperative IOP now undergo trabeculectomies with multiple tightly tied sutures or with releasable sutures in the scleral flap placed to minimize postoperative hypotony. Postoperative argon laser suture lysis or removal of releasable sutures may reduce the likelihood of large postoperative IOP fall and subsequent hypotony.

The FFSS Group recommends the use of subconjunctival 5-FU after trabeculectomy in eyes that have undergone previous cataract surgery or unsuccessful filtering surgery. However, because of a higher risk of late-onset wound leaks, which may increase the risk of endophthalmitis, the study group cautions against the routine use of 5-FU in patients with good prognoses. Preservation of visual function was associated with IOP control in both treatment groups, providing additional evidence to support IOP lowering in patients with glaucoma.

■ TUBE VERSUS TRABECULECTOMY STUDY (TVT)[23,24]

Purpose

To compare the safety and efficacy of nonvalved tube shunt surgery to trabeculectomy with mitomycin C (MMC) in patients with previous intraocular surgery.

Description

It was a multicenter randomized clinical trial conducted at 17 clinical centers. A total of 212 patients were enrolled from 1999 to 2004. Study patients were randomized to undergo placement of a 350-mm^2 Baerveldt glaucoma implant or trabeculectomy with MMC (0.4 mg/mL for 4 minutes).

Inclusion Criteria

Patients 18–85 years of age who had undergone previous trabeculectomy, cataract extraction with intraocular lens implantation, or both and had inadequately controlled glaucoma with IOP ≥18 mm Hg and ≤40 mm Hg on tolerated medical therapy were included.

Study Measures

Intraocular pressure, complication rates, visual acuity, visual field, quality of life, reoperations for glaucoma, and need for supplemental medical therapy were the main outcome measures.

Results

A total of 212 eyes of 212 patients were enrolled, including 107 in the tube group and 105 in the trabeculectomy group.

- At 5 years, IOP (mean ± SD) was 14.4 ± 6.9 mm Hg in the tube group and 12.6 ± 5.9 mm Hg in the trabeculectomy group ($p = 0.12$).
- The number of glaucoma medications (mean ± SD) was 1.4 ± 1.3 in the tube group and 1.2 ± 1.5 in the trabeculectomy group ($p = 0.23$).
- The cumulative probability of failure during 5 years of follow-up was 29.8% in the tube group and 46.9% in the trabeculectomy group ($p = 0.002$; hazard ratio = 2.15; 95% confidence interval = 1.30–3.56).
- The rate of reoperation for glaucoma was 9% in the tube group and 29% in the trabeculectomy group ($p = 0.025$).
- Early postoperative complications occurred in 22 patients (21%) in the tube group and 39 patients (37%) in the trabeculectomy group ($p = 0.012$). Late postoperative complications developed in 36 patients (34%) in the tube group and 38 patients (36%) in the trabeculectomy group during 5 years of follow-up ($p = 0.81$). The rate of reoperation for complications was 22% in the tube group and 18% in the trabeculectomy group ($p = 0.29$). Cataract extraction was performed in 13 phakic eyes (54%) in the tube group and 9 phakic eyes (43%) in the trabeculectomy group ($p = 0.43$).

Conclusion

- Tube shunt surgery had a higher success rate compared to trabeculectomy with MMC during 5 years of follow-up in the TVT Study. Both procedures were associated with similar IOP reduction and use of supplemental medical therapy at 5 years. Additional glaucoma surgery was needed more frequently after trabeculectomy with MMC than tube shunt placement.
- A large number of surgical complications were observed in the TVT Study, but most were transient and self-limited. The incidence of early postoperative complications was higher following trabeculectomy with MMC than tube shunt surgery. The rates of late postoperative complications, reoperation for complications, and cataract extraction were similar with both surgical procedures after 5 years of follow-up.
- Tube-shunt surgery and trabeculectomy with MMC are both viable surgical options for managing glaucoma in patients who have undergone prior cataract and/or failed filtering surgery. Results of the TVT Study support the expanding use of tube shunts beyond refractory glaucomas.

TRABECULECTOMY VERSUS CANALOPLASTY (TVC STUDY) IN THE TREATMENT OF PATIENTS WITH OPEN ANGLE GLAUCOMA: A PROSPECTIVE RANDOMIZED CLINICAL TRIAL[25]

Purpose

To compare the results of canaloplasty and trabeculectomy in patients with open angle glaucoma.

Description

It was a prospective, randomized, interventional clinical trial performed at one surgical center by a single surgeon (2015). 62 eyes of 62 Caucasian patients with uncontrolled open angle glaucoma were enrolled and randomized into trabeculectomy and canaloplasty groups using permuted block randomization.

They considered a null hypothesis, that there was no difference in absolute IOP (± 3 mm Hg) reduction between both groups. Total of 32 trabeculectomies and 30 canaloplasties was performed. Glaucoma was diagnosed based on typical optic nerve head morphology. Baseline standard ophthalmic examination was done. IOP was measured using Goldmann applanation tonometer. Follow-up was done at day 1 and 7, 4 weeks, and 3, 6, 12, and 24 months postoperatively.

Inclusion Criteria

- Male or female patients aged ≥18 years.
- Medically uncontrolled primary or secondary (pseudoexfoliation, pigmentary glaucoma) open angle glaucoma.

Exclusion Criteria

- Previous penetrating or nonpenetrating surgery.
- Patients with angle closure, normal tension, congenital or secondary glaucoma.
- More than 1 laser trabeculoplasty or more than 1 cyclodestructive procedures in the study eye.

Outcome Measures

Primary end point was success rate defined as IOP ≤18 mm Hg (definition 1) or IOP reduction by 20% or more and to ≤21 mm Hg (definition 2).

Criteria for Success

- Eyes with above IOP criteria after 4 weeks.
- Intraocular pressure ≥5 mm Hg after 4 weeks.
- No loss of light perception due to glaucoma.
- Eyes not requiring further glaucoma surgeries.

If the reduction was without any medications then it was termed complete success and if it was irrespective of medications, it was termed qualified success.

Secondary end point was absolute reduction of IOP after 2 years.

Results

Complete success was significantly higher in the trabeculectomy group as per both definitions at 2 years.

Complete success	Trabeculectomy (n, %)	Canaloplasty (n, %)
Definition 1	23, 74.2%	9, 39.1%
Definition 2	21, 67.7%	9, 39.1%

Qualified success was significantly higher in trabeculectomy group as per definition 1 but difference was insignificant as per definition 2.

Qualified success	Trabeculectomy (%)	Canaloplasty (%)	p
Definition 1	96.8	82.6	0.4
Definition 2	90.3	82.6	0.01

Intraocular pressure: Mean IOP reduction was 10.8 ± 6.9 mm Hg in trabeculectomy group and 9.3 ± 5.7 mm Hg in canaloplasty group after 2 years. There was significant reduction in the IOP as compared to preoperative period in both groups but there was no difference between the two groups.

Medication: No patient in trabeculectomy group needed medications up to 4 weeks postoperatively while 5 (16.7%) patients in the canaloplasty group were on antiglaucoma medications. At 2 years, 12 (52.2%) of canaloplasty and 8 (25.8%) of trabeculectomy patients needed antiglaucoma medications.

Visual acuity was not significantly different between the two groups. The number of postoperative complications was significantly higher in the trabeculectomy group.

Conclusion

Trabeculectomy leads to a better reduction in the IOP with lesser medications compared to canaloplasty but at the cost of higher complications and more demanding postoperative care.

■ EFFECTIVENESS OF EARLY LENS EXTRACTION FOR THE TREATMENT OF PRIMARY ANGLE CLOSURE GLAUCOMA (EAGLE): A RANDOMIZED CONTROL TRIAL[26]

Purpose

To assess the efficacy of clear lens extraction over standard of care (laser peripheral iridotomy and topical therapy) in primary angle closure (PAC) glaucoma.

Description

It was a multicentric, comparative effectiveness, randomized, controlled trial. The participants were randomized by a web-based application into the early lens extraction and the standard of care group. All the subjects were started on medical topical therapy at the time of diagnosis and the interventions were performed at day 60.

Clear lens extraction group underwent phacoemulsification with monofocal IOL implantation. IOP measured using Goldmann applanation tonometry and an average of two readings was taken. BCVA was taken on Early Treatment Diabetic Retinopathy Study (ETDRS) chart, gonioscopy was performed and Humphrey 24-2 Swedish Interactive Testing Algorithm (SITA) test was done for visual field analysis. Health status was measured using EQ-5D questionnaire to calculate total quality-adjusted life-years (QALY) at baseline and at 6, 12, 24, and 36 months. To assess the effects of vision problems on vision-targeted functioning and health-related quality of life National Eye Institute Visual Functioning Questionnaire (NEI-VFQ-25) and Glaucoma utility index were used. A target IOP of 15–20 mm Hg was selected and topical medications could be increased to keep IOP in this range. Worsening of the disease was defined as worsening of one or more stages using glaucoma staging system-2.

Need for glaucoma surgery to control IOP was termed as treatment failure.

Inclusion Criteria

- Phakic subjects who were 50 years or older.
- Newly diagnosed PAC (at least 180 degrees of iridotrabecular contact on gonioscopy) with IOP more than 30 mm Hg or primary angle closure glaucoma (PACG) (glaucomatous field defects and/or glaucomatous optic neuropathy and IOP more than 21 mm Hg at least one occasion).

Exclusion Criteria

- Subjects with symptomatic cataract.
- Advanced glaucoma (MD >-15 dB or cup-disc ratio ≥0.9).
- History of previous acute angle closure attack, previous laser or ocular surgery.

Results

419 subjects were included in the study from 30 centers from UK, Malaysia, Singapore, Australia, Taiwan, Hong Kong and China between 2009 and 2011.
- 155 had PAC and 263 PACG. 208 underwent clear lens extraction and 211 received standard of care.
- Mean health status score (EQ-5D) was significantly higher and the IOP (mean: 16.6 ± 3.5 mm Hg) was 1.18 mm Hg ($p = 0.004$) lower in the lens extraction group at 36 months.
- National Eye Institute Visual Functioning Questionnaire-25 and Glaucoma utility index scores were higher in the clear lens extraction group at 36 months.

- The incremental cost-effectiveness ratio was £14,284 for initial lens extraction versus standard care. Clear lens extraction was more cost-effective than laser peripheral iridotomy with topical antiglaucoma therapy.
- Significantly fewer participants in the lens extraction group needed any treatment to control IOP.
- Visual field severity was similar in the two groups.
- Irreversible vision loss was seen in one patient in lens extraction group and in three in standard care group.
- Additional surgeries were needed in three patients of clear lens extraction group and one in standard care group.

Conclusion

Clear lens extraction was found to be more efficacious and cost-effective than laser peripheral iridotomy with topical antiglaucoma drugs and should be considered as first line of treatment.

■ EARLY LENS EXTRACTION WITH INTRAOCULAR LENS IMPLANTATION FOR THE TREATMENT OF PRIMARY ANGLE CLOSURE GLAUCOMA: AN ECONOMIC EVALUATION BASED ON DATA FROM THE EAGLE TRIAL[27]

Purpose

To assess the cost-effectiveness and to evaluate the economics of early lens extraction compared with standard of care in individuals with PAC or PACG.

Description

It was a parallel group randomized control trial. 419 patients were recruited from 30 centers from UK, Malaysia, Singapore, Australia, Taiwan, Hong Kong and China. Patients underwent 1:1 randomization to early lens extraction ($n = 208$) or standard care ($n = 211$).

Economic analysis was carried on from a UK health and social care perspective in patients recruited only from the United Kingdom between June 2009 and August 2012, 145 randomized to early lens extraction and 140 to standard care. Lens extraction group underwent phacoemulsification and intraocular lens implant and standard care group was managed with laser peripheral iridotomy. The worst eye was treated first and subsequently the better eye received the same treatment.

Inclusion Criteria

- Individuals aged ≥50 years with newly diagnosed PAC and IOP ≥30 mm Hg.

- Primary angle closure glaucoma patients either untreated or under medical treatment for 6 months or less.

Exclusion Criteria

- Mean deviation worse than -15 dB.
- Cup disc ratio ≥0.9.
- Previously diagnosed acute angle closure attack in an otherwise eligible eye.
- Increased surgical risk (Fuch's endothelial dystrophy, Pseudoexfoliation syndrome, previous Vitreoretinal surgery, inability to maintain position required for the standard technique).
- Symptomatic cataract in either eye.
- Prior cataract surgery or laser iridotomy in the study eye.
- Axial length <19 mm (nanophthalmos), secondary angle closure glaucoma, retinal ischemia, macular edema, wet age-related macular degeneration, medically unfit for the surgery or completion of the trial.

Study Measures

The primary economic outcome was the incremental cost per QALY gained. QALY was assessed using the EQ-5D 3 level. Costs of primary and secondary healthcare usage [UK National Health Service (NHS) perspective] were used. The costs of surgical or nonsurgical procedures, total medication was estimated. The unit cost per visit to general practitioner, practice nurse consultations, community optometrist visits were valued. All cost elements of the interventions and health services used were summed to generate total cost per patient. Indirect costs such as time costs for accessing health care, time lost due to ill health, time away from paid work, leisure time was evaluated. Markov model was used for extrapolation for longer term cost effectiveness.

Results

- The mean age of participants was 67.5 (8.42), 57.5% were women, 44.6% had both eyes eligible, 1.4% were of Asian ethnicity and 35.4% had PAC.
- The mean adjusted QALYs were higher with early lens extraction: 2.602 versus 2.533.
- The initial cost of the procedure was higher in the lens extraction group (£2467 vs. £1486). But had cost savings due to fewer subsequent procedures and lower medications.
- Incremental cost-effectiveness ratio (ICER) for lens extraction versus standard care was £14 284 per QALY gained at 3 years. Lens extraction had a 67% probability of being cost effective at 3 years.

Conclusion

Lens extraction has a 67–89% chance of being cost effective at 3 years. On extrapolation it may be cost saving by 10 years.

Lens extraction appears likely to offer a cost-effective approach to treatment in patients with newly diagnosed PAC or PACG.

THE AHMED VERSUS BAERVELDT STUDY (AVB STUDY): 5-YEAR TREATMENT OUTCOMES[28]

Purpose

To compare the surgical outcomes of Ahmed Glaucoma valve FP7 and Baerveldt Implant-350.

Description

It was an international, multicenter randomized control trial. Patients were recruited from seven international centers by 10 surgeons between 2005 and 2009. They followed a standardized surgical technique. Follow-up was done on 9 appointments in the first year postoperatively, 2 in the second year and annually through 5 years. IOP, glaucoma medications used, visual acuity and any complications/interventions were noted.

Inclusion Criteria

- Age ≥18 years.
- Intraocular pressure greater than clinical target IOP even after maximal tolerable topical medications and laser therapy.
- Failed trabeculectomy with antimetabolite or conditions associated with high-risk of failure of trabeculectomy.
- Eyes with prior surgery or significant scarring was also included.
- Only one eye was considered.

Exclusion Criteria

- Need for an additional procedure at the time of implantation of the device.
- Unwilling/unable to follow or give consent.

Outcome Measures

Primary outcome was failure of the surgery. It was defined as follows:
- Intraocular pressure more than target range (5–18 mm Hg) or <20% reduction from baseline for 2 consecutive visits after 3 months.
- Need for another glaucoma surgery.
- Removal of implant.
- Severe vision loss related to the surgery.

Success was defined as the absence of failure. It could either be complete or qualified.

Complete success: IOP within target range at all visits after 3 months without use of any antiglaucoma medications, additional surgeries or vision loss.

Qualified success: Nonconsecutive visits could have IOP outside target IOP, use of glaucoma medications and surgical interventions except de novo glaucoma procedures.

Alternate IOP success criteria ≤21 mm Hg and ≤14 mm Hg.

Results

- 238 patients were recruited and randomized.
- 124 into Ahmed valve and 114 to Baerveldt group. Baseline characteristics were similar except higher females in later group.
- The mean baseline IOP of the study group was 31.4 ± 10.8 on a mean of 3.1 ± 1.0 glaucoma medications.
- Intraoperative complications occurred 4% in each group.
- Treatment outcomes at 5 years:
    - Cumulative probability of failure was higher in Ahmed group (53.2%) than Baerveldt group (40.0%). ($p = 0.037$)
    - High IOP was the main cause of failure in both Ahmed (45%) and in Baerveldt group (23%).
    - De novo glaucoma reoperation was needed in 18% of the Ahmed group and 11% in the Baerveldt group and was similar.
    - Hypotony was present in 5 (4%) of the Baerveldt group and none of the Ahmed group.
    - Severe vision loss was present in 7 (6%) of the Ahmed group and 9 (8%) of the Baerveldt group.
    - Complete success was low in both groups; 3 (2%) in Ahmed group and 5 (4%) of Baerveldt group. ($p = 0.49$)
    - Qualified success was seen in 15 (12%) in the Ahmed group and 22 (19%) in the Baerveldt group. ($p = 0.12$)
    - Both neovascular glaucoma (NVG) (56% failure rate, $p = 0.04$) and not having a prior trabeculectomy were a risk factor for failure (52% failure, $p = 0.001$)
    - According to alternate IOP criteria of ≤21 mm Hg, cumulative probability of failure was 49.1% in Ahmed group and 38.3% in the Baerveldt group ($p = 0.057$).
    - When using the alternate criteria of IOP ≤14 mm Hg, the cumulative probability of failure was 83.5% in the Ahmed group and 72.2% in the Baerveldt group ($p = 0.05$).

Intraocular Pressure
- Mean IOP in the Ahmed group reduced from 31.1 ± 10.5 to 16.6 ± 5.9 mm Hg at 5 years (47%). ($p < 0.001$).
- In the Baerveldt group, the mean IOP reduced from 41.9 ± 11 to 13.6 ± 5 at 5 years (57%). ($p < 0.001$)
- Ahmed group had lower mean IOP at day 1, week 1 and week 2. The Baerveldt group had lower mean IOP at all visits after 1 year.
- Baerveldt group has greater reduction in the IOP compared to Ahmed group at all follow ups from the first year to 5 years. ($p = 0.02$)

Glaucoma Medication Uses:
- In the Ahmed group, the mean number of glaucoma medications reduced from 3.1 ± 1 to 1.8 ± 1.5 (44% reduction) at 5 years. ($p < 0.001$)
- In the Baerveldt group, the mean number of glaucoma medications reduced from 3.1 ± 1.0 to 1.2 ± 1.3 (61% reduction) at 5 years. ($p < 0.001$)
- In the early postoperative period, at 1 day, 1 week and 2 weeks, the Ahmed group had lower glaucoma medications whereas, the Baerveldt group had lower medications at all points after 1 month. ($p < 0.05$)
- At 5 years, the Baerveldt group needed a median of 1 glaucoma medication as compared to 2 medications in the Ahmed group. ($p = 0.038$).

Visual Acuity
- In the Ahmed group, the Mean LogMAR visual acuity reduced from 1.3 ± 1.0 to 1.6 ± 1.0 at 5 years ($p < 0.001$)
- In the Baerveldt group, it reduced from 1.2 ± 1.0 to 1.6 ± 1.2 at 5 years ($p < 0.001$).

De Novo Glaucoma Procedure
- The number of patients requiring de novo glaucoma procedures was 17.7% in the Ahmed group and 11% in the Baerveldt group ($p = 0.02$).
- The two groups had comparable IOPs and mean number of antiglaucoma medications when they underwent the de novo procedures.
- Cyclodestruction was the most common de novo procedure used. It was done in 10 (8%) patients in the Ahmed group and 3 (3%) patients in the Baerveldt group.
- Additional shunts (Baerveldt implants) was needed in 7 (6%) patients in the Ahmed group and 4 (4%) patients in the Baerveldt group.
- Gold shunt was needed in 1 (1%) patient in the Ahmed group and 3 (3%) patients in the Baerveldt group.
- Selective laser trabeculoplasty (SLT) was done in 1 patient in each group.

Complications:
- In the Ahmed group, 78 (63%) patients had complications. In the Baerveldt group, 79 (69%) patients had complications. ($p = 0.3$)

- The most common complications were shallow anterior chamber, choroidal effusions, tube complications, persistent corneal edema and persistent iritis.
- Bleb encapsulation was more common in the Ahmed group ($p = 0.023$)
- Refractory hypotony was seen in 1 patient in the Ahmed group and 6 patients in the Baerveldt group. ($p = 0.057$)
- Each group had 1 patient with early postoperative over filtration.

Intervention:
- 64 patients (51%) in the Ahmed group and 58 patients (51%) needed additional interventions.
- The common interventions were anterior chamber reformation, paracentesis, tube related interventions, cataract surgery, vitrectomy and corneal transplantation.
- Three patients in each group had to undergo explantation of the device.

Conclusion
- Both Ahmed glaucoma valve and Baerveldt implant were effective in reducing the IOP and the number of glaucoma medications used.
- The Baerveldt group had lower IOP and lesser use of medications but had a risk of persistent hypotony.
- Both groups were associated with some amount of loss in visual acuity.

A RANDOMIZED, CONTROLLED COMPARISON OF LATANOPROSTENE BUNOD AND LATANOPROST 0.005% IN THE TREATMENT OF OCULAR HYPERTENSION AND OPEN ANGLE GLAUCOMA: THE VOYAGER STUDY[29]

Purpose
- To assess the efficacy and safety of latanoprostene bunod (LBN) as compared to latanoprost 0.005% in reducing IOP in patients with open angle glaucoma and OHT.
- To determine the optimum drug concentration of LBN in reducing IOP.

Description
The study was a multicentric, phase 2, randomized, parallel group, dose ranging study design with investigator masking (2010-2011). They compared four different concentrations of LBN with Xalatan (latanoprost 0.005%). Baseline demographics, ocular and systemic evaluation was done for all patients. The subjects were randomized into 5 groups. LBN of four different concentrations were given 0.006%, 0.012%, 0.024%, and 0.040%. One drop instilled in the conjunctival sac once daily at 20:00 hours for 28 days.

The subjects were followed up for 5 visits on day 1, day 7 ± 1, day 14 ± 1, day 28 ± 1, day 29 ± 1. At all visits, IOP was measured at 8:00, 12:00, and 16:00 using Goldmann applanation tonometry. Adverse events, BCVA, ocular tolerability, ocular signs and vital signs were recorded at each visit. Ocular inflammation and conjunctival hyperemia was recorded. Treatment emergent adverse events were defined as those occurring on or after first dose.

Inclusion Criteria
- Age ≥18 years
- Treatment naïve or currently treated OAG or OHT
- Intraocular pressure of 22–32 mm Hg, and IOP of ≥24 mm Hg in two out of three readings on visit 3, which was after 28-day washout period
- Best-corrected visual acuity of + 0.7 logMAR (20/100) or better in either eye.

Exclusion Criteria
- If the subjects had participated in any other clinical trial within 30 days
- Hypersensitivity or contraindication to latanoprost or any ingredients in the drug under study.
- Contraindication to NO-donating treatment like severe hypotension.
- Unable to discontinue contact lens during visits, during drug administration and for 15 minutes following it.
- Central corneal thickness (CCT) >600 microns.
- Conditions that prevented accurate applanation tonometry.
- Advanced glaucomatous damage.
- Any other significant ocular disease.
- Those taking oral or topical corticosteroids or other drugs that have an effect on IOP.

Outcome Measure
- *Primary efficacy endpoint*: Reduction/change in the mean diurnal IOP at day 28
- *Secondary efficacy endpoint*: Reduction in mean diurnal IOP at day 7, 14, and 29, reduction of IOP at specific time points. And proportion of subjects with IOP ≤18 mm Hg at all-time points.
- *Primary safety endpoints*: Incidence of ocular and systemic adverse events, their severity and relationship to the study drug.

Results
- 413 patients were randomized. 82 in LBN 0.006% group, 85 in 0.012% group, 83 in 0.024% group, 81 in 0.040% group and 82 in latanoprost group.

- All groups had significant reduction in mean diurnal IOP from baseline at all follow up visits. ($p < 0.0001$)
- Intraocular pressure reduction in LBN groups was dose dependent and the effect reached a plateau with 0.024% and 0.040%.
- Latanoprostene bunod 0.024% and 0.040% groups showed significantly higher reduction of IOP from baseline compared to latanoprost group. ($p = 0.005$ and $p = 0.009$) at day 28
- There was significantly greater reduction in the mean diurnal IOP compared to latanoprost at day 7 for LBN 0.024% and 0.040% groups and day 14 for LBN 0.024% group.
- On day 29, there was marginally greater reduction in IOP with LBN 0.024% group.
- At specific time points, there was higher reduction in IOP in LBN 0.024% and 0.040% group at 12:00 and 16:00 hours on day 7, with LBN 0.024% at 08:00 hours and 12:00 hour and with both concentrations at 16:00 hours on day 14, with 0.040% group at 8:00 and both groups at 12:00 hours and 16:00 hours on day 28 and with 0.024% group at 16:00 on day 29.
- There was higher incidence of at least one adverse event with the LBN groups as compared to the latanoprost group.
- The common adverse events reported was pain in the LBN groups.
- Ocular hyperemia was the most common adverse event in the latanoprost group.

Conclusion

Latanoprostene bunod 0.024% in once daily dosing was found to be the most effective least concentration with significantly higher IOP lowering and comparable side effects compared to latanoprost 0.005%.

A PROSPECTIVE, RANDOMIZED, PLACEBO CONTROLLED, DOUBLE-MASKED, THREE-ARMED, MULTICENTER PHASE II/III TRIAL FOR THE STUDY OF A TOPICAL TREATMENT OF ISCHEMIC CENTRAL RETINAL VEIN OCCLUSION TO PREVENT NEOVASCULAR GLAUCOMA—THE STRONG STUDY: STUDY PROTOCOL FOR A RANDOMIZED CONTROLLED TRIAL[30]

Purpose
- To test efficacy and safety of topical antiangiogenic agent Aganirsen to inhibit formation of neovascularization and hence secondary NVG in eyes with ischemic central retinal vein occlusion (CRVO).
- To study the natural course of ischemic CRVO and NVG in a large and well characterized cohort.

- To evaluate the efficacy and safety of Aganirsen
- Of two different doses of the drug when compared to a placebo in terms of the time and intensity of additional investigations, comparing health outcome and quality of life check safety profile of Aganirsen.

Description

Aganirsen is a 25-mer phosphorothioate antisense oligonucleotide of 8,035 Da. It inhibits new vessel formation by blocking Insulin Receptor Substrate- 1 and hence Vascular endothelial growth factor (VEGF) and tumor necrosis factor (TNF)-α. STRONG study is a phase II/III multicenter prospective randomized double masked three-armed controlled study.

333 patients from primary ischemic CRVO or those newly converted to ischemic CRVO (no longer than 4 weeks) were recruited. They were followed up for 30 weeks, 24 weeks treatment phase and a 6 week safety follow-up.
- Arm 1: Had 111 patients. They received Aganirsen (43 µg) daily. 1 drop of 0.86 mg/g emulsion in the morning and placebo in the evening for 24 weeks.
- Arm 2: Had 111 patients. They received high dose Aganirsen (86 µg) daily. 1 drop of 0.86 mg/g emulsion twice daily for 24 weeks.
- Arm 3: Had 111 patients. They received placebo twice daily for 24 weeks.
- Patients were followed up at baseline, the 4, 8, 12, 16, 20, 24, and 30 weeks. Images of the anterior segment and gonioscopic photograph was collected for evaluation.
- Tears and serum sample collected for the biomarker substudy from 200 patients for markers of ischemic CRVO and NVG. 33 eligible patients included in the risk factor substudy.

Inclusion Criteria

- Primary ischemic CRVO or those converted to ischemic CRVO within past 4 weeks.
- Best-corrected visual acuity in ETDRS letter score <35 letters in study eye. (<20/200)
- At least a 10 disc area of retinal capillary obliteration on fundus fluorescein angiography and/or large confluent retinal hemorrhages in the study eye.
- Intraocular pressure ≤21 mm Hg.
- Age ≥18 years.
- Willing to use contraception to prevent pregnancy.
- Willing to sign consent and come for all follow-up visits.

Additionally, at least 4 out of 6 of the following criteria must be fulfilled:
1. A relative afferent pupillary defect with normal other eye.
2. At least 10 cotton-wool spots.
3. Venous tortuosity.

4. Visual field defects corresponding to ischemia. Patient cannot see the I-2e target and has a defective or absent I-4e isopter [Goldmann perimeter or semiautomatic kinetic methods (Humphrey or Octopus visual field analyzer)], targets I-2e, I-4e, V-4e.
5. Engorged vessels over the iris/angle.
6. Anterior chamber flare.

Exclusion Criteria
- Other eye with an ocular condition with bad prognosis compared to the study eye.
- Primary or secondary glaucoma.
- Ranibizumab or Bevacizumab received in the eye in the past 45 days. History of aflibercept injection within the past 60 days. Any anti VEGF treatment in the fellow eye or use of any systemic anti VEGF.
- History of use of intraocular steroid at any time or periocular steroid within 90 days in the study and the fellow eye.
- Idiopathic, autoimmune uveitis.
- Presence of neovascularization of the disc (NVD), neovascularization elsewhere (NVE), neovascularization of the angle (NVA), and neovascularization of the iris (NVI) in the study eye.
- Previous panretinal photocoagulation (PRP), cyclocryophotocoagulation in the study eye.
- Pregnancy and lactation.
- Inability to do a reliable applanation tonometry.
- Intraocular surgery or laser within last 90 days of screening.
- Infectious lesion in the eye.
- Any confounding pathologies in the study eye.
- Inability to perform fundus fluorescein angiography or obtain fundus photographs.
- Hypersensitivity or allergy to drug used or any such similar compound.
- Metabolic dysfunction, breast cancer, medical or psychological diseases.
- Participation in other trials.

Outcomes Compared
- Co-primary efficacy endpoints:
  - Presence of anterior segment neovascularization (NVI/NVA). NVD and/or NVE in the study eye needing PRP or cryotherapy up to week 24.
  - *Intraocular pressure component*: Percentage change ($\geq 20\%$) or more than 21 mm Hg in the study eye is called as "failure".
- Secondary endpoints:
  - Time of development of secondary NVG up to 24 weeks.
  - Time of development of NVI/NVA and also time of development of NVE/NVD needing PRP or cryotherapy.

- Development of change in BCVA.
- Need for retreatment and additional lasers.
- Change in retinal nonperfusion areas.
- National Eye Institute Visual Functioning Questionnaire 25 total score at 24 weeks.
- Changes in EQ-5D questionnaire.
- Changes in CCT in optical coherence tomography (OCT).

GLAUCOMA EPIDEMIOLOGICAL STUDIES IN INDIA

Most data on prevalence of glaucoma in India has been in South India and West Bengal; there is no data available from North India as of now. There have been four prevalence studies from South India:

1. Vellore Eye Study (VES)
2. Andhra Pradesh Eye Disease Study (APEDS)
3. Aravind comprehensive eye survey (ACES)
4. Chennai glaucoma study (CGS).

Though the methodology applied in each of these population-based studies differs widely, all the studies were based on the diagnosis of glaucoma on the appearance of the optic discs and matching visual field defects on automated perimetry. No study relied on measurement of IOP for diagnosis of glaucoma except in situations where optic disc or visual field criteria were unavailable owing to lack of media clarity.

Vellore Eye Study (VES)[31]

Purpose
To estimate the prevalence of POAG and PACG in an urban South Indian population.

Background
Racial variations in the prevalence of primary glaucoma are well known. The VES was the first comprehensive study of the prevalence (and risk factors) for eye diseases using modern examination and diagnostic methods on a random sample of an Indian population.

Description
972 individuals aged 30–60 years were examined. They were chosen using a cluster sampling technique from 12 census blocks of Vellore town.

Visual acuity and refraction were performed by experienced optometrists. A comprehensive ocular examination including slit lamp biomicroscopy, applanation tonometry, gonioscopy, dilated pupil indirect ophthalmoscopy as well as stereo-biomicroscopy of the disc and macula (using a noncontact

+ 78 D lens) was performed in a standard manner. An automated visual field (Humphrey Field Analyzer 30-2 program) was scheduled on the following indications: IOP >21 mm Hg, cup-to-disc-ratio (CDR) ≥0.7 in either eye, difference in CDR >0.2 between the two eyes and/or the presence of glaucomatous features. If an advanced field defect precluded a successful 30-2 examination, the macular program or a 10-2 program was used.

Study Measures

- Primary open-angle glaucoma was defined as the presence of elevated IOP and/or glaucomatous disc changes in the presence of typical glaucomatous field defects, an open angle on gonioscopy and no evidence of a secondary cause.
- The diagnosis of OHT was made based on an IOP >21 mm Hg, absence of glaucomatous disc features, no demonstrable glaucomatous field defects and open angles with no evidence of a secondary cause.
- Primary angle closure glaucoma was considered under the following headings:
  - Acute PACG—defined as an acute painful red eye with a history of loss of vision, dilated pupils, raised IOP and closed angles on gonioscopy in the absence of any secondary cause.
  - Chronic primary angle closure glaucoma (CACG) was considered to be either appositional or synechial. Chronic appositional angle closure was diagnosed in the presence of raised IOP and closed angles on gonioscopy, in the absence of peripheral anterior synechiae (PAS). These angles could always be opened on "manipulation" with the two-mirror gonioscope or by indentation gonioscopy. Chronic synechial angle closure was diagnosed in the presence of PAS with occludable or closed angles on gonioscopy, even in the absence of raised IOP. The presence of glaucomatous field defects or optic disc changes was not considered mandatory for the diagnosis of angle closure glaucoma (ACG). Secondary causes of angle closure were excluded.

Results

- Prevalence (95% confidence interval) of POAG, PACG, and OHT were 4.1 (0.08–8.1), 43.2 (30.14–56.3), and 30.8 (19.8–41.9) per 1,000, respectively, that is, 0.41%, 4.32%, and 3.08% respectively.
- The prevalence of POAG was found to be 0.41% (lower than that reported elsewhere—probably explained by the age of the study population).
- Occludable angles were detected in 10.3%. All the PACG cases detected were of the chronic type.
- The major finding of interest was the prevalence of PACG. Hospital-based data from India had suggested that PACG was at least as common as POAG.

The prevalence of PACG (4.32%) found in this study was almost five times that of POAG. This high prevalence in the present report can be explained by the comprehensive examination protocol that included gonioscopy for all subjects.

Andhra Pradesh Eye Disease Study (APEDS) [32,33]

Purpose

To assess the prevalence and features of OAG and ACG in an urban population in Southern India.

Background

The APEDS (1996) was carried out to assess the magnitude and causes of blindness and moderate visual impairment, prevalence and risk factors for eye diseases, effect of visual impairment on quality of life, and barriers to eye care services perceived by the people, in the urban and rural populations of the southern Indian state of Andhra Pradesh.

Description

A population-based cross-sectional study. A total of 2,522 persons (85.4% of those eligible) of all ages, including 1,399 persons 30 years of age or older, from 24 clusters representative of the population of Hyderabad city participated in the study.

The participants underwent an interview and detailed eye examination that included logarithm of minimum angle of resolution visual acuity, refraction, slit-lamp biomicroscopy, applanation tonometry, gonioscopy, dilatation, cataract grading, and stereoscopic fundus evaluation. Automated Humphrey threshold 24-2 visual fields (Humphrey Instruments Inc., San Leandro, CA) and optic disc photography were performed when indicated by standardized criteria for disc damage or if IOP was 22 mm Hg or more.

Open-angle Glaucoma

Study Measures
- Definite POAG was defined as obvious glaucomatous optic disc damage and visual field loss in the presence of an open-angle
- Suspected POAG was defined as suspected glaucomatous optic disc damage without definite visual field loss.
- Ocular hypertension was defined as IOP of 22 mm Hg or more without glaucomatous optic disc damage or visual field loss in the presence of an open-angle.
- Glaucomatous optic disc damage or IOP of 22 mm Hg or more secondary to an obvious cause and with an open-angle was defined as secondary OAG.

Results

- Definite POAG, suspected POAG, and OHT had an age- and gender-adjusted prevalence (95% confidence interval) of 1.62% (0.77%–2.48%), 0.79% (0.39%–1.41%), and 0.32% (0.10%–0.78%) in those 30 years of age or older, and 2.56% (1.22%–3.91%), 1.11% (0.43%–1.78%), and 0.42% (0.11%–1.12%) in those 40 years of age or older, respectively.
- The prevalence of POAG increased significantly with age.
- Only two of 27 participants (7.4%) with definite POAG had been previously diagnosed and treated, and 66.7% of the previously undiagnosed had IOP less than 22 mm Hg. 14 of 27 participants (51.9%) with definite POAG had severe glaucomatous damage based on optic disc and visual field criteria, of which five participants (18.5%) had at least one blind eye as a result of POAG (all with best-corrected distance visual acuity less than 20/400 or central visual field less than 10°); the other 13 participants (48.1%) had moderate glaucomatous damage. Because visual fields and optic disc photography were not performed on all participants, the prevalence of POAG may have been underestimated.

Conclusion

The prevalence of OAG in this urban population in southern India is at least as much as that reported recently from white populations in developed countries. However, the vast majority of persons with glaucoma were undiagnosed in this population, and a large proportion of those having definite POAG already had severe glaucomatous damage.

Angle Closure Glaucoma

Study Measures

- An occludable angle was defined as pigmented posterior trabecular meshwork not visible by gonioscopy in three quarters or more of the angle circumference.
- Manifest PACG was defined as IOP of 22 mm Hg or more or glaucomatous optic disc damage with visual field loss in the presence of an occludable angle.
- An IOP of 22 mm Hg or more or glaucomatous optic disc damage in the presence of an occludable angle secondary to an obvious cause was defined as secondary ACG.

Results

- Manifest PACG and occludable angles without ACG had an age- and gender-adjusted prevalence (95% confidence interval) of 0.71% (0.34%–1.31%) and 1.41% (0.73%–2.09%) in participants 30 years of age or older,

and 1.08% (0.36%-1.80%) and 2.21% (1.15%-3.27%) in participants 40 years of age or older, respectively.
- With multivariate analysis, the prevalence of these two conditions considered together increased significantly with age; although not statistically significant, these were more common in females and in those belonging to lower socioeconomic strata as compared with middle and upper strata.
- The odds of manifest PACG were higher in the presence of hyperopia of more than 2 diopters.
- Only 4 of 12 participants (33.3%) with manifest PACG had been previously diagnosed, and 1 of 12 (8.3%) had peripheral iridotomy (PI) performed previously. Manifest PACG had caused blindness in one or both eyes in 5 of these 12 participants (41.7%); best-corrected distance visual acuity less than 20/400 in one or both eyes in four patients, and acuity less than 20/200 in one eye in another patient. Most (83.3%) of those with manifest PACG could be classified as having chronic form of the disease. We may have underestimated manifest PACG because visual fields were performed only on those with clinical suspicion of optic disc damage.

Conclusion

The prevalence of PACG in this urban population in southern India is close to that reported recently in a Mongolian population. A large proportion of the PACG in this population was undiagnosed and untreated. Because visual loss resulting from PACG is potentially preventable if peripheral iridotomy or iridectomy is performed in the early stage, strategies for early detection of PACG could reduce the high risk of blindness resulting from PACG seen in this urban population in India.

Aravind Comprehensive Eye Survey (ACES)[34]

Purpose

To determine the prevalence of glaucoma and risk factors for POAG in a rural population of Southern India.

Background

Previous population-based studies from India have reported the prevalence of glaucoma in urban populations. There has been no report on the prevalence of glaucoma in rural populations from India. In addition, in these prior studies, perimetry was limited to those who fulfilled certain conditions, such as elevated IOP or optic disc cupping. This approach offers the potential to miss those who did not meet these criteria but had glaucomatous optic nerve damage. This is the first population-based study from India to attempt threshold perimetric evaluations and dilated fundus examinations on all participants.

Description

A population-based cross-sectional study. A total of 5,150 subjects aged 40 years and older from 50 clusters representative of three southern districts of Tamil Nadu in southern India participated in the study.

All participants had a comprehensive eye examination at the base hospital, including visual acuity using logarithm of the minimum angle of resolution illiterate E charts and refraction, slit-lamp biomicroscopy, gonioscopy, applanation tonometry, dilated fundus examinations, and automated central 24-2 full-threshold perimetry.

Study Measures

- Definite POAG was defined as angles open on gonioscopy and glaucomatous optic disc changes with matching visual field defects.
- Ocular hypertension was defined as IOP greater than 21 mm Hg without glaucomatous optic disc damage and visual field defects in the presence of an open angle.
- Manifest PACG was defined as glaucomatous optic disc damage or glaucomatous visual field defects with the anterior chamber angle partly or totally closed, appositional angle closure or synechiae in the angle, and absence of signs of secondary angle closure.
- Secondary glaucoma was defined as glaucomatous optic nerve damage and/or visual field abnormalities suggestive of glaucoma with ocular disorders that contribute to a secondary elevation in IOP.

Results

- The prevalence (95% confidence interval) of any glaucoma was 2.6% (2.2, 3.0), of POAG it was 1.7% (1.3, 2.1), and if PACG it was 0.5% (0.3, 0.7), and secondary glaucoma excluding pseudoexfoliation was 0.3% (0.2, 0.5).
- On multivariate analysis, increasing age, male gender, myopia greater than 1 diopter, and pseudoexfoliation were significantly associated with POAG.
- After best correction, 18 persons (20.9%) with POAG were blind in either eye because of glaucoma, including 6 who were bilaterally blind and an additional 12 persons with unilateral blindness because of glaucomatous optic neuropathy in that eye. Of those identified with POAG, 93.0% had not been previously diagnosed with POAG.

Conclusion

The prevalence of glaucoma in this population is not lower than that reported for white populations elsewhere. A large proportion of those with POAG had not been previously diagnosed. One-fifth of those with POAG had blindness in one or both eyes from glaucoma. Early detection of glaucoma in this population will reduce the burden of blindness in India.

Chennai Glaucoma Study (CGS)[35-38]

Purpose

To estimate the prevalence and risk factors of POAG, PACG, PAC, and primary angle-closure suspect (PACS) in a rural and in an urban population in southern India.

Background

One of the causes of variations in the prevalence of glaucoma as reported by previous studies could be the different definitions used by each of the studies. The International Society of Geographical and Epidemiologic Ophthalmology (ISGEO) suggested a new classification for the diagnosis of glaucoma in population-based prevalence surveys. In this classification, glaucoma is diagnosed on the grounds of both structural and functional evidence of glaucomatous optic neuropathy. The CGS was started in 2001 to study the prevalence of glaucoma in rural and urban populations of the southern Indian state of Tamil Nadu. Access to ophthalmic care can affect the prevalence of a disease. Ophthalmic care seems to differ in urban and rural India.

Description

Population-based cross-sectional study of subjects 40 years or older.

For the rural population, a total of 3,934 subjects of the 4,800 enumerated (82%) agreed to participate in the study. For the urban population, 3,850 of the 4,800 subjects (80.2%) that were selected using a multistage random cluster sampling procedure in Chennai city participated in the study.

Subjects underwent a complete ophthalmic examination, including logarithm of the minimum angle of resolution visual acuity, applanation tonometry, gonioscopy (including compression gonioscopy), pachymetry, grading of lens opacities, optic disc photography, and automated perimetry.

Study Measures

Glaucoma was diagnosed using the International Society of Geographical and Epidemiological Ophthalmology Classification.

Open-angle Glaucoma (CGS) (Table 1)

Results

The urban population prevalence was more than that of the rural population (1.62%; 95% confidence interval, 1.4%–1.8%; p <0.0001). In both populations, increasing IOP (per mm Hg) and older age were associated with the disease. There was no association with gender, myopia, systemic hypertension, diabetes, or CCT.

Table 1: Results of open-angle glaucoma (CGS).	
Rural population	**Urban population**
Complete data were available for 3,924 subjects for the rural population. In eyes with normal suprathreshold visual fields, the mean IOP was 14.29 ± 3.32 mm Hg (97.5th and 99.5th percentiles, 21 and 25 mm Hg). The mean vertical cup-to-disc ratio (VCDR) was 0.39 ± 0.17 (97.5th and 99.5th percentiles, 0.7 and 0.8).	The distribution of IOP and VCDR was obtained from the right eye of the 2,532 subjects with normal suprathreshold visual fields. Mean IOP was 16.17 ± 3.74 mm Hg (97.5th and 99.5th percentiles, 24 mm Hg and 30 mm Hg). The mean VCDR was 0.43 ± 0.17 (97.5th and 99.5th percentiles, 0.7 and 0.8).
64 subjects had definite POAG (1.62%, 9.5% CI 1.42–1.82); 30 were men and 34 were women.	135 (64 men, 71 women) subjects had POAG (3.51%; 95% confidence interval, 3.04–4.0).
Subjects with POAG (59.85 ± 10.43 years) were older (p <0.001) than the study population (53.78 ± 10.71 years).	POAG subjects (58.4 ± 11.3 years) were older (p <0.0001) than the study population (54.8 ± 10.6 years).
In only one (1.5%) person was POAG diagnosed before the study. Two (3.12%) subjects were blind due to POAG; 21 (32.81%) subjects had a presenting IOP >21 mm Hg, and 43 (67.19%) had an IOP <21 mm Hg.	127 (94%) subjects were diagnosed to have POAG for the first time. Two subjects (1.5%) were bilaterally blind, and 3 (3.3%) were unilaterally blind due to POAG.

(POAG: primary open-angle glaucoma; IOP: intraocular pressure)

Conclusion

- The prevalence of POAG in a ≥40-year-old south Indian rural population was 1.62%. The prevalence increased with age, and 98.5% were not aware of the disease.
- The prevalence of POAG in a ≥40-year-old south Indian urban population was 3.51%, higher than that of the rural population. The prevalence increased with age, and >90% were not aware of the disease.

Angle Closure Glaucoma (CGS) (Table 2)

Study Measures

- Primary angle-closure suspect—an eye in which the posterior trabecular meshwork was not seen for >180° on gonioscopy
- Primary angle closure—an eye with PACS and PAS and/or elevated IOP without glaucomatous damage of the optic disc
- Primary angle closure glaucoma—PACS with evidence of glaucoma as defined by the ISGEO.

Table 2: Results of angle closure glaucoma (CGS).

Rural population	Urban population
Data were analyzed for 3,924 subjects (81.75%). PACG was diagnosed in 34 subjects (0.87%; 95% confidence interval, 0.58–1.16) (27 women, and 7 men).	3,850 (80.2%) responded; 34 subjects (17 female, and 17 male) had PACG (0.88%; 95% confidence interval, 0.60–1.16).
The mean IOP was 20.71 ± 9.24 mm Hg.	The IOP was 26.0 ± 14.9 mm Hg.
One subject (2.94%) was blind.	5 subjects (14.7%) had been previously diagnosed to have glaucoma, 1 of whom had undergone glaucoma surgery and 2 of whom had been diagnosed to have OAG. Two subjects (5.9%) were bilaterally and 3 subjects (8.8%) were unilaterally blind.
28 subjects (0.71%; 95% confidence interval, 0.45–0.98) were diagnosed to have PAC (21 women, and 7 men). 11 subjects (39.3%) had an IOP >21 mm Hg, 13 subjects (46.43%) had peripheral anterior synechiae, and 4 subjects (14.29%) had both.	106 subjects (2.75%; 95% confidence interval, 2.01–3.49) were diagnosed to have PAC (62 female, and 44 male). 39 subjects (36.8%) had presenting IOP >24 mm Hg, 83(78.3%) had peripheral anterior synechiae, and 16 (15.1%) had both.
246 subjects (6.27%; 95% confidence interval, 5.51–7.03) had PACS (168 women, and 78 men).	278 subjects (7.24%; 95% confidence interval, 6.38–8.02) had PACS (183 female, and 95 male).

(PACG: primary angle closure glaucoma; OAG: open-angle glaucoma; IOP: intraocular pressure; PAC: primary angle closure; PACS: primary angle-closure suspect)

Results

Primary angle closure and PACG were positively associated with increasing age and IOP in both populations and were more common in rural women (odds ratio, 4.3; 95% CI, 2.2–8.3). Association with hyperopia was seen only in the urban population (odds ratio, 2.0; 95% CI, 1.4–2.8).

Conclusion

- The overall prevalence of (PAC and PACG) in a rural population of southern India was 1.58%. There was a female preponderance, and the disease tends to be asymptomatic.
- Prevalence of PACG and PACS were similar in the rural and urban populations; PAC was more common in the urban population.
- In both groups, the disease was asymptomatic. Poor detection rates were probably due to lack of gonioscopy as a routine part of an eye examination.

■ OTHER RECENT TRAILS

LiGHT: Laser in Glaucoma and Ocular Hypertension Study (2019)[39]

Purpose

To compare eye drops versus selective laser trabeculoplasty (SLT) as the first line therapy for ocular hypertension and primary open angle glaucoma.

Design

- 718 patients were randomly assigned to receive either eye drops (362 patients) or SLT (356 patients) for 3 years
- First line eye drops were prostaglandin analogues, second line were β-blockers, third and fourth line treatment were topical carbonic anhydrase inhibitors and α agonists.
- *Primary outcome*: Health- related quality of life (HRQoL) at 3 years (EQ-5D)
- *Secondary outcome*: Visual acuity, cost and cost-effectiveness, disease-specific HRQoL, clinical effectiveness, and safety.

Results

- There was no difference in quality of life scores between the eye drops and SLT groups.
- Visual acuity and IOP outcomes were similar between the two groups.
- At 36 months, 95% of patients undergoing SLT were at target IOP with 74.2% of patients off eye drops.
- *Disease progression*: 36 eyes in eye drop group vs 23 eyes in SLT group.
- In the eye drop group 11 patients required incisional glaucoma surgery to lower IOP compared to zero patients in the SLT group.
- Cost analysis showed that the SLT was more cost effective than eye drops.

Conclusion

- SLT is both a clinically effective and cost effective option for first line treatment for primary open angle and ocular hypertensive patients.
- It may spare patients eye drops and reduce the risk of future glaucoma surgery.

The Zhongshan Angle Closure Prevention Trial (2008-2016)[40,41]

Purpose

To assess efficacy and safety of laser peripheral iridotomy prophylaxis against primary angle-closure glaucoma in Chinese people classified as primary angle closure suspects.

Design
- In this randomised controlled trial, bilateral primary angle closure suspects aged 50–70 years were enrolled.
- Eligible patients (889 out of 11991) received laser peripheral iridotomy in one randomly selected eye, with the other remaining untreated.
- The primary outcome was incident primary angle closure disease as a composite endpoint of elevation of intraocular pressure, peripheral anterior synechiae, or acute angle-closure during 72 months of follow-up in an intention-to-treat analysis between treated eyes and contralateral controls.

Results
- Incidence of the primary outcome was 4·19 per 1000 eye-years in treated eyes compared with 7·97 per 1000 eye-years in untreated eyes ($p = 0.024$).
- A primary outcome event occurred in 19 treated eyes and 36 untreated eyes with a statistically significant difference using pair-wise analysis ($p = 0.0041$).
- No serious adverse events were observed during follow-up.

Conclusion
In view of the low incidence rate of outcomes that have no immediate threat to vision, the benefit of prophylactic laser peripheral iridotomy is limited; therefore, widespread prophylactic laser peripheral iridotomy for primary angle-closure suspects is not recommended.

The HORIZON Study[42]

Purpose
To compare cataract surgery with implantation of a Schlemm canal microstent with cataract surgery alone for the reduction of intraocular pressure (IOP) and medication use after 3 years.

Design
- Subjects with concomitant primary open-angle glaucoma (POAG), visually significant cataract, and washed-out modified diurnal IOP (MDIOP) between 22 and 34 mm Hg.
- Subjects were randomized 2:1 to receive a single Hydrus Microstent (HMS-369 eyes) in the Schlemm canal or no stent after (NMS-187 eyes) uncomplicated phacoemulsification.

Results
- At 3 years, IOP was 16.7 ± 3.1 mm Hg in the HMS group and 17.0 ± 3.4 mm Hg in the NMS group ($p = 0.85$)

- The number of glaucoma medications was 0.4 ± 0.8 in the HMS group and 0.8 ± 1.0 in the NMS group ($p < 0.001$),
- The HMS group included a higher proportion of eyes with IOP of 18 mm Hg or less without medications compared with the NMS group (56.2% vs. 34.6%; $p < 0.001$), as well as IOP reduction of at least 20%, 30%, or 40% compared with NMS group.
- 73% of HMS group eyes were medication free compared with 48% in the NMS group ($p < 0.001$)
- There were no serious ocular adverse events in both group.

Conclusion

There was superior reduction in MDIOP and medication use among subjects with mild-to-moderate POAG who received a Schlemm canal microstent combined with phacoemulsification compared with phacoemulsification alone.

COMPASS Trial (2011-2015)[43]

Purpose

To evaluate 2-year safety and efficacy of supraciliary microstenting (CyPass Micro-Stent) for treating mild-to-moderate primary open-angle glaucoma (POAG) in patients undergoing cataract surgery.

Design

- *Participants*: POAG with mean diurnal unmedicated intraocular pressure (IOP) 21-33 mm Hg and undergoing phacoemulsification cataract surgery.
- After completing cataract surgery, subjects were intraoperatively randomized to phacoemulsification only (control-131) or supraciliary microstenting with phacoemulsification (microstent-374) groups (1:3 ratio).
- Microstent implantation via an ab interno approach to the supraciliary space allowed concomitant cataract and glaucoma surgery.

Results

- At 2 years, 60% of controls versus 77% of microstent subjects achieved ≥20% unmedicated IOP lowering ($p = 0.001$)
- Mean IOP reduction was ↓7.4 mm Hg for the microstent group versus ↓5.4 mm Hg in controls ($p < 0.001$)
- 59% of control versus 85% of microstent subjects were medication free.
- No vision-threatening microstent-related AEs occurred. Visual acuity was high in both groups through 24 months.

Conclusion

This RCT demonstrated safe and sustained 2-year reduction in IOP and glaucoma medication use after microinterventional surgical treatment for mild-to-moderate POAG.

The JUPITER Study[44]

Purpose

To evaluate the long-term safety and intraocular pressure (IOP)-lowering efficacy of Latanoprostene bunod 0.024% (LBN; Vyzulta, a novel nitric oxide (NO)-donating prostaglandin F2α analog) over 1 year.

Design

- Japanese subjects with open-angle glaucoma (OAG) or ocular hypertension (OHT).
- One drop of LBN 0.024% was instilled in the affected eye(s) (both study and fellow eye) once daily in the evening for 52 weeks and were evaluated every 4 weeks.
- 130 subjects were enrolled and 121 (93.1%) completed the study.

Results

- Mean reductions from baseline in IOP of 22.0% and 19.5% were achieved by week 4 in study and treated fellow eyes, respectively.
- In both study eyes and treated fellow eyes, the most common adverse events were conjunctival hyperemia, growth of eyelashes, eye irritation, and eye pain.
- ≥ 1 adverse events: Study eye- 58.5%, treated fellow eye- 61.9%
- 9% of treated eyes had an increase in iris pigmentation

Conclusion

- Once daily LBN ophthalmic solution 0.024% was safe and well-tolerated.
- Long-term treatment with LBN ophthalmic solution 0.024% provided significant and sustained IOP reduction.

APOLLO and LUNAR Trial[45]

Purpose

To compare the diurnal intraocular pressure (IOP)-lowering effect of latanoprostene bunod (LBN) 0.024% with timolol maleate 0.5% in subjects with open-angle glaucoma (OAG) or ocular hypertension (OHT).

Design

- Adults with OAG or OHT were randomized 2:1 to double-masked treatment with LBN once daily (qd) or timolol twice daily (bid) for

3 months followed by open-label LBN treatment for 3 (LUNAR) or 9 (APOLLO) months.
- IOP was measured at 8 AM, 12 PM, and 4 PM at week 2, week 6, and months 3, 6, 9, and 12.

Results

- Of the 840 subjects randomized, 774 (LBN, n = 523; timolol crossover to LBN, n = 251) completed the efficacy phase, and 738 completed the safety extension phase.
- Mean IOP was significantly lower with LBN versus timolol at all 9 evaluation timepoints during the efficacy phase ($p < 0.001$).
- A significantly greater proportion of LBN-treated subjects attained a mean IOP ≤18 mm Hg and IOP reduction ≥25% from baseline versus timolol-treated subjects ($p < 0.001$).
- Both treatments were well tolerated, and there were no safety concerns with long-term LBN treatment.

Conclusion

LBN 0.024% qd provided greater IOP-lowering compared with timolol 0.5% bid and maintained lowered IOP through 12 months.

ROCKET Trial[46]

Purpose

The purpose of this study was to assess the efficacy and safety of the Rho kinase inhibitor netarsudil (Rhopressa) in patients with open-angle glaucoma or ocular hypertension.

Design

Pooled analysis of data from the ROCKET-1 to 4 phase III studies of once-daily (PM) netarsudil or twice-daily timolol in patients with open-angle glaucoma or ocular hypertension.

Results

- In the pooled primary efficacy population (netarsudil, n = 494; timolol, n = 510), once-daily netarsudil was noninferior to twice-daily timolol at all 9 time points through month 3.
- Mean treated IOP ranged from 16.4 to 18.1 mm Hg among netarsudil-treated patients and 16.8 to 17.6 mm Hg among timolol-treated patients.

- The most common ocular AE, conjunctival hyperemia (netarsudil, 54.4%; timolol, 10.4%), was graded as mild in 77.6% (354/456) of affected netarsudil-treated patients.

Conclusion

Once-daily netarsudil resulted in IOP lowering that was noninferior to twice-daily timolol, with tolerable ocular AEs that were generally mild and self-resolving.

MERCURY Trial[47]

Purpose

Two phase 3 superiority studies compared a fixed-dose combination (FDC) of netarsudil and the prostaglandin latanoprost with each active component for IOP-lowering efficacy.

Design

- Pooled efficacy and safety data were analyzed from MERCURY-1 and -2 studies in patients with OAG or OHT.
- Patients instilled one drop of netarsudil (0.02%)/latanoprost (0.005%) FDC (n = 483), netarsudil (0.02%, n = 499), or latanoprost (0.005%, n = 486) into each eye once-daily between 20:00 and 22:00.
- IOP was measured at 08:00, 10:00, and 16:00 at weeks 2, 6, and the primary endpoint at month 3.

Results

- Baseline mean diurnal IOP was 23.6, 23.6, and 23.5 mm Hg in netarsudil/latanoprost FDC, netarsudil, and latanoprost groups, respectively.
- Mean diurnal IOP in each group was 15.8, 18.4, and 17.3 mm Hg at week 12.
- The netarsudil/latanoprost FDC met criteria for superiority compared with each active component ($p < 0.0001$ for all nine time points).
- Among patients randomized to netarsudil/latanoprost FDC or netarsudil or latanoprost, 30.9% vs 5.9% ($p < 0.0001$) vs 8.5% ($p < 0.0001$) achieved at least a 40% reduction from baseline in mean diurnal IOP.

Conclusion

Once-daily netarsudil/latanoprost FDC produced statistically significant and clinically relevant reductions in mean IOP that were statistically superior to IOP reductions achieved by netarsudil and latanoprost monotherapy.

Table 3: Summary of landmark trials in glaucoma.

Titles	No. of patients	Inclusion criteria	Description	Follow-up	IOP reduction	Results	Conclusion
EMGT (NEI) 1992–97	255	OAG (IOP <30 mm Hg)	Treatment (Betaxolol + ALT) vs. observation	4 years	25% (average)	% progression - 45% versus 62%	Early treatment reduces and delays glaucoma progression
CIGTS (NEI) 1993–97	607	OAG	Medical treatment versus surgery	5 years	Medical—38% Surgery—46%	No progression	With aggressive therapy aimed at IOP lowering, visual field loss is minimal
OHTS (NEI) 1994–2009	1637	OHT (IOP 24–32 mm Hg; normal disc and fields)	Medical treatment versus observation	5 years	Target—20% reduction/<24 mm Hg. Average IOP drop—22.5% versus 4%	Probability of OAG—4.4% versus 9.5%	Medical therapy is effective in delaying/preventing onset of OAG in elevated IOP
EGPS	1,077	OHT (IOP 22–29 mm Hg; normal disc and fields)	E/D dorzolamide versus placebo	5 years	15–22% reduction with dorzolamide	13.4% in dorzolamide group had visual field defects vs. 14.1% with placebo	Failed to establish role of dorzolamide in reducing the incidence of POAG among OHT
CNTGS (GRF) 1998	145	NTG (no IOP >24 mm Hg)	Medical treatment ± surgery versus observation	7 years	Target—30% reduction	% progression — 12% versus 35%	Lowering IOP reduces risk of vision loss in NTG

Contd...

Contd...

Titles	No. of patients	Inclusion criteria	Description	Follow-up	IOP reduction	Results	Conclusion
AGIS (NEI) 1988–92	789	OAG unresponsive to medical treatment	TAT versus ATT	10 years	Target—<18 mm Hg	No progression	Consistently low IOP is associated with reduced progression of visual field defects. ATT is preferable in blacks and TAT in whites

(NEI: National Eye Institute; GRF: Glaucoma Research Foundation; IOP: intraocular pressure; EMGT: Early Manifest Glaucoma Trial; OHT: ocular hypertension: OAG: open-angle glaucoma; TAT: trabeculectomy–ALT–trabeculectomy; ATT: ALT–trabeculectomy–trabeculectomy; ALT: argon laser trabeculoplasty; CNTGS: collaborative normal tension glaucoma study; CIGTS: collaborative initial glaucoma treatment study; EGPS: European Glaucoma Prevention Study; POAG: primary open-angle glaucoma; NTG: normal-tension glaucoma)

Table 4: Epidemiological studies of glaucoma in India.

Name/Date of published results	Purpose	Description	Study measures	Results	Conclusion
Vellore Eye Study (VES)/1998	Prevalence of POAG and PACG in an urban South Indian population	972 individuals aged 30–60 years were examined	POAG, OHT, PACG—acute and chronic	POAG—0.41%, PACG (all chronic)—4.32%, OHT—3.08%	Hitherto unsuspected high prevalence of PACG
Andhra Pradesh Eye Disease Study (APEDS)/2000	Prevalence and features of OAG and ACG in an urban South Indian population	Population-based cross-sectional study of 2,522 persons, including 1,399 persons ≥30 years	Definite POAG, suspected POAG, and OHT (OAG) Occludable angles and manifest PACG (ACG)	Definite POAG — 1.62%, suspected POAG— 0.79% and OHT— 0.32% in ≥30 years, and 2.56%, 1.11% and 0.42% in ≥40 years. Manifest PACG —0.71% and occludable angles 1.41% in ≥30 years, and 1.08% and 2.21% in ≥40 years	Majority of persons with glaucoma were undiagnosed and untreated. Prevalence of glaucoma increased with age
Aravind Comprehensive Eye Survey (ACES)/2003	Prevalence of glaucoma and risk factors for POAG in a rural South Indian population	Population-based cross-sectional study of 5,150 subjects ≥40 years	Definite POAG, OHT, manifest PACG, secondary glaucoma	Prevalence of any glaucoma— 2.6%, POAG —1.7%, PACG— 0.5%, secondary glaucoma excluding pseudoexfoliation— 0.3%	A large proportion of POAG were previously undiagnosed. One-fifth of POAG had blindness in one or both eyes.
Chennai Glaucoma Study (CGS)/2008	Prevalence and risk factors of POAG and PACG, PAC and PACS in rural and urban South Indian population and their comparison	Population-based cross-sectional study of 3,924 (rural) and 3850 (urban) subjects ≥40 years	Glaucoma was diagnosed using the International Society of Geographical and Epidemiological Ophthalmology Classification	Prevalence of POAG (rural)—1.62% (urban) —3.51%. 98.5% (rural) and >90% (urban) were not aware of the disease. Prevalence of PACG, PAC and PACS–(rural)–0.87%, 0.71%, 6.27%; (urban)–0.88%, 2.75%, 7.24%	POAG and PAC were more in the urban population; PACG and PACS rates were similar. Detection rates were low in both groups

(PACG: primary angle closure glaucoma; POAG: primary open-angle glaucoma; OHT: ocular hypertension: OAG: open-angle glaucoma; PAC: primary angle closure; ACG: angle closure glaucoma; PACS: primary angle-closure suspect)

REFERENCES

1. Leske MC, Heijl A, Hyman L, Bengtsson B. Early Manifest Glaucoma Trial: Design and baseline data. Ophthalmology. 1999;106(11):2144-53.
2. Heijl A, Leske MC, Bengtsson B, Hyman L, Bengtsson B, Hussein M, et al. Reduction of intraocular pressure and glaucoma progression: Results from the Early Manifest Glaucoma Trial. Arch Ophthalmol. 2002;120(10):1268-79.
3. Lichter PR, Musch DC, Gillespie BW, Guire KE, Janz NK, Wren PA, et al. Interim Clinical Outcomes in the Collaborative initial Glaucoma Treatment Study (CIGTS) comparing initial treatment randomized to medications or surgery. Ophthalmology. 2001;108(11):1943-53.
4. Janz NK, Wren PA, Lichter PR, Musch DC, Gillespie BW, Guire KE, et al. The Collaborative Initial Glaucoma Treatment Study (CIGTS): interim quality of life findings following initial medical or surgical treatment of glaucoma. Ophthalmology. 2001;108(11):1954-65.
5. Parrish RK 2nd, Feuer WJ, Schiffman JC, Lichter PR, Musch DC. Five-year follow-up optic disc findings of the Collaborative Initial Glaucoma Treatment Study. Am J Ophthalmol. 2009;147(4):717-24.e1.
6. Kass MA, Heuer DK, Higginbotham EJ, Johnson CA, Keltner JL, Miller JP, et al. The Ocular Hypertension Treatment Study: a randomized trial determines that topical ocular hypotensive medication delays or prevents the onset of primary open-angle glaucoma. Arch Ophthalmol. 2002;120(6):701-13.
7. Gordon MO, Beiser JA, Brandt JD, Heuer DK, Higginbotham EJ, Johnson CA, et al. The Ocular Hypertension Treatment Study: baseline factors that predict the onset of primary open-angle glaucoma. Arch Ophthalmol. 2002;120(6):714-20.
8. Miglior S, Zeyen T, Pfeiffer N, Cunha-Vaz J, Torri V, Adamsons I. Results of the European Glaucoma Prevention Study. Ophthalmology. 2005;112(3):366-75.
9. Collaborative Normal-Tension Glaucoma Study Group. Comparison of glaucomatous progression between untreated patients with normal-tension glaucoma and patients with therapeutically reduced intraocular pressures. Am J Ophthalmol. 1998;126(4):487-97.
10. Collaborative Normal-Tension Glaucoma Study Group. The effectiveness of intraocular pressure reduction in the treatment of normal-tension glaucoma. Am J Ophthalmol. 1998;126(4):498-505.
11. Drance S, Anderson DR, Schulzer M; Collaborative Normal-Tension Glaucoma Study Group. Risk factors for progression of visual field abnormalities in normal-tension glaucoma. Am J Ophthalmol. 2001;131(6):699-708.
12. AGIS Investigators. The Advanced Glaucoma Intervention Study (AGIS): 4. Comparison of treatment outcomes within race. Seven year results. Ophthalmology. 1998;105(7):1146-64.
13. Schwartz AL, Van Veldhuisen PC, Gaasterland DE, Ederer F, Sullivan EK, Cyrlin MN. The Advanced Glaucoma Intervention Study (AGIS): 5. Encapsulated bleb after initial trabeculectomy. Am J Ophthalmol. 1999;127(1):8-19.
14. AGIS (Advanced Glaucoma Intervention Study) Investigators. The Advanced Glaucoma Intervention Study: 8. Risk of cataract formation after trabeculectomy. Arch Ophthalmol. 2001;119(12):1771-9.
15. Gaasterland DE, Blackwell B, Dally LG, Caprioli J, Katz LJ, Ederer F. The Advanced Glaucoma Intervention Study (AGIS): 10. Variability among academic glaucoma subspecialists in assessing optic disc notching. Trans Am Ophthalmol Soc. 2001;99:177-84.
16. AGIS Investigators. Advanced Glaucoma Intervention Study (AGIS): 11. Risk factors for failure of trabeculectomy and argon laser trabeculoplasty. Am J Ophthalmol. 2002;134(4):481-98.

17. AGIS Investigators. Advanced Glaucoma Intervention Study (AGIS): 12. Baseline risk factors for sustained loss of visual field and visual acuity in patients with advanced glaucoma. Am J Ophthalmol. 2002;134(4):499-512.
18. Ederer F, Gaasterland DA, Dally LG, Kim J, VanVeldhuisen PC, Blackwell B, et al. The Advanced Glaucoma Intervention Study (AGIS): 13. Comparison of treatment outcomes within race: 10-year results. Ophthalmology. 2004;111(4):651-64.
19. Glaucoma Laser Trial Research Group:. 2. Results of argon laser trabeculoplasty versus topical medicines. The Glaucoma Laser Trial (GLT). Ophthalmology. 1990;97(11):1403-13.
20. The Glaucoma Laser Trial (GLT) and glaucoma laser trial follow-up study: 7. Results. Glaucoma Laser Trial Research Group. Am J Ophthalmology. 1995;120(6):718-31.
21. The Fluorouracil Filtering Surgery Study Group: Five-year follow-up of the Fluorouracil Filtering Surgery Study. Am J Ophthalmol. 1996;121(4):349-66.
22. The Fluorouracil Filtering Surgery Study Group: Risk factors for suprachoroidal hemorrhage after filtering surgery. Am J Ophthalmol. 1992;113(5):501-7.
23. Gedde SJ, Schiffman JC, Feuer WJ, Herndon LW, Brandt JD, Budenz DL. Treatment outcomes in the Tube Versus Trabeculectomy (TVT) study after five years of follow-up. Am J Ophthalmol. 2012;153(5):789-803.e2.
24. Gedde SJ, Herndon LW, Brandt JD, Budenz DL, Feuer WJ, Schiffman JC. Postoperative complications in the Tube Versus Trabeculectomy (TVT) study during five years of follow-up. Am J Ophthalmol. 2012;153(5):804-14.e1.
25. Matlach J, Dhillon C, Hain J, Schlunck G, Grehn F, Klink T. Trabeculectomy versus canaloplasty (TVC study) in the treatment of patients with open-angle glaucoma: a prospective randomized clinical trial. Acta Ophthalmol. 2015;93(8):753-61.
26. Azuara-Blanco A, Burr J, Ramsay C, Cooper D, Foster PJ, Friedman DS, et al. Effectiveness of early lens extraction for the treatment of primary angle-closure glaucoma (EAGLE): a randomised controlled trial. Lancet. 2016;388(10052):1389-97.
27. Javanbakht M, Azuara-Blanco A, Burr JM, Ramsay C, Cooper D, Cochran C, et al. Early lens extraction with intraocular lens implantation for thetreatment of primary angle closure glaucoma: an economic evaluation based on datafrom the EAGLE trial. BMJ Open. 2017;7(1):e013254.
28. Christakis PG, Kalenak JW, Tsai JC, Zurakowski D, Kammer JA, Harasymowycz PJ, et al. The Ahmed Versus Baerveldt Study: five-Year Treatment Outcomes. Ophthalmology. 2016;123(10):2093-102.
29. Weinreb RN, Ong T, Scassellati Sforzolini B, Vittitow JL, Singh K, Kaufman PL. A randomised, controlled comparison of latanoprostene bunod and latanoprost 0.005% in the treatment of ocular hypertension and open angle glaucoma: the VOYAGER study. Br J Ophthalmol. 2015;99(6):738-45.
30. Lorenz K, Scheller Y, Bell K, Grus F, Ponto KA, Bock F, et al. A prospective, randomised, placebo-controlled, double-masked, three-armed, multicentre phase II/III trial for the Study of a Topical Treatment of Ischaemic Central Retinal Vein Occlusion to Prevent Neovascular Glaucoma—the STRONG study: study protocol for a randomised controlled trial. Trials. 2017;18(1):128.
31. Jacob A, Thomas R, Koshi SP, Braganza A, Muliyil J. Prevalence of primary glaucoma in an urban south Indian population. Indian J Ophthalmol. 1998;46(2):81-6.
32. Dandona L, Dandona R, Srinivas M, Mandal P, John RK, McCarty CA, et al. Open-angle glaucoma in an urban population in southern India: the Andhra Pradesh eye disease study. Ophthalmology. 2000;107(9):1702-9.
33. Dandona L, Dandona R, Mandal P, Srinivas M, John RK, McCarty CA, et al. Angle-closure glaucoma in an urban population in southern India. The Andhra Pradesh eye disease study. Ophthalmology. 2000;107(9):1710-6.
34. Ramakrishnan R, Nirmalan PK, Krishnadas R, Thulasiraj RD, Tielsch JM, Katz J, et al. Glaucoma in a rural population of southern India: the Aravind comprehensive eye survey. Ophthalmology. 2003;110(8):1484-90.

35. Vijaya L, George R, Paul PG, Baskaran M, Arvind H, Raju P, et al. Prevalence of open-angle glaucoma in a rural south Indian population. Invest Ophthalmol Vis Sci. 2005;46(12):4461-7.
36. Vijaya L, George R, Baskaran M, Arvind H, Raju P, Ramesh SV, et al. Prevalence of primary open-angle glaucoma in an urban south Indian population and comparison with a rural population. The Chennai Glaucoma Study. Ophthalmology. 2008;115(4):648-54.e1.
37. Vijaya L, George R, Arvind H, Baskaran M, Paul PG, Ramesh SV, et al. Prevalence of angle-closure disease in a rural southern Indian population. Arch Ophthalmol. 2006;124(3):403-9.
38. Vijaya L, George R, Arvind H, et al. Prevalence of primary angle-closure disease in an urban south Indian population and comparison with a rural population. The Chennai Glaucoma Study. Ophthalmology. 2008;115(4):655-60.e1.
39. Konstantakopoulou E, Gazzard G, Vickerstaff V, On behalf of the LiGHT Trial Study Group, et al. The laser in glaucoma and ocular hypertension (LiGHT) trial. A multicentre randomised controlled trial: baseline patient characteristics. Br J Ophthalmol. 2018;102:599-603.
40. Jiang Y, Friedman DS, He M, Huang S, Kong X, Foster PJ. Design and methodology of a randomized controlled trial of laser iridotomy for the prevention of angle closure in southern China: the Zhongshan angle Closure Prevention trial. Ophthalmic Epidemiol. 2010;17(5):321-32.
41. He M, Jiang Y, Huang S, Chang DS, Munoz B, Aung T, et al. Laser peripheral iridotomy for the prevention of angle closure: a single-centre, randomised controlled trial. Lancet. 2019;393(10181):1609-18.
42. Samuelson TW, Chang DF, Marquis R, Flowers B, Lim KS, Ahmed IIK, et al. A Schlemm canal microstent for intraocular pressure reduction in primary open-angle glaucoma and cataract: The HORIZON Study. Ophthalmology. 2019;126(1):29-37.
43. Vold S, Ahmed II, Craven ER, Mattox C, Stamper R, Packer M, Brown RH, Ianchulev T; CyPass Study Group. Two-year COMPASS Trial results: Supraciliary microstenting with phacoemulsification in patients with open-angle glaucoma and cataracts. Ophthalmology. 2016;123(10):2103-12.
44. Kawase K, Vittitow JL, Weinreb RN, Araie M, JUPITER Study Group. Long-term safety and efficacy of latanoprostene bunod 0.024% in Japanese subjects with open-angle glaucoma or ocular hypertension: The JUPITER Study. Adv Ther. 2016;33(9):1612-27.
45. Weinreb RN, Liebmann JM, Martin KR, Kaufman PL, Vittitow JL. Latanoprostene bunod 0.024% in subjects with open-angle glaucoma or ocular hypertension: Pooled Phase 3 Study Findings. J Glaucoma. 2018;27(1):7-15.
46. Singh IP, Fechtner RD, Myers JS, Kim T, Usner DW, McKee H, et al. Pooled efficacy and safety profile of Netarsudil ophthalmic solution 0.02% in patients with open-angle glaucoma or ocular hypertension. J Glaucoma. 2020;29(10):878-84.
47. Asrani S, Bacharach J, Holland E, McKee H, Sheng H, Lewis RA, et al. Fixed-dose combination of Netarsudil and Latanoprost in ocular hypertension and open-angle glaucoma: Pooled efficacy/safety analysis of Phase 3 MERCURY-1 and -2. Adv Ther. 2020;37(4):1620-31.

Clinical Trials in Diabetic Retinopathy-I

Neha Goel, Vinod Kumar

■ WISCONSIN EPIDEMIOLOGICAL STUDY OF DIABETIC RETINOPATHY (WESDR)[1-8]

Purpose

- To describe the prevalence, incidence, and progression of diabetic retinopathy and its component lesions and to determine the incidence of visual impairment in a large population-based cohort.
- To determine the relationships between incidence and progression of diabetic retinopathy and risk factors in this cohort.
- To provide information on healthcare delivery and quality of life in persons with diabetes.

Background

Population-based epidemiologic data on the incidence and progression of diabetic retinopathy are important in developing approaches to preventing diabetic retinopathy, in medical counseling and rehabilitative services.

Description

The WESDR was an epidemiological study of a cohort of diabetic patients receiving their medical care in an 11-county area in Southern Wisconsin (Health Service Area 1) from 1979 to 1980. 452 of the 457 physicians who provided primary care to diabetic patients in this area participated in the study. The 452 physicians kept lists of all their diabetic patients for whom they provided primary care from July 1, 1979, to June 30, 1980. During this 1-year period, 10,135 diabetic patients were identified. A sample of 2,990 persons were selected for the baseline examination. This sample was composed of two groups:

1. The first consisted of all patients with diabetes diagnosed before 30 years of age who took insulin (1,210 patients); this group was referred to as "*younger onset.*"
2. The second group consisted of a probability sample of 1,780 persons of the 5,431 patients who met the eligibility criteria of having diabetes

diagnosed at 30 years of age or older and who had the diagnosis confirmed by a casual or a postprandial serum glucose level of at least 11.1 mM or a fasting serum glucose level of at least 7.8 mM on at least two occasions. This group was referred to as "*older onset.*" The latter group was stratified by the duration of disease (<5 years, 576 persons; 5–14 years, 579 persons; and >15 years, 625 persons). Of these, 824 were taking insulin and 956 were not.

Of the 2,990 eligible patients, 2,366 (79.1%) participated in the baseline examination from 1980 through 1982. The younger-onset cohort was re-examined in 1984–1986, 1990–1992, 1994–1996, and 2000–2002, whereas the older-onset cohort was re-examined in 1984–1986 and 1990–1992 and interviewed in 1994–1996. Stereoscopic photographs of the Diabetic Retinopathy Study's seven standard fields were taken of each eye.

Results

- In the WESDR, 71% of younger-onset persons had retinopathy, 23% had proliferative diabetic retinopathy (PDR), and 10% had Diabetic Retinopathy Study high-risk characteristics (DRS-HRC) for severe visual loss.[1] Data from the WESDR also showed that diabetic retinopathy was infrequent before puberty. When adjustment was made for other factors, such as duration of diabetes, glycemic control, and blood pressure, younger-onset subjects who were postmenarchal in the WESDR were 3.2 times as likely to have diabetic retinopathy as those who were premenarchal.
- In the older-onset group, 50% had retinopathy, 5% had PDR, and 2% had DRS-HRC.[2]
- Six percent of the younger- and 5% of the older-onset subjects had clinically significant macular edema (CSME).[3]
- In younger- and older-onset persons, both the frequency and the severity of retinopathy and CSME increased with increasing duration of diabetes.[3]
- Glycated hemoglobin (HbA1c) was associated with the incidence and progression of diabetic retinopathy, progression to PDR, and the incidence of CSME.[6] The incidence and progression in each quartile of HbA1c were similar in both younger- and older-onset participants. This suggested that it was the level of glycemia and not the type of diabetes that is important in determining the risk of progression of retinopathy. A 1% increase in HbA1c was also associated with a 25–40% higher risk of incident visual loss, gross proteinuria, lower-extremity amputation, and ischemic heart disease death in both the younger- and the older-onset groups.
- Data from the WESDR have shown associations of high blood pressure, lipid levels, and the presence of gross proteinuria with retinopathy.

Conclusion

The WESDR provided population-based estimates of the prevalence and incidence of diabetic retinopathy. The associations of glycemia and other traditional risk factors with the incidence and progression of retinopathy have been quantitated, and the findings have shown the need for better general medical and eye care delivery for persons with diabetes. These findings have resulted in the development of guidelines and health education programs directed at prevention, and earlier treatment, of diabetic retinopathy.

The findings from the WESDR provided the rationale for the development of guidelines for dilated eye examination by eye doctors experienced in detection and treatment of diabetic retinopathy: at the time of diagnosis in older-onset persons and yearly thereafter and after 5 years' duration of diabetes in younger-onset persons and yearly thereafter. When diabetes is diagnosed before puberty, the first dilated eye examinations should begin after puberty, and if no retinopathy is present, yearly thereafter.

Epidemiologic studies such as the WESDR cannot determine whether reduction of HbA1c would result in lowered risk of progression of retinopathy and other complications with an acceptable risk–benefit ratio. These questions were addressed by two large randomized therapeutic trials of metabolic control: (1) Diabetes Control and Complications Trial (DCCT) and (2) UK Prospective Diabetes Study (UKPDS). These prospective clinical trials demonstrated the efficacy of intensive treatment of diabetes in preventing diabetic retinopathy and other microvascular complications.

■ DIABETES CONTROL AND COMPLICATIONS TRIAL (DCCT)[9]

Purpose

To assess the effect of tight glycemic control on complications of diabetes (nephropathy, neuropathy, and diabetic retinopathy) for persons with type 1 diabetes.

Background

Long-term microvascular and neurologic complications cause major morbidity and mortality in patients with insulin-dependent diabetes mellitus (IDDM). This trial examined whether intensive treatment with the goal of maintaining blood glucose concentrations close to the normal range could decrease the frequency and severity of these complications.

Description

This multicenter study was conducted from 1983 to 1993 and funded by the National Institute of Diabetes and Digestive and Kidney Diseases. A total of 1,441 patients with type 1 diabetes—726 with no retinopathy at baseline (primary-prevention cohort) and 715 with mild retinopathy (secondary-intervention cohort), were randomly assigned to intensive therapy administered either with an external insulin pump or by three or more daily insulin injections and guided by frequent blood glucose monitoring or to conventional therapy with one or two daily insulin injections. The patients were followed up for a mean of 6.5 years, and the appearance and progression of retinopathy and other complications were assessed regularly.

Inclusion Criteria

The major criteria for eligibility included insulin dependence, as evidenced by deficient C-peptide secretion; an age of 13–39 years; and the absence of hypertension, hypercholesterolemia, and severe diabetic complications or medical conditions.

To be eligible for the primary-prevention cohort, patients were required to have had IDDM for 1–5 years, to have no retinopathy as detected by seven-field stereoscopic fundus photography, and to have urinary albumin excretion of <40 mg per 24 hours.

To be eligible for the secondary-intervention cohort, the patients were required to have IDDM for 1–15 years, to have very-mild to moderate nonproliferative retinopathy, and to have urinary albumin excretion of <200 mg per 24 hours.

Results

- In the primary-prevention cohort, intensive therapy (mean HbA1c 7.2%) reduced the risk for the development of retinopathy by 76% as compared with conventional therapy (mean HbA1c 9.0%).
- In the secondary-intervention cohort, intensive therapy slowed the progression of retinopathy by 54% and reduced the development of proliferative or severe nonproliferative retinopathy by 47%.
- In the two cohorts combined, intensive therapy reduced the occurrence of microalbuminuria (urinary albumin excretion of 40 mg per 24 hours) by 39%, that of albuminuria (urinary albumin excretion of 300 mg per 24 hours) by 54%, and that of clinical neuropathy by 60%.
- The chief adverse event associated with intensive therapy was a two-to-three-fold increase in severe hypoglycemia. Because of this risk, DCCT researchers do not recommend intensive therapy for children under the age of 13 years, people with heart disease or advanced complications, older adults, and people with a history of frequent severe hypoglycemia. Persons in the intensive management group also gained a modest amount of weight, suggesting that intensive treatment may not be appropriate for people with diabetes who are overweight.
- DCCT researchers estimate that intensive management doubles the cost of managing diabetes because of increased visits to a healthcare

professional and the need for more frequent blood testing at home. However, this cost is offset by the reduction in medical expenses related to long-term complications and by the improved quality of life of people with diabetes.

Conclusion

Intensive therapy effectively delays the onset and slows the progression of microvascular complications of diabetes, namely diabetic retinopathy, nephropathy, and neuropathy in patients with IDDM.

■ EPIDEMIOLOGY OF DIABETES INTERVENTIONS AND COMPLICATIONS (EDIC)[10]

Purpose

To examine the persistence of the original treatment effects 10 years after the DCCT in the follow-up EDIC study.

Background

The DCCT demonstrated the powerful impact of glycemic control on the early manifestations of microvascular complications. Contemporary prospective data on the evolution of macrovascular and late microvascular complications of type 1 diabetes are limited.

Description

EDIC was a multicenter, longitudinal, observational study designed to use the well-characterized DCCT cohort of >1,400 patients to determine the long-term effects of prior separation of glycemic levels on micro- and macrovascular outcomes. EDIC is in its 13th year of follow-up. The study is expecting to last until 2016.

Using a standardized annual history and physical examination, 28 EDIC clinical centers that were DCCT clinics followed the EDIC cohort for 10 years. Annual evaluation also included resting electrocardiogram, Doppler ultrasound measurements of ankle/arm blood pressure, and screening for nephropathy. At regular intervals, a timed 4-hour urine sample was collected and lipid profiles were obtained. In addition, dual B-mode Doppler ultrasound scans of the common and internal carotid arteries were performed at years 1 and 6 and at study end. Retinopathy was evaluated by stereoscopic fundus photography in 1,211 subjects at EDIC year 10. Further, three-step progression on the Early Treatment Diabetic Retinopathy Study scale from DCCT closeout was the primary outcome.

Inclusion Criteria

Patients aged 19–45 years, who were participants of the DCCT, were eligible.

Results
After 10 years of EDIC follow-up, there was no significant difference in mean HbA1c levels (8.07% vs. 7.98%) between the original treatment groups. Nevertheless, compared with the former conventional treatment group, the former intensive group had significantly lower incidences from DCCT close of further retinopathy progression and proliferative retinopathy or worse (hazard reductions, 53–56%; $p < 0.001$). The risk (hazard) reductions at 10 years of EDIC were attenuated compared with 70–71% over the first 4 years of EDIC ($p < 0.001$). The persistent beneficial effects of the former intensive therapy were largely explained by the difference in HbA1c levels during DCCT.

Conclusion
The persistent difference in diabetic retinopathy between former intensive and conventional therapy ("metabolic memory") continues for at least 10 years but may be waning.

■ UNITED KINGDOM PROSPECTIVE DIABETES STUDY (UKPDS)[11,12]

Purpose
- To determine whether the risk of cardiovascular and microvascular complications in type 2 diabetes can be reduced by intensive blood glucose control.
- In patients with high blood pressure, to determine whether the risk of complications can be reduced by tight control of blood pressure.
- To determine if any specific treatment for type 2 diabetes such as sulfonylureas (first or second generation), metformin, or insulin or antihypertensives such as angiotensin-converting-enzyme (ACE) inhibitor (captopril) or β-blocker (atenolol) confer any particular benefit.

Background
Improved blood-glucose control decreases the progression of diabetic microvascular disease, but the effect on macrovascular complications was unknown. Although a higher incidence of microvascular disease has been shown at fasting glucose concentrations >140 mg/dL, epidemiological studies have suggested that the glycemic threshold for an increased risk of cardiovascular disease may be much lower, possibly near the upper limit of the normal range (110 mg/dL). There were no prospective clinical trials that provided firm data indicating whether intensive therapy of type 2 diabetes was advantageous. There was concern that sulfonylureas may increase cardiovascular mortality in patients with type 2 diabetes and that high insulin concentrations (from sulfonylureas or insulin therapy) may enhance atheroma formation.

The objective of the UKPDS, initiated in 1977, was set up to determine whether improved blood glucose control in people with type 2 diabetes will prevent the complications of diabetes. The UKPDS was also designed to determine whether there are differences between conventional policy (diet therapy) and three different regimens of intensive treatment policy, based on sulfonylurea, metformin, or insulin. A final study report was issued in September 1998, when the median duration of therapy was 11 years.

Description

The UKPDS was a multicenter, randomized, controlled trial. A total of 5,102 people with newly diagnosed type 2 diabetes were enrolled in the UKPDS from 1977 to 1991.

After an initial treatment with diet alone for 3 months, people with raised fasting blood glucose were randomly allocated to one of various treatment policies. People with fasting plasma glucose < 6 mmol/L, who were asymptomatic, were allocated to a *conventional* policy, primarily with diet alone. When marked hyperglycemia developed, they were allocated to *nonintensive* pharmacological therapy. People with fasting plasma glucose 6.1–15 mmol/L, who were asymptomatic, were allocated to an *intensive* policy group aiming for near-normal glucose control, with two different sulfonylureas tablets, or to insulin. Overweight people could also be randomized to metformin, as an additional option.

People with raised blood pressure as well as diabetes were randomly allocated to a policy aiming for *tight* blood pressure control (<150/85 mm Hg), using two treatments, an ACE inhibitor (captopril) or beta-blocker (atenolol), or to a *less tight* blood pressure control (<180/105 mm Hg).

Inclusion Criteria

Subjects with fasting plasma glucose concentrations of >108 mg/dL (6.0 mmol/L) on two occasions were eligible.

Study Measures

These included follow-up of patients to major fatal and nonfatal clinical endpoints and recording of surrogate endpoints, namely clinical and biochemical markers, e.g., urine albumin, retinal photographs, and visual acuity.

Results

- Intensive blood glucose control reduces the risk of progression of diabetic retinopathy by 17%, need for laser photocoagulation surgery by 29%, development of vitreous hemorrhage by 23%, and risk of legal blindness by 16% and early kidney disease by 33%. In addition, there was some evidence, albeit inconclusive, that it reduced the risk of myocardial infarction and it reduced the risk of requiring a cataract extraction.

- All three therapies were similarly effective in reducing HbA1c and had equivalent risk reduction for major clinical outcomes compared with conventional policy.
- Better blood pressure control reduces the risk of death from long-term complications of diabetes by a third, strokes by more than a third, and serious deterioration of vision by more than a third. In addition, improved blood pressure also decreased the progression of the small blood vessel disease of diabetes.
- ACE inhibitors and beta-blockers were each shown to be effective in reducing the risk of any diabetes-related endpoint, diabetes-related deaths, and microvascular endpoints.

Conclusion

The complications of type 2 diabetes, previously often regarded as inevitable, could be reduced by improving blood glucose and/or blood pressure control. Intensive blood glucose control and tight blood pressure control reduce the risk of diabetic complications, the greatest effect being on microvascular complications.

APPROPRIATE BLOOD PRESSURE CONTROL IN NIDDM (ABCD)[13,14]

Purpose

- To compare the effects of intensive blood pressure control with moderate control on the prevention and progression of diabetic nephropathy, retinopathy, cardiovascular disease, and neuropathy in non-insulin-dependent diabetes mellitus (NIDDM).
- To determine the equivalency of the effects of a calcium channel blocker (nisoldipine) and an ACE inhibitor (enalapril) as a first-line antihypertensive agent in the prevention and/or progression of these diabetic vascular complications.

Description

ABCD was a prospective, controlled, randomized, double-blinded clinical trial of 950 patients with NIDDM conducted from 1993 to 1998. All patients were seen at the Colorado Prevention Center, the site of the ABCD trial, for follow-up visits.

The study consisted of two study populations aged 40–74 years, 470 hypertensive patients (diastolic blood pressure of ≥ 90.0 mm Hg at the time of randomization) and 480 normotensive patients (diastolic blood pressure of 80.0 mm Hg at the time of randomization). Patients were randomized to receive either intensive antihypertensive drug therapy (target diastolic pressure of 75 mm Hg) or moderate antihypertensive drug therapy (target diastolic pressure of 80–89 mm Hg). Patients were also randomized to nisoldipine or enalapril, with open-label medications added if further blood pressure control was necessary.

Inclusion Criteria

Hypertensive subjects, defined as having a baseline diastolic blood pressure of ≥90 mm Hg, were included.

Study Measures

The primary outcome measure was glomerular filtration rate as assessed by 24-hour creatinine clearance. Secondary outcome measures were urinary albumin excretion, left ventricular hypertrophy, retinopathy, and neuropathy. Cardiovascular morbidity and mortality were also evaluated.

Results

The mean blood pressure achieved was 132/78 mm Hg in the intensive group and 138/86 mm Hg in the moderate control group.

- During the 5-year follow-up period, no difference was observed between intensive versus moderate blood pressure control and those randomized to nisoldipine versus enalapril with regard to the change in creatinine clearance.
- Intensive therapy demonstrated a lower overall incidence of deaths, 5.5 versus 10.7%, $p = 0.037$. Over a 5-year follow-up period, there was no difference between the intensive and moderate groups with regard to the progression of diabetic retinopathy and neuropathy.
- Analysis of the 470 patients in the trial who had hypertension (baseline diastolic blood pressure, >90 mm Hg) showed similar control of blood pressure, blood glucose and lipid concentrations, and smoking behavior in the nisoldipine group (235 patients) and the enalapril group (235 patients) throughout 5 years of follow-up. Using a multiple logistic-regression model with adjustment for cardiac risk factors, it was found that nisoldipine was associated with a higher incidence of fatal and nonfatal myocardial infarctions (total of 25) than enalapril (total of 5) (risk ratio, 9.5; 95% confidence interval, 2.3–21.4). However, the use of nisoldipine versus enalapril had no differential effect on diabetic retinopathy and neuropathy.

Conclusion

Blood pressure control of 138/86 or 132/78 mm Hg with either nisoldipine or enalapril as the initial antihypertensive medication appeared to stabilize renal function in hypertensive type 2 diabetic patients without overt albuminuria over a 5-year period. The more intensive blood pressure control decreased all-cause mortality.

Table 1: Summary of epidemiological studies in diabetic retinopathy.

Title	Purpose	No of patients	Inclusion criteria	Outcome measure	Result/conclusion
WESDR (1979)	Prevalence, incidence, and progression of diabetic retinopathy and its component lesions along with visual loss	2,990	Patients with diabetes diagnosed before 30 years of age Diabetics diagnosed at 30 years of age or older	—	71% of younger-onset persons had retinopathy In the older-onset group, 50% had retinopathy 6% of the younger- and 5% of the older-onset subjects had CSME Both the frequency and the severity of retinopathy and CSME increased with increasing duration of diabetes
DCCT (1983)	Effect of tight glycemic control on complications of diabetes for persons with type 1 diabetes	1,441	IDDM, age 13–39 years, absence of hypertension, hypercholesterolemia, and severe diabetic complications	Appearance and progression of retinopathy and other complications over 6.5 years	Intensive therapy delays the onset and slows the progression of microvascular complications of diabetes (diabetic retinopathy, nephropathy, and neuropathy) in IDDM
EDIC	To examine the persistence of the original treatment effects 10 years after the DCCT	1,400	Patients aged 19–45 years, who were participants of the DCCT	Appearance of micro- and macrovascular complications (presently in 13th year follow-up)	The persistent difference in diabetic retinopathy between former intensive and conventional therapy continues for at least 10 years but may be waning

Contd...

Contd...

Title	Purpose	No of patients	Inclusion criteria	Outcome measure	Result/conclusion
UKPDS (1977)	Improved blood glucose and blood pressure control in type 2 diabetes for preventing the complications of diabetes	5,102	Newly diagnosed type 2 diabetes patients	Follow-up of patients to major fatal and nonfatal clinical endpoints	Intensive blood glucose control and tight blood pressure control reduce the risk of diabetic complications, the greatest effect being on microvascular complications
ABCD (1993)	Intensive blood pressure control versus moderate control in the prevention and progression of nephropathy, retinopathy, cardiovascular disease, and neuropathy in NIDDM	950	Hypertensive subjects with NIDDM were included	Glomerular filtration rate as assessed by 24-hour creatinine clearance	The more intensive blood pressure control decreased all-cause mortality

(ABCD: Appropriate blood pressure control in NIDDM; CSME: clinically significant macular edema; DCCT: Diabetes Control and Complications Trial; EDIC: Epidemiology of Diabetes Interventions and Complications; IDDM: insulin-dependent diabetes mellitus; NIDDM: non-insulin-dependent diabetes mellitus; UKPDS: UK Prospective Diabetes Study; WESDR: Wisconsin Epidemiological Study of Diabetic Retinopathy)

REFERENCES

1. Klein R, Klein BE, Moss SE, Davis MD, DeMets DL. The Wisconsin epidemiologic study of diabetic retinopathy. II. Prevalence and risk of diabetic retinopathy when age at diagnosis is less than 30 years. Arch Ophthalmol. 1984;102:520-6.
2. Klein R, Klein BE, Moss SE, Davis MD, DeMets DL. The Wisconsin epidemiologic study of diabetic retinopathy. III. Prevalence and risk of diabetic retinopathy when age at diagnosis is 30 or more years. Arch Ophthalmol. 1984;102:527-32.
3. Klein R, Klein BE, Moss SE, Davis MD, DeMets DL. The Wisconsin epidemiologic study of diabetic retinopathy. IV. Diabetic macular edema. Ophthalmology. 1984;91:1464-74.
4. Klein R, Klein BE, Moss SE, Davis MD, DeMets DL. The Wisconsin epidemiologic study of diabetic retinopathy. IX. Four-year incidence and progression of diabetic retinopathy when age at diagnosis is less than 30 years. Arch Ophthalmol. 1989;107:237-43.
5. Klein R, Klein BE, Moss SE, Davis MD, DeMets DL. The Wisconsin epidemiologic study of diabetic retinopathy. X. Four-year incidence and progression of diabetic retinopathy when age at diagnosis is 30 years or more. Arch Ophthalmol. 1989;107:244-9.
6. Klein R, Klein BE, Moss SE, Cruickshanks KJ. Relationship of hyperglycemia to the long-term incidence and progression of diabetic retinopathy. Arch Intern Med. 1994;154:2169-78.
7. Klein R, Klein BE, Moss SE, Cruickshanks KJ. The Wisconsin epidemiologic study of diabetic retinopathy. XIV. Ten-year incidence and progression of diabetic retinopathy. Arch Ophthalmol. 1994;112:1217-28.
8. Klein R, Klein BE, Moss SE, Cruickshanks KJ. The Wisconsin epidemiologic study of diabetic retinopathy: XVII. The 14-year incidence and progression of diabetic retinopathy and associated risk factors in type 1 diabetes. Ophthalmology. 1998;105:1801-15.
9. The Diabetes Control and Complications Trial Research Group: The effect of intensive treatment of Diabetes on the development and progression of long-term complications in Insulin-Dependent Diabetes Mellitus. N Engl J Med. 1993;329:977-86.
10. White NH, Sun W, Cleary PA, Danis RP, Davis MD, Hainsworth DP, et al. Prolonged effect of intensive therapy on the risk of retinopathy complications in patients with type 1 diabetes mellitus: 10 years after the Diabetes Control and Complications Trial. Arch Ophthalmol. 2008;126:1707-15.
11. Turner RC. The U.K. Prospective Diabetes Study. A review. Diabetes Care. 1998;21(Suppl 3):C35-8.
12. UK Prospective Diabetes Study Group: Risks of progression of retinopathy and vision loss related to tight blood pressure control in type 2 diabetes mellitus: UKPDS 69. Arch Ophthalmol. 2004;122:1631-40.
13. Estacio RO, Jeffers BW, Gifford N, Schrier RW. Effect of blood pressure control on diabetic microvascular complications in patients with hypertension and type 2 diabetes. Diabetes Care. 2000;23(Suppl 2):B54-64.
14. Estacio RO, Jeffers BW, Hiatt WR, Biggerstaff SL, Gifford N, Schrier RW. The effect of nisoldipine as compared with enalapril on cardiovascular outcomes in patients with non-insulin-dependent diabetes and hypertension. N Engl J Med. 1998;338:645-52.

Clinical Trials in Diabetic Retinopathy-II

Neha Goel, Vinod Kumar

■ DIABETIC RETINOPATHY STUDY (DRS)[1-4]

Purpose

- To determine if photocoagulation helps in preventing severe visual loss from proliferative diabetic retinopathy (PDR).
- To determine if difference exists in the efficacy and safety of argon versus xenon photocoagulation for PDR.

Background

The use of photocoagulation to treat proliferative retinopathy gained widespread use in ophthalmic practice following its introduction in 1959. However, only a few studies of photocoagulation incorporated any of the basic principles of controlled clinical trials, and these involved inadequate numbers of patients. Consequently, there was inadequate evidence of the actual value of the procedure. Because of the clinical importance of diabetic retinopathy and the increasing use of photocoagulation in its management, the DRS was begun in 1971.

Description

The DRS was a randomized controlled clinical trial sponsored by the National Eye Institute (NEI) to evaluate photocoagulation treatment for PDR. 1,758 patients were enrolled at 15 centers between 1972 and 1975. Patient eligibility criteria were presence of PDR in at least one eye or severe nonproliferative diabetic retinopathy (NPDR) in both eyes. One eye of each patient was randomly assigned to immediate photocoagulation and the other to follow-up without treatment, regardless of the course followed by either eye. The eye chosen for photocoagulation was randomly assigned to either of two treatment techniques, one using an argon laser and the other a xenon arc photocoagulator.

Treatment was usually completed in one or two sittings and included scatter [panretinal photocoagulation (PRP)] photocoagulation extending to or beyond the vortex vein ampullae. The argon treatment technique specified 800–1,600, 500-μm scatter burns of 0.1-second duration and direct treatment of new vessels whether on or within 1 disc diameter of the optic disc [neovascularization of the disc (NVD)] or outside this area [neovascularization elsewhere (NVE)]. Focal treatment was also applied to microaneurysms or other lesions thought to be causing macular edema (although such treatment was not routinely carried out within 1 disc diameter of the foveal center or in the papillomacular bundle). The xenon technique was similar, but scatter burns were fewer in number, generally of longer duration, and stronger and direct treatment was applied only to NVE on the surface of the retina. Follow-up treatment was applied as needed at 4-month intervals.

Patients were followed up at 4-month intervals according to a protocol that provided for measurement of the best corrected visual acuity and photographs of the seven standardized fundus fields and Goldmann visual fields.

In 1976, there was a protocol change which allowed photocoagulation of eyes originally randomized to the control group and a preference for argon photocoagulation. Also, laser application to elevated NVE and NVD was not required or used.

Inclusion Criteria

Patients were eligible if they had the best corrected visual acuity of 20/100 or better in each eye and the presence of PDR in at least one eye or severe NPDR in both eyes. Severe NPDR was defined as the presence of at least three of the four following lesions:
1. Extensive retinal hemorrhages and/or microaneurysms
2. Cotton-wool spots
3. Intraretinal microvascular abnormalities (IRMA)
4. Venous beading

Patients could not have had prior treatment with photocoagulation or pituitary ablation, and both eyes had to be suitable for photocoagulation. Patients with a macula threatening tractional retinal detachment were excluded. All eligible patients were younger than 70 years, and the examining physician assessed the outlook for survival and availability for 5 years of follow-up to be good.

Study Measures

The primary outcome measure was the development of *severe vision loss* (SVL), defined as visual acuity < 5/200 at two consecutively completed 4-monthly follow-up visits. Secondary outcome measures included regression of diabetic retinopathy and documentation of side effects associated with treatment.

Results

Primary Outcomes
- Both argon and xenon photocoagulation reduced the risk of severe visual loss by 50% or more compared with no treatment. In 1976, the DRS

protocol was modified to allow eyes randomized to indefinite deferral of photocoagulation to receive photocoagulation.
- The study identified a stage of retinopathy, termed *high-risk PDR*, where the benefits of photocoagulation definitely outweighed the risks (5-year rate of SVL in such eyes was reduced from 50% without treatment to 20% with treatment). No clear benefit was demonstrated for PRP in eyes with severe NPDR or in eyes with PDR without high-risk characteristics.

High-risk PDR was defined as three or more of the following high-risk characteristics (HRCs):
1. Presence of vitreous hemorrhage or preretinal hemorrhage
2. Presence of new vessels
3. Location of new vessels on or within 1 disc diameter of the optic disc (NVD)
4. Severe new vessels (NVD ≥ 1/3 disc area or NVE ≥ 1/2 disc area)

Secondary Outcomes

- *Progression of retinopathy*: Scatter photocoagulation with both argon and xenon reduced the rate of progression of eyes to more severe stages of PDR compared to no treatment.
- The common practice of supplemental photocoagulation for eyes with nonregressing neovascularization was supported by the high statistical significance found for treatment density.
- *Risks of treatment*: These include small reductions in visual acuity or visual field. Harmful effects of argon laser treatment were less than those seen with xenon arc treatment. In the argon laser treatment group, a decrease in visual acuity of one or more lines was seen in 11% of eyes; visual field loss was seen in 5%.

Xenon treatment conveyed a higher risk if significant visual loss (five or more lines) was noticed in eyes with severe fibrovascular proliferation. In patients with retinal elevation, xenon treatment resulted in larger areas of retinal detachment.

Despite these deleterious treatment effects, the beneficial reduction in severe visual loss of xenon treatment at 4 years overshadowed its immediate harmful effects. Argon treatment demonstrated an equally beneficial effect without the harmful vitreoretinal traction effects associated with xenon treatment.
- *Macular edema*: *Macular edema* defined in the DRS encompassed thickening of the retina within 1 disc diameter of the foveal center. Eyes with macular edema were almost twice as likely to have lost two or more lines of vision as similarly treated eyes without macular edema. The presence of macular edema became an important predictor of visual loss to 20/200 or worse after treatment.
- *Intraocular pressure (IOP)*: PRP reduced the risk of elevated IOP, possibly preventing the development of neovascular glaucoma. However, the DRS

could not evaluate the early effects of PRP in IOP because IOP results were not reported between entry and 8 months follow-up.

Conclusion

Data from DRS showed that both xenon and argon laser photocoagulation inhibited the progression of retinopathy. These beneficial effects were noted to some degree in all those stages of diabetic retinopathy. Some side effects including losses of visual acuity and constriction of peripheral visual field were also found. The risk of these harmful effects was considered acceptable in eyes with retinopathy in the moderate or severe proliferative stage when the risk of severe visual loss without treatment was great. Thus, eyes with high-risk PDR should receive prompt treatment with PRP. For eyes with less severe retinopathy, DRS findings do not provide a clear choice between prompt treatment and deferral unless progression to these more severe stages occurs.

■ EARLY TREATMENT DIABETIC RETINOPATHY STUDY (ETDRS)[5-10]

Purpose

- To evaluate the effectiveness of argon laser photocoagulation in delaying or preventing progression of early diabetic retinopathy to more severe stages of visual loss and blindness.
- To help determine the best time to initiate PRP treatment in diabetic retinopathy.
- To determine if photocoagulation is effective in the management of diabetic macular edema.
- To evaluate the effectiveness of aspirin treatment in altering the course of diabetic retinopathy.

Background

The DRS did not address the question of timing or extent of PRP in diabetic retinopathy nor did it clarify the role of laser photocoagulation in NPDR and in early PDR.

While several studies had reported a beneficial effect of xenon-arc or argon laser photocoagulation in diabetic macular edema, they were inconclusive for several reasons including small number of patients, lack of randomization, lack of a reliable and standard measurement of pretreatment and post-treatment visual acuity, insufficient consideration of coexistent proliferative retinopathy requiring PRP, lack of detailed and standardized treatment techniques, little or no consideration of baseline visual acuity, and effects of laser photocoagulation on other visual functions such as color vision and visual field.

Previous observations of diabetic patients who were taking large doses of aspirin for rheumatoid arthritis showed that the prevalence of retinopathy in this group was lower than the prevalence that would be expected in the diabetic population at large. Evidence suggested that diabetic patients have altered platelet aggregation and disaggregation, which may contribute to the capillary closure seen in retinopathy. This abnormality is reversed by aspirin in vitro. However, because of aspirin's other possible mechanisms of action and its well-known side effects, such as allergic, idiosyncratic, and intolerance reactions, the use of this therapy in the ETDRS was carefully controlled and monitored.

Description

The ETDRS was a multicenter, randomized clinical trial designed to evaluate argon laser photocoagulation and aspirin treatment in the management of patients with NPDR or early PDR. A total of 3,711 patients were recruited to be followed up for a minimum of 4 years to provide long-term information on the risks and benefits of the treatments under study. Recruitment began in December 1979 and was completed in July 1985.

- Eyes with moderate-to-severe NPDR or early PDR and no macular edema had one eye randomly assigned to immediate photocoagulation (further randomized to either full scatter or mild scatter PRP) and the other eye to deferral of photocoagulation (careful follow-up) until high-risk PDR developed.
- Eyes with diabetic macular edema and "less severe" retinopathy were assigned to immediate or deferred focal photocoagulation (direct laser for focal leaks and grid laser for diffuse leaks), with immediate or deferred mild scatter PRP. Eyes with diabetic macular edema and "more severe" retinopathy were assigned to immediate or deferred focal photocoagulation, with immediate mild scatter or full scatter PRP.
- The trial use of aspirin therapy was based on clinical observation and on aspirin's possible mechanisms of action. Patients were assigned randomly to aspirin (650 mg daily) or placebo.

Scatter photocoagulation was performed with argon blue-green or argon-green wavelength. The extent of the scatter treatment was just outside the major arcades superiorly and inferiorly, 500 μm from the nasal disc margin nasally, and 2 disc diameters from the center of the macula temporally. *Full scatter* consisted of 1,200–1,600 spots of moderately intense white burns spaced no more than 1 burn-width apart. The protocol allowed no more than 900 burns in a single treatment and no more than 5 weeks to complete the initial full scatter treatment. The sessions were placed at least 2 weeks apart. *Mild scatter* consisted of 450–600 burns spaced more than 1 burn-width apart. When both scatter and focal/grid had to be performed, the protocol suggested focal/grid and nasal PRP in the first session and deferral of temporal PRP for at least 2 weeks. Additional scatter treatment (supplemental PRP) was performed if high-risk characteristics developed during the follow-up.

Laser photocoagulation for macular edema was generally performed with argon-green wavelength. Focal photocoagulation or direct treatment of focal fluorescein leakage was aimed to close or obliterate the microaneurysms producing focal areas of hyperfluorescence. Grid pattern photocoagulation or treatment of diffuse macular edema aimed to decrease leakage secondary to permeability abnormalities within the dilated macular capillaries. Retreatment for clinically significant macular edema (CSME) was considered if documented CSME persisted at the 4-month follow-up or later.

Patients were randomized and treated within the first 5 weeks of the initial visit, examined 6 weeks and 4 months from the initial visit, and then every 4 months thereafter. The initial evaluation included a complete ocular examination, best corrected visual acuity with a standardized ETDRS visual acuity chart, standardized stereoscopic fundus photography, and a fluorescein angiogram. To assess visual fields, Goldmann perimetry employing I/4e and I/2e test objects was done at baseline and 48 months after enrolment, respectively.

Inclusion Criteria

Men and women between the ages of 18 and 70 years with moderate or severe NPDR or mild PDR in both eyes, with no previous photocoagulation treatment, and with visual acuity of 20/40 or better (20/200 or better if macular edema is present) were eligible for this study. Patients with high-risk PDR were excluded.

Terminology used in the Study

- *Macular edema*: Thickening of the retina and/or hard exudates within 1 disc diameter of the center of the macula
- *Clinically significant macular edema (CSME)*: One or more of the following:
  - Retinal thickening at or within 500 μm of the center of the macula
  - Hard exudates at or within 500 μm of the center of the macula if associated with adjacent retinal thickening
  - A zone or zones of retinal thickening one disc area in size at least part of which is within 1 disc diameter of the center of the fovea
- *Nonproliferative diabetic retinopathy* (NPDR):
  - *Mild NPDR*: At least one microaneurysm, but not as severe as "moderate" NPDR
  - *Moderate NPDR*: Extensive intraretinal hemorrhages and/or microaneurysms and/or cotton wool spots, venous beading, or IRMA definitely present but not as severe as "severe" NPDR
  - *Severe NPDR*: Defined as the presence of any one of the following (4-2-1 rule):
    - Intraretinal hemorrhages in four quadrants
    - Venous beading present in two quadrants
    - Severe IRMA in one quadrant

- *Early proliferative retinopathy*: PDR without DRS high-risk characteristics
- *Less severe retinopathy*: Mild or moderate NPDR
- *More severe retinopathy*: Severe NPDR or early PDR.

Study Measures

- *To assess the benefits of early photocoagulation*: Severe visual loss (visual acuity < 5/200 at two consecutive follow-up visits) and vitrectomy rate
- *To assess the effect of photocoagulation on macular edema*: Moderate visual loss (loss of 15 or more letters on the ETDRS visual acuity chart, equivalent to a doubling of the initial visual angle)
- *To assess the role of aspirin*: Mortality, development of cardiovascular disease, progression to high-risk retinopathy, development of vitreous hemorrhage, and development of cataract.

Results

Development of High-risk Proliferative Diabetic Retinopathy

Both early scatter and deferral were followed by low rates of severe visual loss (5-year rates in deferral subgroups were 2–10%; in early photocoagulation groups, these rates were 2–6%). There was a statistically significant reduction in severe visual loss for eyes with early treatment, especially for those patients with type 2 diabetes. However, the reduction was small and the risk was low in the deferral group.

Macular Edema

- For eyes with macular edema and "less severe" retinopathy, the most effective strategy was immediate focal with delayed scatter initiated only when more severe retinopathy developed. For eyes with macular edema and "more severe" retinopathy, the most effective strategy was immediate focal combined with immediate mild scatter. The worst outcome strategy involved immediate full-scatter photocoagulation and deferred focal photocoagulation.
- Focal photocoagulation reduced the risk of moderate vision loss (defined as doubling of visual angle) by 50% or more and increased the chance of a small improvement in visual acuity, especially for those eyes with macular edema that involved or threatened the center of the macula. The principal benefit of focal treatment in CSME was to reduce the risk of further visual loss rather than to improve vision.
- Although the ETDRS was not designed to determine the timing of focal photocoagulation in diabetic macular edema, a clear benefit of immediate focal laser was found, particularly when the thickening involved or threatened the center of the macula.

- Visual prognosis was worse for eyes with worse vision at baseline, although the magnitude of treatment benefit increased as the baseline visual acuity decreased.
- Fluorescein leakage was not a sufficient indication for laser treatment in the absence of CSME. Such eyes should be observed closely at 4-month intervals.

Visual Field

Significant visual field loss occurred with the I/4e object in the immediate full-scatter subgroup compared to the deferred and immediate mild-scatter subgroups at the 4-month follow-up. Eyes with macular edema assigned to deferral were more likely to develop scotomas with the I/2e object at 4 months. Eyes with no macular edema assigned to immediate full-scatter treatment also had significant scotomas.

Accommodative Amplitude

Full-scatter photocoagulation produced a transient reduction in accommodative amplitude, which was prominent at 4 months. Older age and longer duration of diabetes also presented risk factors for reduced accommodative amplitude regardless of photocoagulation.

Vitrectomy

The ETDRS studied the occurrence and outcome of vitrectomy and reported baseline and previtrectomy characteristics and visual outcome in these eyes. Overall, the vitrectomy rate was 5.6% at 5 years. Patients undergoing vitrectomy were typically white, type 1 diabetics, younger at onset of diabetes, more likely to have proteinuria and higher glycated hemoglobin at study entry, and more likely to have severe NPDR or worse at baseline. The visual outcome was not altered by the treatment assignment to immediate or deferred photocoagulation or by the preoperative presence of a retinal detachment.

Aspirin

Aspirin use did not affect the progression of retinopathy to the high-risk proliferative stage in eyes assigned to deferral of photocoagulation. However, aspirin did not increase the risk of vitreous hemorrhage, did not affect vision or reduce the risk of cataract, and was associated with a decreased risk of cardiovascular disease.

Conclusion

- Scatter treatment is not indicated for eyes with mild-to-moderate NPDR, provided that careful follow-up could be maintained. As the retinopathy

progresses to the severe NPDR or early PDR, scatter treatment should be considered, especially for patients with type 2 diabetes and it should be performed without delay for virtually all eyes with high-risk PDR.
- Focal photocoagulation is recommended for eyes with CSME and mild-to-moderate NPDR. It should also be considered for eyes with CSME and severe NPDR or early PDR.
- For patients with mild-to-severe NPDR or early PDR, aspirin has no clinically important beneficial effect on the progression of retinopathy. However, since aspirin also has no clinically important harmful effects for diabetic patients with retinopathy, there are no ocular contraindications to aspirin use when required for cardiovascular disease or other medical indications.

■ DIABETIC RETINOPATHY VITRECTOMY STUDY (DRVS)[11-13]

Purpose
- To compare two therapies, early vitrectomy and conventional management, for recent severe vitreous hemorrhage secondary to diabetic retinopathy.
- To compare early vitrectomy and conventional management in eyes that have good vision but a poor prognosis because they are threatened with hemorrhage or retinal detachment from very severe proliferative retinopathy.
- To study the natural history of severe PDR.

Background
Vitrectomy may not only remove vitreous hemorrhage but also prevent or relieve traction on the retina from contraction of the fibrovascular membranes that characterize severe PDR. It is important to determine whether early intervention with vitrectomy has a better visual outcome or instead produces a rate of serious complications higher than the rate associated with conventional management. Conventional management includes vitrectomy if hemorrhage fails to clear during a waiting period of 6–12 months or if retinal detachment involving the center of the macula develops at any time.

Description
Two randomized trials were carried out in the DRVS among patients aged 18–70 years who had either insulin-dependent or non-insulin-dependent diabetes. Patients were recruited between October 1976 and June 1983.

Group H: Early Vitrectomy for Severe Vitreous Hemorrhage
In the first trial, the 616 patients who were recruited had severe visual loss from recent (within 6 months prior to randomization) severe vitreous

hemorrhage in at least one eye. Eligible eyes were randomly assigned either to early vitrectomy or to conventional management. In the conventional management group, vitrectomy was carried out 1 year later if hemorrhage persisted; vitrectomy was carried out sooner if retinal detachment involving the center of the macula occurred.

Group N: Course of Visual Acuity in Severe PDR with Conventional Management

A total of 744 eyes of 622 patients with severe PDR were enrolled in the trial. The study was designed to follow these patients over a 2-year period to determine their visual outcome. It also ascertained whether a subgroup could be identified in which prognosis with conventional management was so poor that a randomized trial of vitrectomy in eyes still retaining useful vision was justified.

Group NR: Early Vitrectomy for Severe PDR in Eyes with Useful Vision

In the second trial, 381 patients were recruited, all of whom had severe fibrovascular proliferations and useful vision in at least one eye. Eligible eyes were assigned either to early vitrectomy or to conventional management. Conventional management included photocoagulation when indicated, with vitrectomy if a severe vitreous hemorrhage occurred and failed to clear spontaneously during a 6-month waiting period or if retinal detachment involving the center of the macula occurred.

After randomization and treatment, all patients were examined at 6-month intervals for 2 years and annually thereafter, for a total of 4 years. Comparisons of visual acuity distributions between experimental and control groups were made.

Inclusion Criteria

Group H

Men and women eligible for the vitreous hemorrhage group had at least one eye with recent severe vitreous hemorrhage (within 6 months) and visual acuity of 5/200 or less. Vitreous hemorrhage obscured the macula and retina within 15° from the center of the macula, so that no major vessel or other landmark could be followed continuously for a distance as great as 3 disc diameters with binocular indirect ophthalmoscopy.

Group NR

Patients eligible had extensive active neovascular or fibrovascular proliferations and visual acuity of 10/200 or better. Patients with neovascularization of the iris, angle or neovascular glaucoma, retinal detachment involving the center of the macula, previous vitrectomy, or severe renal disease were excluded.

Study Measures

The primary outcome measure was visual acuity. Visual acuity of 10/20 or better was considered "good vision" while <5/200 was "poor vision." Complications were tabulated as "untoward events."

Results

- In *Group H*, 2-year results showed that recovery of good vision (10/20 or better) was more frequent in the early vitrectomy group (25% vs. 15% in the conventional management group) and the advantage was more apparent in type 1 diabetics who were younger, with disease duration < 20 years and more severe fibrovascular proliferations (36% with visual acuity of 10/20 or better in the early vitrectomy group vs. 12% with conventional management). In type 1 diabetics, the risk of loss of light perception was the same in two groups (28% and 26%, respectively) but in type 2 diabetics, there was a trend toward more frequent loss of light perception in the early group (25% vs. 19%). These benefits remained at least as great after 4 years of follow-up as it was at 2 years.
- In *Group N*, change in vision was greater between baseline and year 1 than between years 1 and 2. Both the initial visual acuity and the activity of retinopathy predicted further visual loss. The prognosis of eyes with tractional retinal detachment not involving the macula did not justify surgical intervention for this indication, independent of the activity of retinopathy. The data analysis allowed definition of Group NR, a subgroup of eyes with sufficiently poor prognosis to justify a randomized trial of vitrectomy in eyes still retaining useful vision.
- In *Group NR*, after 4 years of follow-up, the percentage of eyes with visual acuity of at least 10/20 was 44% in the early vitrectomy group and 28% in the conventional management group, although the proportion with poor visual outcome was similar in the two groups. There was an increased chance of poor vision at the 4-year visit as baseline vision decreased. Prior photocoagulation increased the chances of good vision.

Conclusion

- In eyes with recent severe vitreous hemorrhage causing significant reduction of vision, early vitrectomy provided a greater chance of prompt recovery of visual acuity, especially in type 1 diabetics and if vision is poor in the fellow eye although a greater early risk of visual acuity of no light perception must be kept in mind.
- In eyes with severe, active neovascular proliferation and moderate or no vitreous hemorrhage, early vitrectomy is of benefit especially in those with both fibrous proliferations and at least moderately severe new vessels, in which extensive scatter photocoagulation has been carried out or is precluded by vitreous hemorrhage.

Table 1: Summary of landmark trials in diabetic retinopathy.

Title	Purpose	No of patients	Inclusion criteria	Outcome measure	Result/conclusion
DRS (1971)	• Photocoagulation in preventing severe visual loss from PDR • Efficacy and safety of argon versus xenon	1,758	BCVA of 20/100 or better in each eye and the presence of PDR in at least one eye or severe NPDR in both eyes	Development of *severe vision loss* at two consecutive 4-month follow-ups	• Photocoagulation reduced the risk of severe visual loss by 50% compared with no treatment • Xenon laser resulted in more harmful effects than argon laser • Defined *high-risk* PDR. Eyes with high-risk PDR should receive prompt PRP
ETDRS (1979)	• Determine the best time to initiate PRP in DR • Efficacy of photocoagulation in DME • Effectiveness of aspirin in altering course of DR	3,711	Patients with moderate or severe NPDR or mild PDR in both eyes and with visual acuity of 20/40 or better (20/200 or better if macular edema was present)	• Benefits of early photocoagulation—severe visual loss and vitrectomy rate • Effect of photocoagulation on macular edema—(MVL)	• Scatter treatment is not indicated for eyes with mild-to-moderate NPDR. Scatter treatment should be considered in severe NPDR or early PDR. Scatter treatment should be performed without delay for high-risk PDR • Focal photocoagulation is recommended for eyes with CSME (reduces risk of MVL to half) • Aspirin had no effect on DR
DRVS (1976)	• Early vitrectomy versus conventional management for recent severe vitreous hemorrhage • Early vitrectomy vs conventional management for eye with good vision but a poor prognosis	1,741	• At least one eye with recent severe vitreous hemorrhage and visual acuity of 5/200 or less • Extensive active neovascular or fibrovascular proliferations and visual acuity of 10/200 or better	Visual acuity was the main outcome measure. Visual acuity of 10/20 or better was considered "good vision" while <5/200 was "poor vision"	• Early vitrectomy provided a greater chance of prompt recovery of visual acuity, especially in type 1 diabetics and if vision is poor in the fellow eye • Early vitrectomy is of benefit, especially in those with both fibrous proliferations and at least moderately severe new vessels, in which extensive scatter photocoagulation has been carried out or is precluded by vitreous hemorrhage

(BCVA: best corrected visual acuity; CSME: clinically significant macular edema; DME: diabetic macular edema; DR: diabetic retinopathy; DRS: Diabetic Retinopathy Study; DRVS: Diabetic Retinopathy Vitrectomy Study; ETDRS: Early Treatment Diabetic Retinopathy Study; MVL: moderate visual loss; NPDR: nonproliferative diabetic retinopathy; PDR: proliferative diabetic retinopathy)

REFERENCES

1. The Diabetic Retinopathy Study Research Group. Photocoagulation treatment of proliferative diabetic retinopathy: The second report of diabetic retinopathy study findings. Ophthalmology. 1978;85:82-106.
2. The Diabetic Retinopathy Study Research Group. Four risk factors for severe visual loss in diabetic retinopathy: The third report from the diabetic retinopathy study. Arch Ophthalmol. 1979;97:654-5.
3. The Diabetic Retinopathy Study Research Group. Photocoagulation treatment of proliferative diabetic retinopathy: Clinical applications of Diabetic Retinopathy Study (DRS) findings. DRS Report No. 8. Ophthalmology. 1981;88:583-600.
4. Ferris FL III, Podgor MJ, Davis MD, and the Diabetic Retinopathy Study Research Group. Macular edema in Diabetic Retinopathy Study patients: Diabetic Retinopathy Study Report No. 12. Ophthalmology. 1987;94:754-60.
5. Photocoagulation for diabetic macular edema. Early Treatment Diabetic Retinopathy Study report number 1. Early Treatment Diabetic Retinopathy Study research group. Arch Ophthalmol. 1985;103:1796-806.
6. Techniques for scatter and local photocoagulation treatment of diabetic retinopathy: Early Treatment Diabetic Retinopathy Study Report no. 3. The Early Treatment Diabetic Retinopathy Study Research Group. Int Ophthalmol Clin. 1987;27:254-60.
7. Photocoagulation for diabetic macular edema: Early Treatment Diabetic Retinopathy Study Report no. 4. The Early Treatment Diabetic Retinopathy Study Research Group. Int Ophthalmol Clin. 1987;27:265-72.
8. Effects of aspirin treatment on diabetic retinopathy. ETDRS report number 8. Early Treatment Diabetic Retinopathy Study Research Group. Ophthalmology. 1991;98:757-65.
9. Early photocoagulation for diabetic retinopathy. ETDRS report number 9. Early Treatment Diabetic Retinopathy Study Research Group. 1991;98:766-85.
10. Flynn HW, Chew EY, Simmons BD, Barton FB, Remaley NA, Ferris FL. Pars plana vitrectomy in the Early Treatment Diabetic Retinopathy Study. ETDRS report number 17. The Early Treatment Diabetic Retinopathy Study Research Group. Ophthalmology. 1992;99:1351-7.
11. Two-year course of visual acuity in severe proliferative diabetic retinopathy with conventional management. Diabetic Retinopathy Vitrectomy Study (DRVS) report #1. Ophthalmology. 1985;92:492-502.
12. Early vitrectomy for severe proliferative diabetic retinopathy in eyes with useful vision. Results of a randomized trial—Diabetic Retinopathy Vitrectomy Study Report 3. The Diabetic Retinopathy Vitrectomy Study Research Group. Ophthalmology. 1988;95:1307-20.
13. Early vitrectomy for severe vitreous hemorrhage in diabetic retinopathy. Four-year results of a randomized trial: Diabetic Retinopathy Vitrectomy Study Report 5. Arch Ophthalmol. 1990;108:958-64.

Clinical Trials in Diabetic Retinopathy - III

Neha Goel, Brijesh Takkar, Pooja Shah

DIABETIC RETINOPATHY CLINICAL RESEARCH NETWORK (DRCR.NET)

The Diabetic Retinopathy Clinical Research Network (DRCR.net) is a collaborative network dedicated to facilitating multicenter clinical research of diabetic retinopathy (DR), diabetic macular edema (DME), and associated conditions. The DRCR.net supports the identification, design, and implementation of multicenter clinical research initiatives focused on diabetes-induced retinal disorders. The DRCR.net was formed in September 2002 with principal emphasis on clinical trials. It is funded by the National Eye Institute (NEI), a part of the National Institutes of Health. Its main protocols and their clinical relevance are described in the following text.

Protocol A: Pilot Study of Laser Photocoagulation for DME[1]

Purpose

To compare two laser photocoagulation (LP) techniques for treatment of DME: (1) modified Early Treatment Diabetic Retinopathy Study (mETDRS) technique and (2) mild macular grid (MMG) technique.

Methods

263 subjects with previously untreated DME were randomly assigned to receive laser by the mETDRS (162 eyes) or the MMG (161 eyes) technique. MMG burns are lighter, more diffuse in nature, and are distributed throughout the macula in both areas of thickened and unthickened retina. Microaneurysms are not directly photocoagulated. In contrast, mETDRS direct/grid photocoagulation is comprised of treating only areas of thickened retina (and areas of retinal nonperfusion) and leaking microaneurysms. The modification to the original ETDRS protocol is that the laser burns are less intense (gray) and smaller (50 µm). Visual acuity (VA), fundus photographs, and optical coherence tomography (OCT) measurements were obtained at baseline and after 3.5, 8, and 12 months. The main outcome measure was change in OCT measures at 12 months.

Results

From baseline to 12 months, central subfield thickening [central macular thickness (CMT)] decreased by an average of 88 μm in the mETDRS group and decreased by 49 μm in the MMG group. At 12 months, the mean change in VA was 0 letters in the mETDRS group and 2 letters worse in the MMG group.

Conclusion

At 12 months after treatment, the MMG technique was less effective at reducing retinal thickening than the current mETDRS LP approach. *However, the VA outcome with both approaches was not considerably different.* Given these findings, a larger long-term trial of the MMG technique was not justified.

 Application to Clinical Practice

Modified ETDRS photocoagulation should continue as a standard approach to treating DME.

Protocol B: Randomized Trial Comparing Intravitreal Triamcinolone Acetonide and Laser Photocoagulation for DME[2-4]

Purpose

To evaluate the efficacy and safety of 1- and 4-mg doses of intravitreal triamcinolone acetonide (IVTA) in comparison with focal/grid photocoagulation (LP) for DME.

Methods

This multicenter randomized clinical trial involved 840 study eyes of 693 subjects with DME involving the fovea and VA 2 of 0/40 to 20/320. Eyes were randomized to LP (330), 1-mg IVTA (256), or 4-mg IVTA (254). Retreatment was given for persistent or new edema at 4-month intervals. The outcome measures were ETDRS VA, OCT-macular thickness, and safety at 3 years.

Results

- At 4 months, the mean VA was better in the 4-mg TA group than the other two groups. By 1 year, there were no significant differences among groups in mean VA. At 2 and 3 years, the mean VA was better in the laser group than in the other two groups. Treatment group differences in the VA outcome could not be attributed solely to cataract formation.
- OCT results paralleled the VA results.
- Intraocular pressure (IOP) was increased from baseline by ≥10 mm Hg at any visit in 4%, 16%, and 33% of eyes in the three treatment groups, respectively, and cataract surgery was performed in 31%, 46%, and 83% of eyes in the three treatment groups, respectively.

Conclusion

Over a 2- as well as a 3-year period, LP was more effective and had fewer side effects than 1-or 4-mg doses of IVTA for most patients with DME. Most eyes receiving 4 mg of IVTA were likely to require cataract surgery.

Though IVTA (4 mg) appeared to reduce the risk of progression of DR, use of this treatment merely to reduce the rates of progression of proliferative DR (PDR) did not seem warranted.

  Application to Clinical Practice

The results of this study also support that focal/grid photocoagulation currently should be the benchmark of treatment of DME.

Protocol C: Temporal Variation in Optical Coherence Tomography Measurements of DME[5]

Purpose

To evaluate diurnal variation in OCT-measured retinal thickness in center-involving DME.

Methods

Serial OCT measurements were performed in 156 eyes of 96 subjects with DME and OCT central subfield retinal thickness (CMT) ≥ 225 µm at 8 am. CMT was measured from retinal thickness maps over a single day between 8 am and 4 pm.

Results

At 8 am, the mean CMT was 368 µm and the mean VA was 66 letters. The mean change in relative CMT between 8 am and 4 pm was a decrease of 6% and the mean absolute change was a decrease of 13 µm.

Conclusion

Although on average there are slight decreases in retinal thickening during the day, *most eyes with DME have little meaningful change in OCT CMT between 8 am and 4 pm.*

  Application to Clinical Practice

The clinical impact of diurnal variation of macular edema is likely to be small and not significant.

Protocol D: Evaluation of Vitrectomy for DME[6,7]

Purpose

To evaluate vitrectomy for DME in eyes with at least moderate vision loss and vitreomacular traction (VMT).

Methods

It was a prospective cohort study. The primary cohort included 87 eyes with DME and VMT, VA 20/63 to 20/400, OCT CMT > 300 µm, and no concomitant cataract extraction at the time of vitrectomy. Surgery was performed according to the investigator's usual routine. Follow-up visits were performed after 3 months, 6 months, and 1 year. The main outcome measures were VA, OCT retinal thickening, and surgical complications.

Results

At baseline, the median VA in the 87 eyes was 20/100 and the median OCT thickness was 491 µm. During vitrectomy, additional procedures included epiretinal membrane (ERM) peeling in 61%, internal limiting membrane (ILM) peeling in 54%, panretinal photocoagulation (PRP) in 40%, and injection of corticosteroids at the close of the procedure in 64%. At 6 months, the median OCT CMT decreased by 160 µm. The VA improved by 10 or more letters in 38% and deteriorated by 10 or more letters in 22%. Postoperative surgical complications through 6 months included vitreous hemorrhage (VH; 5 eyes), elevated IOP requiring treatment (7 eyes), retinal detachment (3 eyes), and endophthalmitis (1 eye). Little changes in results were noted between 6 months and 1 year.

Conclusion

Following vitrectomy performed for DME and VMT, retinal thickening was reduced in most eyes. Between 28% and 49% of eyes were likely to have improvement of VA, while between 13% and 31% of eyes were likely to have worsened. The results suggested that removal of ERM may favorably affect the visual outcome after vitrectomy. The surgical complication rate is low.

 Application to Clinical Practice

Vitrectomy performed for eyes with at least moderate vision loss and VMT usually results in a reduction in macular thickening. VA results are less consistent with some eyes improving and some eyes worsening.

Protocol E: A Randomized Trial of Peribulbar Triamcinolone Acetonide with and without Focal Photocoagulation for Mild DME: A Pilot Study[8]

Purpose

To provide data on the safety and efficacy of anterior or posterior subtenon's injections of TA either alone or in combination with focal photocoagulation in the treatment of mild DME.

Methods

It was a prospective phase 2, multicenter randomized clinical trial involving 129 eyes with mild DME and VA 20/40 or better. The participants were randomly assigned to receive either focal photocoagulation (38), 20-mg anterior subtenon's injection of TA ($n = 23$), 20-mg anterior subtenon's injection followed by focal photocoagulation after 4 weeks ($n = 25$), 40-mg posterior subtenon's injection of TA ($n = 21$), or 40-mg posterior subtenon's injection followed by focal photocoagulation after 4 weeks ($n = 22$). Follow-up visits were performed at 4, 8, 17, and 34 weeks. The main outcome measures included change in VA and retinal thickness.

Results

Changes in retinal thickening and in VA were not significantly different among the five groups at 34 weeks. There was a suggestion of a greater proportion of eyes having a central subfield thickness < 250 µm at 17 weeks when the peribulbar TA was combined with focal photocoagulation. Elevated IOP and ptosis were adverse effects attributable to the injections.

Conclusion

In cases of DME with good VA, peribulbar TA, with or without focal photocoagulation, is unlikely to be of substantial benefit. Based on these results, a phase 3 trial to evaluate the benefit of these treatments for mild DME was not justified.

Application to Clinical Practice

It is unlikely that significant clinical benefit exists for peribulbar TA in cases of DME with good VA.

Protocol F: Observational Study of the Development of DME Following Scatter Laser Photocoagulation[9]

Purpose

To compare the effects of single-sitting versus four-sitting PRP on macular edema in subjects with severe nonproliferative DR (NPDR) or early PDR with relatively good VA and no or mild center-involved macular edema.

Method

Subjects were treated with one sitting or four sittings of PRP in a nonrandomized, prospective, multicentric clinical trial. The main outcome measure was CMT on OCT.

Results

Central macular thickness was slightly greater in the one-sitting group than in the four-sitting group at the 3-day and 4-week visits. At 34 weeks, the slight differences had reversed. VA differences paralleled OCT differences.

Conclusion

Clinically meaningful differences are unlikely in OCT thickness or VA following application of PRP in one sitting compared with four sittings in subjects in this cohort.

 Application to Clinical Practice

Panretinal photocoagulation for DR can be safely administered in a single sitting in patients with relatively good VA and no or mild preexisting center-involved DME.

Protocol G: Subclinical DME Study[10]

Purpose

To determine the rate of progression of eyes with subclinical DME to clinically apparent DME or DME necessitating treatment during a 2-year period.

Methods

43 eyes from 39 study participants with subclinical DME were enrolled. Eyes were evaluated annually for up to 2 years for the primary outcome, which was an increase in OCT CMT of at least 50 μm from baseline and a CMT of at least 300 μm, or treatment for DME (performed at the discretion of the investigator).

Results

The cumulative probability of meeting an increase in OCT CMT of at least 50 μm from baseline and a CMT of at least 300 μm, or treatment for DME was 27% by 1 year and 38% by 2 years.

Conclusion

Although subclinical DME may be uncommon, this study suggests that between *one-quarter and one-half of eyes with subclinical DME will progress to more definite thickening or be judged to need treatment for DME within 2 years after its identification.*

 Application to Clinical Practice

Patients with subclinical DME should be monitored more closely for progression.

Protocol H: Phase 2 Randomized Clinical Trial of Intravitreal Bevacizumab for DME[11]

Purpose

To provide data on the short-term effect of intravitreal bevacizumab (IVB) for DME.

Methods

It was a randomized phase 2 clinical trial. 121 eyes of 121 subjects with DME and VA ranging from 20/32 to 20/320 were enrolled and randomly assigned to one of five groups:
1. Focal photocoagulation at baseline ($n = 19$, Group A),
2. 1.25-mg IVB at baseline and 6 weeks ($n = 22$, Group B),
3. 2.5-mg IVB at baseline and 6 weeks ($n = 24$, Group C),
4. 1.25-mg IVB at baseline and sham injection at 6 weeks ($n = 22$, Group D), or
5. 1.25-mg IVB at baseline and 6 weeks with photocoagulation at 3 weeks ($n = 22$, Group E).

The main outcome measures were CMT on OCT and VA measured at baseline and after 3, 6, 9, 12, 18, and 24 weeks.

Results

Compared with Group A, Groups B and C had a greater reduction in CMT at 3 weeks and about one line better median VA over 12 weeks. There were no meaningful differences between Groups B and C. Combining focal photocoagulation with bevacizumab resulted in no apparent short-term benefit or adverse outcomes.

Conclusion

These results demonstrate that *IVB can reduce DME in some eyes*, but the study was not designed to determine whether treatment is beneficial.

Protocol I: Laser-Ranibizumab-Triamcinolone Study for DME[12]

Purpose

To evaluate intravitreal 0.5-mg ranibizumab or 4-mg triamcinolone combined with focal/grid laser compared with focal/grid laser alone for treatment of DME.

Background

At the time of this study, anti-vascular endothelial growth factor (VEGF) agents were largely being used for age-related macular degeneration (ARMD) and focal/grid laser was the standard of care for management of DME. Few studies reported benefit of intravitreal steroids for DME. This protocol clearly established the role of intravitreal anti-VEGF therapy as first-line treatment for center involving DME.

Methods

This multicenter, randomized clinical trial enrolled a total of 854 eyes of 691 participants with VA of 20/32 to 20/320 and DME involving the fovea. Eyes were randomized to one of the four groups:
1. Sham injection + prompt laser ($n = 293$)
2. 0.5-mg ranibizumab + prompt laser ($n = 187$)
3. 0.5-mg ranibizumab + deferred (≥24 weeks) laser ($n = 188$)
4. 4-mg triamcinolone + prompt laser ($n = 186$)

Retreatment followed an algorithm facilitated by a web-based system. The main outcome measures were best-corrected visual acuity (BCVA) and safety at 1 year.

Results

At 1 year
- The mean change in the VA from baseline was significantly greater in the Ranibizumab + prompt laser group and Ranibizumab + deferred laser group but not in the Triamcinolone + prompt laser group compared with the sham + prompt laser group.
- The reduction in mean CMT in the Triamcinolone + prompt laser group was similar to both Ranibizumab groups and greater than in the sham + prompt laser group.
- Three eyes (0.8%) had injection-related endophthalmitis in the Ranibizumab groups whereas elevated IOP and cataract surgery were more frequent in the Triamcinolone + prompt laser group.

Extension study
- At 2 years, VA results were similar to 1-year results.[12]
- At 3 years, amongst intravitreal ranibizumab (IVR) groups, the median numbers of injections were 12 and 15 in prompt and deferral group results, respectively. However, the number of letters gained were slightly more in the deferred laser group (9.7 vs. 6.8, $p = 0.02$). More eyes had >10-letter gain in the deferred laser group (56% vs. 42%, $p = 0.02$). One third of eyes in both groups had time-domain OCT (TDOCT) CMT > 250 μm while half of eyes in the deferred group did not need laser at all.[13]
- At 5 years, most eyes of both groups maintained vision gains obtained at year 1, with little additional treatment after 3 years. Adding laser at initiation of ranibizumab was no better than deferring laser at least 24 weeks. The median number of injections was 13 versus 17 in the IVR with prompt and deferral groups.[14]

Conclusion

Intravitreal ranibizumab with prompt or deferred laser had a superior VA outcomes at 1 and 5 years compared with prompt laser alone for the treatment of DME involving the central macula.

Application to Clinical Practice

Ranibizumab should be considered for patients with DME including vision impairment with DME involving the center of the macula.

Protocol J: Intravitreal Ranibizumab or Triamcinolone Acetonide as Adjunctive Treatment to PRP and Focal Laser for PDR with DME[15]

Purpose

To evaluate 14 weeks of IVR or TA in eyes receiving LP for DME and PRP.

Methods

345 eyes with a VA of 20/320 or better, center-involved DME receiving LP, and DR receiving prompt PRP were randomly assigned to sham ($n = 123$), 0.5-mg ranibizumab ($n = 113$) at baseline and 4 weeks, and 4-mg triamcinolone at baseline and sham at 4 weeks ($n = 109$). Treatment was at the investigator's discretion from 14 to 56 weeks.

Results

Mean changes in VA score from baseline were significantly better in the ranibizumab and triamcinolone groups compared with those in the sham group at the 14-week visit, mirroring retinal thickening results. These differences were not maintained when study participants were followed up for 56 weeks for safety outcomes.

Conclusion

The addition of one IVTA or two ranibizumab injections in eyes receiving LP for DME and PRP is associated with better VA and decreased DME by 14 weeks. Whether continued long-term intravitreal treatment is beneficial or not could not be determined from this study.

Application to Clinical Practice

The risk of short-term exacerbation of macular edema and associated VA loss following prompt PRP in eyes also receiving focal/grid laser for DME can be reduced by intravitreal triamcinolone or ranibizumab.

Protocol K: The Course of Response to Focal Photocoagulation for DME[16]

Purpose

To determine whether eyes with center-involved DME, and treated with LP, in which there is a reduction in CMT measured with OCT after 16 weeks, will continue to improve if retreatment is deferred.

Methods

This is a prospective, multicenter, observational, single group LP study of 122 eyes with center-involved DME (OCT CMT ≥ 250 μm). At the 16-week visit and continuing every 8 weeks, eyes were assessed for retreatment and additional laser was deferred if the VA letter score improved ≥5 letters or OCT CMT decreased ≥10% compared with the visit 16 weeks prior.

Results

Of the 115 eyes that completed the 16-week visit, 54 (47%) had a decrease in CMT by ≥10% compared with baseline. Of these, 26 (48%) had a CMT ≥ 250 μm at 16 weeks and were evaluable at 32 weeks. 11 of the 26 eyes had a further decrease in CMT ≥ 10% from 16 to 32 weeks without further treatment.

Conclusion

Sixteen weeks following LP for DME, in eyes with a definite reduction, but not resolution, of central edema, 23–63% will continue to improve without additional treatment.

Application to Clinical Practice

Eyes undergoing focal/grid laser, especially eyes with greater macular thickening, may continue to have improvement in VA and macular thickness even after 16 weeks.

Protocol L: Evaluation of Visual Acuity Measurements in Eyes with DME[17]

Purpose

To compare autorefraction (AR) with manual refraction in patients with DME.

Methods

Autorefraction measured and manually measured visual scores using predefined protocols were assessed using electronic ETDRS charts. Test–retest variability was assessed.

Results

878 eyes of 456 participants were evaluated. Manual results were slightly better automated across the range of VA. Variability between automated and manual testing was substantially more than repeated manual refractions.

Conclusion

Current autorefractors are not a good substitute for manual refraction for trials.

Application to Clinical Practice
Manual refraction is a more accurate and gold standard for DME patients.

Protocol M: Effect of Diabetes Education during Retinal Ophthalmology Visits on Diabetes Control[18]

Purpose

To assess the utility of point-of-care glycated hemoglobin (HbA1c) measurements and personalized risk factor scaling during ophthalmic visits.

Methods

Annual follow-up visitors were compared with more frequent visitors. HbA1c, disease severity, and progression risks were evaluated. Diabetic education was provided with immediate assessment of patient understanding.

Results

No significant difference was observed between the two groups in terms of long-term change in HbA1c.

Conclusion

Personalized education and risk assessment during retinal ophthalmology visits did not help in the overall betterment of diabetic control.

 Application to Clinical Practice
Glycemic control endured over a long term is challenging despite best efforts of patient education.

Protocol N: Intravitreal Ranibizumab for Vitreous Hemorrhage from PDR Study[19]

Purpose

To compare IVR with saline for the need of vitrectomy rates in VH due to PDR.

Methods

A PRP laser was not possible in all study eyes. Eyes were randomized to receive IVR and saline for three doses at 1 month apart.

Results

12% IVR eyes needed surgery (cumulative probability) at 16 weeks in comparison to 17% of eyes receiving saline. Complete PRP could be done in 44% of eyes receiving IVR in comparison to 31% of saline. Recurrent VH occurred in 6% of IVR group versus 17% of saline group.

Conclusion

Little benefit of IVR and saline on the rate of vitrectomy in study eyes has been seen. Short-term benefits such as VA improvement, higher PRP completion rates, and reduction of recurrent VH may be seen with IVR. Long-term effects are not known.

 Application to Clinical Practice

Long-term results of this study at 1 year again showed no benefit of IVR over saline in vitrectomy rates or visual gain at 1 year.[20] Hence, it is of no benefit for this indication.

Protocol O: Time-domain/Spectral-domain OCT Comparison and Reproducibility[21]

Purpose

To compare between TDOCT and spectral-domain OCT (SDOCT) for utility in measurement of retinal thickness.

Methods

Stratus OCT has been compared with Cirrus or Spectralis OCT. Two cohorts were enrolled: (1) center-involving DME and (2) no DME.

Results

The Bland–Altman coefficient of repeatability for relative change in retinal thickness was lowest on Spectralis (7%) than Stratus (12–15%) or Cirrus (14%) OCT.

Conclusion

Spectralis OCT showed the best reproducibility over all machines tested. Retinal thickness measurements >10% on the same machine or >20% after switching machines are likely to be due to actual change in retinal thickness rather than observation variability.

 Application to Clinical Practice

Newer SDOCTs are more reproducible and large changes in retinal thickness measurements are due to actual changes.

Protocol P: Cataract Surgery with Center-involved DME Study[22]

The conclusions of this study were considered limited by the authors due to lack of standardization.

 Application to Clinical Practice

Vision outcomes may not be uniform in patients with DR. Half of the eyes may have worsening of vision or no gain in vision.

Protocol Q: An Observational Study in Individuals with Diabetic Retinopathy without Center-involved DME Undergoing Cataract Surgery[23]

Purpose
To assess the occurrence of center-involving DME after cataract surgery in eyes without prior DME preoperatively.

Methods
293 eyes with (1) no topical treatment for ME and (2) CMT > 250 μm (TDOCT) or 310 μm (SDOCT) with >1-step logCMT increase at 16 weeks from surgery or >2-step logOCT increase at 16 weeks from surgery were used.

Results
44% eyes had previous treatment for DME. No eye without prior DME ($n = 17$) developed central DME at 16 weeks from surgery, while 10% of 97 eyes with prior noncentral DME and 12% of 147 eyes with "possible" prior central DME progressed to have central DME at 16 weeks of surgery.

Conclusion
The presence of noncentral DME or a history of previous treatment for DME increases the chances for central DME after cataract surgery.

 Application to Clinical Practice

The risk of occurrence of central DME should be counselled if there is previous DME, noncentral or treated DME. An anti-VEGF agent may be considered at the time of cataract surgery.

Protocol R: A Phase II Evaluation of Topical NSAIDs in Eyes with Non-central-involved DME[24]

Purpose
To evaluate the effect of topical nepafenac in eye with noncentral DME.

Methods
Eyes with good vision and noncentral DME (definite retinal thickening by clinical examination, due to DME within 3,000 μm of center but not involving it) were randomized to receive topical nepafenac (0.1% TDS) or placebo for 1 year. The change in OCT retinal volume at 1 year was measured.

Results
The change in macular volume or development of center-involving DME was similar in both groups statistically.

Conclusion

Topical nepafenac does not affect retinal volume in eyes with noncentral DME.

 Application to Clinical Practice

Topical nonsteroidal anti-inflammatory drugs (NSAIDs) should not be advised to patients with noncentral DME and good vision.

Protocol S: Prompt Panretinal Photocoagulation versus Intravitreal Ranibizumab with Deferred Panretinal Photocoagulation for Proliferative Diabetic Retinopathy Study[25]

Purpose

To determine if VA outcomes at 2 years in eyes with (PDR that receive anti-VEGF therapy with deferred PRP are noninferior to those in eyes that receive standard prompt PRP therapy.

Background

Panretinal photocoagulation is the standard of care for high-risk PDR. PRP is efficacious in preventing severe vision loss in high-risk PDR albeit it has disadvantages such as loss of peripheral vision, delayed dark adaptation, and risk of development of macular edema. Pharmacotherapy with IVR offers a lucrative alternative as it is less destructive and can cause a regression in retinopathy severity.

Description

This was a randomized controlled trials of 394 eyes, comparing 2-year results of PRP versus repeated IVR. 203 eyes received one to three sessions of PRP and 191 eyes received IVR (0.5 mg) at baseline, followed by every 4 weeks for 6 months, unless resolution was achieved after four injections. After 6 months, injections could be deferred if neovascularization was stable over three consecutive visits. Eyes with DME received IVR in both groups. Retreatment in both groups was determined by OCT and clinical examination. PRP was deferred in the IVR group till failure criteria were met.

Inclusion Criteria

Patients with PDR, VA of 20/320 or better, and no previous PRP were included. Center-involving DME at baseline was allowed in both groups, which was treated as per protocol I.

Study Measures

The study measures were mean change in VA, eyes with ≥10-letter vision gain, cumulative score on HVF, eyes with regressed neovascularization, DME, and VH.

Results

At baseline, the groups were well balanced with respect to age, sex, duration of diabetes, mean A1C level, and no prior PRP. The mean baseline vision was 75 letters (20/32) in both groups, and the mean OCT central subfield thickness was 262 in the ranibizumab group and 249 in the PRP group. Center-involving DME was present at baseline in 22% (IVR) and 23% (PRP) of eyes.

At 2 years
- There was no difference in terms of the final level of neovascularization. The number of eyes without active or regressed neovascularization on fundus photography at 2 years was 44 in prompt PRP group and 49 in IVR group.
- The mean change in VA from baseline was slightly better in the IVR group (2.8 letters) than the PRP (0.2 letters) group ($p = 0.001$).
- *PRP group*
  - It had worse mean peripheral visual field sensitivity loss [−23 vs. −422 dB; difference, 372 dB; 95% confidence interval (CI), 213–531 dB; $p < .001$]
  - DME was more common (28% vs. 9%).
  - Vitrectomy was required more frequently (15% vs. 4%).
  - Supplemental PRP for worsening PDR was needed in 45% patients at a median of 7 months from baseline.
- *IVR group*
  - The median number of injections without baseline DME ($n = 133$) was 10 versus 14 in eyes with baseline DME ($n = 36$).
  - 6% eyes required rescue PRP over 2 years usually during vitrectomy.
- Only three eyes in the IVR group met the criteria for failure to receive PRP.
- Baseline characteristics had no impact on the benefit of IVR over PRP.
- One case in IVR group developed endophthalmitis.

Conclusion

Intravitreal ranibizumab is at least as effective as PRP for PDR patients.

At 5 years[26]
- Loss to follow-up was relatively high. The 5-year visit was completed by 184 of 277 participants (66% excluding deaths).
- VA in most study eyes was very good at 5 years and was similar in both groups. The mean change in VA letter score was 3.1 (IVR) and 3.0 (PRP) letters (95% CI, −2.3 to 3.5; $p = 0.68$).

- Severe vision loss or serious PDR complications were uncommon with PRP or ranibizumab.
- The IVR group had lower rates of developing vision-impairing DME and less visual field loss. The mean change in cumulative visual field was −330 (IVR) versus −527 (PRP) dB. Vision-impairing DME developed in 27 (IVR) and 53 (PRP) eyes.
- The mean requirement of injections was 19.2 injections in the IVR group and 5.4 injections in the PRP group.

Conclusion

Patient-specific factors, including anticipated visit compliance, cost, and frequency of visits, should be considered when choosing treatment for patients with PDR.

Application to Clinical Practice

When DME is present, IVR is a more suitable option than PRP in patients with PDR. However, continuous access to IVR is necessary for such a line of management.

Protocol T: A Comparative Effectiveness Study of Intravitreal Aflibercept, Bevacizumab, and Ranibizumab for DME[27]

Purpose

To compare between aflibercept, bevacizumab, and ranibizumab for DME.

Methods

660 adults with center-involving DME were randomized to receive intravitreal aflibercept (IVA; 2 mg), IVB (1.25 mg), or IVR (0.3 mg). The baseline VA was between 20/32 and 20/320 (approximately). OCT was used to define center-involving DME, and no patient had received an anti-VEGF injection in the past 12 months. Patients with BP > 180/110 mm Hg, significant renal disease, and thromboembolic event in the last 4 months were excluded. The minimum dosing interval was 4 weeks, and dosage scheduling was done on the basis of a predefined protocol. For the first 24 weeks, the study drugs were injected at baseline and then every 4 weeks unless VA was 20/20 or better and a CMT below the eligibility threshold. After 24 weeks, irrespective of VA and CMT, an injection was withheld if there was no improvement or worsening after two consecutive injections. Laser was allowed only after the 24-week visit, if clinically significant macular edema (CSME) was present, CMT > 250 (TD) or equivalent, and the eye had not improved with either OCT or vision as per the last two consecutive visits. Follow-up visits occurred every 4 weeks up to the 1-year visit. After 1 year, visits occurred every 4–16 weeks depending on disease progression and treatment administered. The primary outcome measure was mean change in vision at 1 year.

Results

The mean change in visual letters from baseline to 1 year was 13.3 letters with IVA, 11.2 with IVR, and 9.7 with IVB. However, this difference was considered to be due to different baseline visual acuities across the groups ($p < 0.001$). Hence, analysis was done after stratification on the basis of baseline VA. In patients with baseline vision below 20/50 (approximately), mean change in visual letters was 18.9 letters were with IVA, 11.8 with IVB, and 14.2 with IVR ($p < 0.001$ for IVA vs. IVB, $p = 0.003$ for IVA vs. IVR, and $p = 0.21$ for IVR vs. IVB). In eyes with baseline vision better than 20/40, the mean improvement was 8.0 letters with IVA, 7.5 with IVB, and 8.3 with IVR ($p > 0.50$ for each). All drugs were similar in terms of side effects.

Conclusion

All drugs were found to be effective and safe in central DME. The trend of visual improvement was driven by baseline vision, and IVA was better than other drugs at worse levels of baseline vision. In eyes with mild vision loss, the efficacy was similar.

Application to Clinical Practice

In eyes with mild vision loss, if treatment is being contemplated for center-involving DME, IVA, IVB and IVR are similar. In patients with poor baseline vision, IVA is a better option.

In 2-year results, the median numbers of injections in year 2 and over 2 years were almost similar numerically in the three groups.[28] A 2-year post-hoc analysis of this study found VA to remain stable at 2 years in all the groups. However, IVA was found to be significantly beneficial only to IVB and not IVR, though average letter gain with IVA was more than either IVB or IVR. IVA was found to be quicker in action in terms of letter improvement. At 1 year, reduction in CMT was less in IVB and at 2 years the change in CMT was similar in all the groups. Laser was seen to help only in IVB-treated eyes. Anti-Platelet Trialists' Collaboration (APTC) events were highest with IVR.[28,29]

Another analysis showed low rates of worsening of DR while on anti-VEGF treatment for DME. While eyes with NPDR receiving treatment showed improvement, IVB was less effective in the short-term than others. IVA was better in terms of reducing PDR than other drugs. Concomitant DR status may also affect the choice of anti-VEGF therapy as per the study data.[30] A further analysis of plasma-free levels of VEGF found greater reduction in VEGF levels by IVB and IVA as compared to IVR. No correlation was found, however, between plasma-free VEGF levels and systemic factors. The difference of VEGF levels between IVB and IVR was significant throughout the study. The reason for differences could be attributed to either the drug or an actual change.[31] 5-year extension results are awaited.

Protocol U: Short-term Evaluation of Combination Corticosteroid + Anti-VEGF Treatment for Persistent Central-involved DME Following Anti-VEGF Therapy[32]

Purpose
To evaluate continued IVR versus IVR with intravitreous dexamethasone implant (IDI) in eyes with persistent DME.

Methods
Persistent DME was defined as eyes with vision of 20/32 to 20/320, treated with at least three IVRs and a maintenance phase of additional IVR injections, and persisting DME on OCT. Eyes were randomized to receive IDI or sham in addition to IVR. The primary measure was vision at 6 months and the secondary measure was CMT on OCT.

Results
116 patients were included. The adjusted treatment group difference was 0.5 letters, and the difference was statistically insignificant. The adjusted treatment group difference for CMT was 52 letters ($p < 0.001$). 29% of eyes in the IDI group needed IOP management.

Conclusion
A combination of IDI and IVR did not help in improving vision in comparison to IVR alone in eyes with persistent DME.

 Application to Clinical Practice

While addition of IDI for persistent DME may lead to increase in IOP and eyes may have better OCT findings, it is not helpful in visual outcomes. Hence, combination therapy with the two agents may not be useful.

Protocol V: Treatment for Central-involved Diabetic Macular Edema in Eyes with Very Good Visual Acuity[33]

Purpose
To compare visual decline at 2 years in patients treated with IVA, laser, and observation in central-involved DME with very good baseline vision.

Methods
A randomized controlled trial was done at multiple sites of the network in 702 adults with type 1 or 2 diabetes mellitus. Only one eye of each patient with BCVA > 20/25 was recruited. For eyes randomized to laser or observation, loss of >10 letters or 5–9 letters at two consecutive visits was considered an

indication for shift to IVA. The main outcome measure was visual decline of >5 letters at 2 years.

Results

The analysis included 625 adults. 25% of the laser group and 34% of the observation group required shift to IVA during 2 years. 16% of IVA, 17% of laser, and 19% of observation group dropped significant vision at 2 years, which was statistically insignificant. APTC events occurred in 7%, 5%, and 3% of IVA, laser, and observation, respectively.

Conclusion

The authors concluded no difference in the three groups for managing central-involved DME.

 Application to Clinical Practice

Central-involved DME with good baseline VA need not be treated. If VA in such a patient would decline during follow-up, he/she may be shifted to IVA with no negative impact on the outcome.

Protocol AA: Peripheral Diabetic Retinopathy Lesions on Ultrawide-field Fundus Images and Risk of Diabetic Retinopathy Worsening Over Time[34]

Purpose

To compare the findings of ETDRS (7-field imaging) and ultrawide-field (UWF) imaging for DR.

Methods

A cross-sectional analysis of the modified ETDRS method and UWF imaging was used. Agreement between observers for ETDRS imaging, UWF masked for only ETDRS 7-field area, and UWF imaging was evaluated.

Results

764 eyes were included. On comparing only the 7-field images (ETDRS and UWF) for agreement after open evaluation by a senior grader, perfect agreement was found in 59.0% and agreement within 1 step in 96.9% eyes (κ, 0.77; 95% CI = 0.73–0.82). UWF imaging changed grading in overall 12.5% of cases with at least 1 step change in grading. Predominantly peripheral lesions were noted in 41% of eyes.

Conclusion

The two imaging systems have moderate-substantial agreement, and both may be equally better or worse.

> **Application to Clinical Practice**
> UWF and modified ETDRS 7-field grading system are equitable in grading DR. The implications of missing predominantly peripheral disease are unknown.

Other upcoming research protocols from the network include:

- *Protocol GEN*: Genes in Diabetic Retinopathy Project
- *Protocol W*: Intravitreous Anti-VEGF Treatment for Prevention of Vision Threatening Diabetic Retinopathy in Eyes at High Risk
- *Protocol AB*: Intravitreous Anti-VEGF versus Prompt Vitrectomy for Vitreous Hemorrhage from Proliferative Diabetic Retinopathy
- *Protocol AC*: Randomized Trial of Intravitreous Aflibercept versus Intravitreous Bevacizumab + Deferred Aflibercept for Treatment of Central-involved Diabetic Macular Edema
- *Protocol AD*: PROMINENT-Eye Ancillary Study: Diabetic Retinopathy Outcomes in a Randomized Trial of Pemafibrate versus Placebo
- *Protocol AG*: Randomized Clinical Trial Assessing the Effects of Pneumatic Vitreolysis on Vitreomacular Traction
- *Protocol AH*: Single-Arm Study Assessing the Effects of Pneumatic Vitreolysis on Macular Hole.

OTHER IMPORTANT CONCLUSIONS OF VARIOUS DRCR.NET STUDIES

- There is a decline in best-corrected ETDRS VA after dilation in diabetic subjects. The post-dilation ETDRS VA should not be used as a substitute for undilated VA.
- There is a modest correlation of OCT-measured center point thickness with VA and modest correlation of changes in retinal thickening and VA following focal laser treatment for DME. However, CIs are large and a wide range of VA may be observed for a given degree of retinal edema.[35]
- Central subfield mean thickness is the preferred OCT measurement for the central macula because of its higher reproducibility and correlation with other measurements of the central macula. The total macular volume may be preferred when the central macula is less important.
- A low rate of endophthalmitis (for intravitreal injections) can be achieved using topical povidone-iodine and using a sterile lid speculum and topical anesthetic but does not require topical antibiotics.
- Transformation of OCT retinal thickness data to logOCT may assist in the assessment of clinically meaningful changes in retinal thickness just as use of the logMAR scale has helped assess clinically meaningful changes in VA.

Clinical Trials in Diabetic Retinopathy - III

Table 1: Summary of various protocols of DRCR.net.

Title	Purpose	No. of patients	Inclusion criteria	Outcome measure	Result/conclusion
Protocol A	mETDRS technique versus mild macular grid technique of laser for DME	263	Patients with previously untreated DME	Change in OCT measures at 12 months	At 12 months, the MMG technique was less effective at reducing retinal thickening than the current mETDRS laser photocoagulation approach with similar visual acuity.
Protocol B	IVTA (1 mg, 4 mg) versus laser for DME	840	DME involving the fovea and VA 20/40 to 20/320	ETDRS VA, OCT macular thickness and safety at 3 years	Over a 2- as well as 3-year period, LP was more effective and had fewer side effects than 1- or 4 mg doses of IVTA for most patients with DME.
Protocol C	Diurnal variation in OCT-measured retinal thickness in center-involving DME	156	DME and OCT CMT ≥225 μm at 8 am	CMT was measured from retinal thickness maps over a single day between 8 am and 4 pm.	Most eyes with DME have little meaningful change in OCT CMT between 8 am and 4 pm.
Protocol D	Vitrectomy for DME	87	DME with at least moderate vision loss and VMT	VA, OCT retinal thickening, and surgical complications	Following vitrectomy, retinal thickening was reduced in most eyes with less consistent VA results, some eyes improving and some eyes worsening.
Protocol E	Peribulbar triamcinolone acetonide (TA) with and without focal photocoagulation for mild DME	129	Mild DME and VA 20/40 or better	Change in VA and retinal thickness	In DME with good VA, peribulbar TA, with or without focal photocoagulation, is unlikely to be of substantial benefit.
Protocol F	Development of DME following scatter laser photocoagulation	155	Severe NPDR or early PDR with good VA and no or mild DME	OCT CMT at day 3 and week 4	Clinically meaningful differences are unlikely in OCT thickness or VA following application of PRP in one sitting compared with four sittings in subjects

Contd...

Contd...

Title	Purpose	No. of patients	Inclusion criteria	Outcome measure	Result/conclusion
Protocol G	To determine the rate of progression of eyes with subclinical DME to clinically apparent DME or DME necessitating treatment during a 2-year period	43	Subclinical DME	Increase in OCT CMT of at least 50 µm from baseline and a CMT of at least 300 µm, or treatment for DME	Cumulative probability of meeting an increase in OCT CMT of at least 50 µm from baseline and a CMT of at least 300 µm, or treatment for DME was 27% by 1 year and 38% by 2 years.
Protocol H	Phase 2 randomized clinical trial of IVB for DME	121	DME and VA ranging from 20/32 to 20/320	CMT on OCT and VA was measured at baseline and after 3, 6, 9, 12, 18, and 24 weeks	IVB can reduce DME in some eyes.
Protocol I	Compare treatment of DME with ranibizumab or triamcinolone with focal or grid laser versus focal or grid laser alone	854 eyes	Patients with type 1 or 2 diabetes with visual acuity between 20/32 and 20/320 and DME involving fovea were included	BCVA at 1 year	Ranibizumab with prompt or deferred laser was superior to TA + laser and laser alone in treatment of DME at the end of 1 year. In pseudophakic eyes subset, visual acuity improvement was similar in TA + laser groups and both Ranibizumab + laser groups with an increased risk of elevation of IOP in TA group.
Protocol J	Intravitreal ranibizumab or triamcinolone acetonide as adjunctive treatment to PRP and focal laser for PDR with DME	345	VA of 20/320 or better, center-involved DME receiving LP, and DR	Changes in VA score	Addition of one IVTA or two ranibizumab injections in eyes receiving LP for DME and PRP is associated with better VA and decreased DME by 14 weeks.

Contd...

Title	Purpose	No. of patients	Inclusion criteria	Outcome measure	Result/conclusion
Protocol K	Course of response to focal photocoagulation for DME	122	LP for center-involved DME, OCT CMT ≥ 250 µm	VA letter score, OCT CMT decrease ≥10%	16 weeks following LP for DME, in eyes with a definite reduction, but not resolution, of central edema, 23–63% will continue to improve without additional treatment.
Protocol L	Comparison of AR with manual refraction in patients with DME	878	AR measured and manually measured visual scores using predefined protocols were assessed using electronic ETDRS charts	ETDRS VA	Current autorefractors are not a good substitute for manual refraction for trials.
Protocol M	To assess utility of point-of-care HbA1c measurements and personalized risk factor scaling during ophthalmic visits		Annual follow-up visitors were compared with more frequent visitors	Long-term change in HbA1c	Personalized education and risk assessment during retinal ophthalmology visits did not help in the overall betterment of diabetic control
Protocol N	Intravitreal ranibizumab versus saline for vitreous hemorrhage from PDR	261	Vitreous hemorrhage precluding PRP in eyes with PDR	Rate of vitrectomy, VA improvement, PRP completion rate, recurrent VH	• Little benefit of IVR and saline was observed on the rate of vitrectomy. Short-term benefits such as visual acuity improvement, higher PRP completion rates, and reduction of recurrent VH may be seen with IVR. • Long-term results at 1 year again showed no benefit of IVR over saline in vitrectomy rates or visual gain at 1 year.

Contd...

Title	Purpose	No. of patients	Inclusion criteria	Outcome measure	Result/conclusion
Protocol O	Comparison between time-domain and spectral-domain OCT for utility in measurement of retinal thickness		Center-involving DME and no DME	Bland–Altman coefficient of repeatability for relative change in retinal thickness	Spectralis OCT showed the best reproducibility over all machines tested. Retinal thickness measurements > 10% on the same machine or >20% after switching machines are likely to be due to actual change in retinal thickness rather than observation variability.
Protocol Q	Observational study in individuals with diabetic retinopathy without center-involved DME undergoing cataract surgery	293	Individuals with DR without center-involved DME undergoing cataract surgery	CMT > 250 µm (TDOCT) or 310 µm (SDOCT) with >1-step or 2-step logCMT increase at 16 weeks from surgery	No eye without prior DME (n = 17) developed central DME at 16 weeks from surgery, while 10% of 97 eyes with prior noncentral DME and 12% of 147 eyes with "possible" prior central DME progressed to have central DME at 16 weeks of surgery.
Protocol R	Phase II evaluation of topical NSAIDs in eyes with non-central-involved DME		Eyes with good vision and noncentral DME	Change in OCT CMT	Topical nepafenac does not affect retinal volume in eyes with noncentral DME.
Protocol S	Ranibizumab versus PRP in treatment of PDR	394 eyes of 304 patients	PDR with vision ≥20/320 and no prior PRP	Efficacy in terms of BCVA and CFT and safety at 24 months	Ranibizumab is noninferior to PRP in PDR.
Protocol T	Aflibercept versus bevacizumab versus ranibizumab in treatment of DME	660 eyes	Eyes with center-involving DME and visual acuity between 20/32 and 20/320	Efficacy in terms of BCVA and CFT and safety at 24 months	In eyes with mild visual loss at baseline, there was no significant difference in the efficacy of the three drugs. In eyes with more marked visual loss at baseline, aflibercept had superior efficacy than bevacizumab and ranibizumab at the end of 1 year. Aflibercept and ranibizumab had similar efficacy at the end of 2 years and were still superior to bevacizumab.

Contd...

Contd…

Title	Purpose	No. of patients	Inclusion criteria	Outcome measure	Result/conclusion
Protocol U	Addition of dexamethasone to continued ranibizumab therapy in patients with persistent central-involving DME	129 eyes	Eyes with persistent central-involving diabetic macular edema	Change in mean visual acuity and central subfield thickness at the end of 24 weeks	Addition of dexamethasone over ranibizumab in treatment of persistent center-involving diabetic macular edema provided no additional benefit in visual acuity improvement.
Protocol V	Observation versus laser versus aflibercept for center-involving DME in eyes with very good visual acuity	702 eyes	Eyes with center-involving DME having visual acuity ≥ 20/25	Compare % of eyes that lost at least 5 letters over a period of 2 years in the three groups	At the end of 2 years, there was no difference in visual outcomes of the three groups.
Protocol AA	Peripheral diabetic retinopathy lesions on ultrawide-field fundus images and risk of DR worsening over time	764	Eyes with DR	Agreement between observer for DR grading based on ETDRS (7-field imaging) and ultrawide-field imaging	Ultrawide-field and modified ETDRS 7-field grading system are equitable in grading DR. Implications of missing predominantly peripheral disease are unknown.

(DRCR.net: The Diabetic Retinopathy Clinical Research Network; AR: autorefraction; BCVA: best-corrected visual acuity; CFT: central foveal thickness; CMT: central macular thickness; DME: diabetic macular edema; DR: diabetic retinopathy; IVB: intravitreal bevacizumab; IVR: intravitreal ranibizumab; IVTA: intravitreal triamcinolone acetonide; LP: laser photocoagulation; mETDRS: modified Early Treatment Diabetic Retinopathy Study; MMG: mild macular grid; NPDR: nonproliferative diabetic retinopathy; NSAIDs: nonsteroidal anti-inflammatory drugs; OCT: optical coherence tomography; PDR: proliferative diabetic retinopathy; PRP: panretinal photocoagulation; SDOCT: spectral-domain OCT; TDOCT: time-domain OCT; VA: visual acuity; VH: vitreous hemorrhage; VMT: vitreomacular traction;)

REFERENCES

1. Writing Committee for the Diabetic Retinopathy Clinical Research Network; Fong DS, Strauber SF, Aiello LP, Beck RW, Callanan DG, et al. Comparison of the modified Early Treatment Diabetic Retinopathy Study and mild macular grid laser photocoagulation strategies for diabetic macular edema. Arch Ophthalmol. 2007;125:469-80.
2. Diabetic Retinopathy Clinical Research Network. A randomized trial comparing intravitreal triamcinolone acetonide and focal/grid photocoagulation for diabetic macular edema. Ophthalmology. 2008;115:1447-9.
3. Diabetic Retinopathy Clinical Research Network. Three-year follow-up of a randomized trial comparing focal/grid photocoagulation and intravitreal triamcinolone for diabetic macular edema. Arch Ophthalmol. 2009;127:245-51.
4. Bressler NM, Edwards AR, Beck RW, Flaxel CJ, Glassman AR, et al; Diabetic Retinopathy Clinical Research Network. Exploratory analysis of diabetic retinopathy progression through 3 years in a randomized clinical trial that compares intravitreal triamcinolone acetonide with focal/grid photocoagulation. Arch Ophthalmol. 2009;127:1566-71.
5. Diabetic Retinopathy Clinical Research Network; Danis RP, Glassman AR, Aiello LP, Antoszyk AN, Beck RW, et al. Diurnal variation in retinal thickening measurement by optical coherence tomography in center-involved diabetic macular edema. Arch Ophthalmol. 2006;124:1701-7.
6. Flaxel CJ, Edwards AR, Aiello LP, Arrigg PG, Beck RW, Diabetic Retinopathy Clinical Research Network. Factors associated with visual acuity outcomes after vitrectomy for diabetic macular edema. Retina. 2010;30:1488-95.
7. Diabetic Retinopathy Clinical Research Network Writing Committee on behalf of the DRCR.net; Haller JA, Qin H, Apte RS, Beck RR, Bressler NM, et al. Vitrectomy outcomes in eyes with diabetic macular edema and vitreomacular traction. Ophthalmology. 2010;117:1087-93.e3.
8. Chew E, Strauber S, Beck R; Diabetic Retinopathy Clinical Research Network. Randomized trial of peribulbar triamcinolone acetonide with and without focal photocoagulation for mild diabetic macular edema: a pilot study. Ophthalmology. 2007;114:1190-6.
9. Diabetic Retinopathy Clinical Research Network; Brucker AJ, Qin H, Antoszyk AN, Beck RW, Bressler NM, et al. . Observational study of the development of diabetic macular edema following pan-retinal (scatter) photocoagulation given in 1 or 4 sittings. Arch Ophthalmol. 2009;127:132-40.
10. Diabetic Retinopathy Clinical Research Network; Bressler NM, Miller KM, Beck RW, Bressler SB, Glassman AR, et al. Observational Study of Subclinical Diabetic Macular Edema. Eye (Lond). 2012;26:833-40.
11. Diabetic Retinopathy Clinical Research Network; Scott IU, Edwards AR, Beck RW, Bressler NM, Chan CK, et al. A phase II randomized clinical trial of intravitreal bevacizumab for diabetic macular edema. Ophthalmology. 2007;114:1860-7.
12. Diabetic Retinopathy Clinical Research Network; Elman MJ, Bressler NM, Qin H, Beck RW, Ferris 3rd FL, et al. Expanded 2-year follow-up of ranibizumab plus prompt or deferred laser or triamcinolone plus prompt laser for diabetic macular edema. Ophthalmology. 2011;118:609-14.
13. Diabetic Retinopathy Clinical Research Network; Elman MJ, Qin H, Aiello LP, Beck RW, Bressler NM, et al. Intravitreal ranibizumab for diabetic macular edema with prompt versus deferred laser treatment: three-year randomized trial results. Ophthalmology. 2012;119(11):2312-8.
14. Diabetic Retinopathy Clinical Research Network; Elman MJ, Ayala A, Bressler NM, Browning D, Flaxel CJ, et al. Intravitreal ranibizumab for diabetic macular edema with prompt versus deferred laser treatment: 5-year randomized trial results. Ophthalmology. 2015;122(2):375-81.

15. Diabetic Retinopathy Clinical Research Network; Googe J, Brucker AJ, Bressler NM, Qin H, Aiello LP, et al. Randomized trial evaluating short-term effects of intravitreal ranibizumab or triamcinolone acetonide on macular edema following focal/grid laser for diabetic macular edema in eyes also receiving panretinal photocoagulation. Retina. 2011;31:1009-27.
16. Diabetic Retinopathy Clinical Research Network. The course of response to focal/grid photocoagulation for diabetic macular edema. Retina. 2009;29:1436-43.
17. Sun JK, Qin H, Aiello LP, Melia M, Beck RW, Andreoli CM, et al. Evaluation of visual acuity measurements after autorefraction vs manual refraction in eyes with and without diabetic macular edema. Arch Ophthalmol. 2011;130(4):470-9.
18. Diabetic Retinopathy Clinical Research Network; Aiello LP, Ayala AR, Antoszyk AN, Arnold-Bush B, Baker C, et al. Assessing the effect of personalized diabetes risk assessments during ophthalmologic visits on glycemic control: a randomized clinical trial. JAMA Ophthalmol. 2015;133(8):888-96.
19. Diabetic Retinopathy Clinical Research Network. Randomized clinical trial evaluating intravitreal ranibizumab or saline for vitreous hemorrhage from proliferative diabetic retinopathy. JAMA Ophthalmol. 2013;131(3):283-93.
20. Diabetic Retinopathy Clinical Research Network; Bhavsar AR, Torres K, Glassman AR, Jampol LM, Kinyoun JL, Evaluation of results 1 year following short-term use of ranibizumab for vitreous hemorrhage due to proliferative diabetic retinopathy. JAMA Ophthalmol. 2014;132(7):889-90.
21. Chalam KV, Bressler SB, Edwards AR, Berger BB, Bressler NM, Glassman AR, et al. Retinal thickness in people with diabetes and minimal or no diabetic retinopathy: Heidelberg Spectralis optical coherence tomography. Invest Ophthalmol Vis Sci. 2012;53(13):8154-61.
22. Diabetic Retinopathy Clinical Research Network Authors/Writing Committee; Bressler SB, Baker CW, Almukhtar T, Bressler NM, et al. Pilot study of individuals with diabetic macular edema undergoing cataract surgery. JAMA Ophthalmol. 2014;132(2):224-6.
23. Diabetic Retinopathy Clinical Research Network Authors/Writing Committee; Baker CW, Almukhtar T, Bressler NM, Glassman AR, Grover S, et al. Macular edema after cataract surgery in eyes without preoperative central-involved diabetic macular edema. JAMA Ophthalmol. 2013;131(7):870-9.
24. Friedman SM, Almukhtar TH, Baker CW, Glassman AR, Elman MJ, Bressler NM, et al. Topical nepafenec in eyes with noncentral diabetic macular edema. Retina. 2015;35(5):944-56.
25. Writing Committee for the Diabetic Retinopathy Clinical Research Network; Gross JG, Glassman AR, Jampol LM, Inusah S, Aiello LP, et al. Panretinal photocoagulation vs intravitreous ranibizumab for proliferative diabetic retinopathy: A randomized trial. JAMA. 2015;314(20):2137-46.
26. Gross JG, Glassman AR, Liu D, Sun JK, Antoszyk AN, Baker CW, et al. Five-year outcomes of panretinal photocoagulation vs intravitreous ranibizumab for proliferative diabetic retinopathy: A randomized clinical trial. JAMA Ophthalmol. 2018;136(10):1138-48.
27. Diabetic Retinopathy Clinical Research Network; Wells JA, Glassman AR, et al. Aflibercept, bevacizumab, or ranibizumab for diabetic macular edema. N Engl J Med. 2015;372(13):1193-203.
28. Diabetic Retinopathy Clinical Research Network; Wells JA, Glassman AR, Ayala AR, Jampol LM, Aiello LP, et al. Aflibercept, bevacizumab, or ranibizumab for diabetic macular edema: two-year results from a comparative effectiveness randomized clinical trial. Ophthalmology. 2016;123(6):1351-9.
29. Jampol LM, Glassman AR, Bressler NM, Wells JA, Ayala AR, Diabetic Retinopathy Clinical Research Network. Anti-vascular endothelial growth factor comparative

effectiveness trial for diabetic macular edema: additional efficacy post hoc analyses of a randomized clinical trial. JAMA Ophthalmol. 2016;134(12):10.1001/jamaophthalmol.2016.3698.
30. Bressler SB, Liu D, Glassman AR, Blodi BA, Castellarin AA, Jampol LM, et al. Change in diabetic retinopathy through 2 years: Secondary analysis of a randomized clinical trial comparing aflibercept, bevacizumab, and ranibizumab. JAMA Ophthalmol. 2017;135(6):558-68.
31. Jampol LM, Glassman AR, Liu D, Aiello LP, Bressler NM, Duh EJ, et al. Plasma vascular endothelial growth factor concentrations after intravitreous anti–vascular endothelial growth factor therapy for diabetic macular edema. Ophthalmology. 2018;125(7):1054-63.
32. Maturi RK, Glassman AR, Liu D, Beck RW, Bhavsar AR, Bressler NM, et al. Effect of adding dexamethasone to continued ranibizumab treatment in patients with persistent diabetic macular edema: A DRCR network phase 2 randomized clinical trial. JAMA Ophthalmol. 2017;136(1):29-38.
33. DRCR Retina Network; Baker CW, Glassman AR, Beaulieu WT, Antoszyk AN, Browning DJ, et al. Effect of initial management with aflibercept vs laser photocoagulation vs observation on vision loss among patients with diabetic macular edema involving the center of the macula and good visual acuity: A randomized clinical trial. JAMA. 2019;321(19):1880-94.
34. Aiello LP, Odia I, Glassman AR, Melia M, Jampol LM, Bressler NM, et al. Comparison of early treatment diabetic retinopathy study standard 7-field imaging with ultrawide-field imaging for determining severity of diabetic retinopathy. JAMA Ophthalmol. 2019;137(1):65-73.
35. Browning DJ, Glassman AR, Aiello LP et al. Diabetic Retinopathy Clinical Research Network. The relationship between optical coherence tomography-measured central retinal thickness and visual acuity in diabetic macular edema. Ophthalmology. 2007;114:525-36.

Clinical Trials in Diabetic Retinopathy-IV

Neha Goel, Saurabh Verma, Shorya Azad

■ INTRODUCTION

Vascular endothelial growth factor (VEGF) levels are elevated in the vitreous of eyes with diabetic retinopathy making anti-VEGF treatment an attractive therapeutic modality in diabetic macular edema (DME). Pegaptanib (Macugen; Eyetech Pharmaceuticals Inc. New York, NY, USA) is a pegylated aptamer that targets only the VEGF 165 isoform and is currently approved for the treatment of neovascular age-related macular degeneration (AMD). Intravitreal bevacizumab (IVB; Avastin; Genentech Inc. San Francisco, CA, USA) is a full-length humanized antibody that binds to all types of VEGF. It is used in and licensed for tumor therapy. Ranibizumab (RBZ; Lucentis; Genentech Inc.; marketed by Novartis in Europe) comes from the same parent molecule as IVB; however, it is a humanized monoclonal antibody fragment that binds all active forms of VEGF-A and is currently approved for AMD and DME. Regeneron's VEGF Trap-Eye (Eylea, aflibercept) is Food and Drug Administration (FDA) approved for AMD and DME. Aflibercept (AFB) is a fully human, soluble VEGF receptor fusion protein that binds all forms of VEGF-A along with another vascular growth factor, the placental growth factor (PlGF). VEGF Trap-Eye is a specific and highly potent blocker of VEGF-A and PlGF that has been demonstrated in preclinical models to bind these growth factors with greater affinity than their natural receptors. A newer addition, Brolucizumab (RTH258, Beovu, Novartis), is the smallest active unit of antibody allowing concentrated molar dosing of 22 times that of RBZ and more than 11 times that of AFB. Brolucizumab has FDA approval for AMD while trials for DME are underway.

Corticosteroids may have multiple mechanisms of action in the treatment of DME. In addition to their anti-inflammatory properties, corticosteroids have been reported to reduce the activity of VEGF. Intravitreal triamcinolone acetonide injection was the first agent used which was not formulated for ocular use and had problems of cataract formation and elevated intraocular pressure (IOP). To reduce the need for repeated intravitreal injections, several extended-release corticosteroid delivery systems have been studied. Sustained-release fluocinolone acetonide (FA; Iluvien, Alimera Sciences) consists of a tiny, cylindrical polyimide tube that contains 190 µg of FA.

Biodegradable sustained-release micronized dexamethasone implant (Ozurdex, Allergen) consisting of 0.35- and 0.7-mg dexamethasone in the Novadur solid polymer drug delivery system is now FDA approved for use in DME and is available as a single-use preloaded rod-shaped implant for injection in vitreous cavity.

■ RANIBIZUMAB FOR EDEMA OF THE MACULA IN DIABETES: A PHASE 2 STUDY (READ-2)[1-3]

Purpose

To compare RBZ with focal/grid laser or a combination of both in DME. This comprises the following:
1. To obtain data on the bioactivity and dose interval effects of intravitreal RBZ alone, as well as in combination with laser photocoagulation, on retinal thickness and visual acuity in subjects with DME.
2. To obtain additional safety and bioactivity data to aid in the design of a phase 3 clinical trial to evaluate RBZ as a therapeutic option for patients with DME.

Description

READ-2 is a phase 2, prospective, randomized, interventional, multicenter clinical trial that began in December, 2006. The study consisted of a 2-week screening period, a 6-month treatment period with a primary time endpoint, and an 18-month follow-up and treatment period with secondary time endpoints. Consented subjects entered the 14-day screening period to determine eligibility. Serum chemistry and hematology testing, urinalysis, and pregnancy testing were performed. Screening also included best-corrected visual acuity (BCVA), ophthalmic examination, macular thickness measurements based on optical coherence tomography (OCT), and fundus fluorescein angiography (FFA) entry criteria.

A total of 126 patients with DME were randomized 1:1:1 to receive 0.5 mg of RBZ at baseline and months 1, 3, and 5 (group 1, 42 patients), focal/grid laser photocoagulation at baseline and month 3 if needed (group 2, 42 patients), or a combination of 0.5 mg of RBZ and focal/grid laser at baseline and month 3 (group 3, 42 patients). Starting at month 6, if retreatment criteria were met, all subjects could be treated with RBZ. Patients who agreed to participate between months 24 and 36 (RBZ, 28 patients; laser, 22; and RBZ + laser, 24) returned monthly and received RBZ, 0.5 mg, if foveal thickness (FTH, center subfield thickness) was 250 μm or greater.

Inclusion Criteria

Patients who meet the following eligibility criteria were enrolled in the study:
- Foveal thickening from macular edema secondary to diabetes (type 1 or 2)

- Early Treatment Diabetic Retinopathy Study (ETDRS) visual acuity of 20/40 or worse but better than or equal to 20/320
- Baseline FTH by OCT at least 250 µm. This level is often associated with visual acuity of 20/40 or worse and provides sufficient thickening so that a treatment effect is easily detectable.
- Only one eye was treated in the study. If both eyes were eligible, the investigator selected the eye to be enrolled. Visual acuity in the nonstudy eye must be greater than 20/800.

Patients with prior laser photocoagulation (macular or panretinal) within 3 months of study entry, use of periocular or intraocular steroids within 3 months of study entry, or use of antiangiogenic drugs within 2 months of study entry were excluded. The presence of proliferative diabetic retinopathy, vitreomacular traction, or epiretinal membrane in the study eye was also an exclusion criteria.

Study Measures

The primary outcome measure was the change from baseline in BCVA—improvement in vision of 15 or more letters, or achievement of a final vision of 50 letters (20/25), or better if baseline visual acuity was 40 letters (20/40). Secondary outcome measures included several outcomes related to OCT measurements (reduction in FTH between months 24 and 36) and FFA.

Results

- At month 6, the mean gain in BCVA was significantly greater in group 1 (+7.24 letters, $p = 0.01$, analysis of variance) compared with group 2 (−0.43 letters). The mean gain in group 3 (+3.80 letters) was not statistically different from group 1 or 2. For patients with data available at 6 months, improvement of 3 lines or more occurred in 8 of 37 (22%) in group 1 compared with 0 of 38 (0%) in group 2 ($p = 0.002$, Fisher exact test) and 3 of 40 (8%) in group 3. Excess FTH was reduced by 50%, 33%, and 45% in groups 1, 2, and 3, respectively.
- After the primary endpoint at month 6, most patients in all groups were treated only with RBZ, and the mean number of injections was 5.3, 4.4, and 2.9 during the 18-month follow-up period in groups 1, 2, and 3, respectively. For the 33 patients in group 1, 34 patients in group 2, and 34 patients in group 3 who remained in the study through 24 months, the mean improvement in BCVA was 7.4, 0.5, and 3.8 letters at the 6-month primary endpoint, compared with 7.7, 5.1, and 6.8 letters at month 24, and the percentage of patients who gained 3 lines or more of BCVA was 21, 0, and 6 at month 6, compared with 24, 18, and 26 at month 24. The percentage of patients with 20/40 or better Snellen equivalent at month 24 was 45% in group 1, 44% in group 2, and 35% in group 3. The mean FTH, defined as center subfield thickness, at month 24 was 340, 286, and

258 μm for groups 1, 2, and 3, respectively, and the percentage of patients with center subfield thickness of 250 μm or less was 36%, 47%, and 68%, respectively.
- At 3 years, the mean improvement from the baseline BCVA in group 1 was 10.3 letters at month 36 versus 7.2 letters at month 24 (ΔBCVA letters = 3.1, $p = 0.009$), and FTH at month 36 was 282 μm versus 352 μm at month 24 (ΔFTH = 70 μm, $p = 0.006$). Changes in BCVA and FTH in group 2 (–1.6 letters and –36 μm, respectively) and group 3 (+2.0 letters and –24 μm) were not statistically significant. The mean number of RBZ injections was significantly greater in group 1 compared with group 2 (5.4 vs. 2.3 injections, $p = 0.008$) but not compared with group 3 (3.3, $p = 0.11$).

Conclusion

- During a span of 6 months, RBZ injections by the current protocol had a significantly better visual outcome than focal/grid laser treatment in patients with DME.
- Intraocular injections of RBZ provided benefit for patients with DME for at least 2 years, and when combined with focal or grid laser treatments, the amount of residual edema was reduced, as were the frequency of injections needed to control edema, without impairment of visual acuity. The 2-year follow-up also showed that RBZ is associated with significant improvement in patients who previously received only laser photocoagulation.
- More aggressive treatment with RBZ during year 3 resulted in a reduction in mean FTH and improvement in BCVA in the RBZ group. More extensive focal/grid laser therapy in the other two groups may have reduced the need for more frequent RBZ injections to control edema.

Application to Clinical Practice

Long-term visual outcomes for treatment of DME with RBZ are excellent, but many patients require frequent injections to optimally control edema and maximize vision.

A STUDY OF RANIBIZUMAB INJECTION IN SUBJECTS WITH CLINICALLY SIGNIFICANT MACULAR EDEMA WITH CENTER INVOLVEMENT SECONDARY TO DIABETES MELLITUS (RISE AND RIDE)[4,5]

Purpose

To evaluate the efficacy and safety of intravitreal RBZ in DME patients.

Background

Ranibizumab (Lucentis) is the first and only medicine approved by the US FDA for treatment of DME, a condition for which the standard of care has not changed significantly in more than 25 years. The standard of care for DME has been laser, which slows the rate of vision loss and helps stabilize vision but has demonstrated only limited ability to restore lost vision. The approval of Lucentis in DME was based on Genentech's phase III trials, RIDE and RISE.

Description

RISE and RIDE were Genentech's phase III trials, identically designed, parallel, double-masked, multicenter, 3-year clinical trials, which were sham-treatment controlled for 24 months. A total of 759 patients were randomized into three groups (1:1:1 randomization, one eye per subject) to receive monthly treatment with 0.3-mg RBZ ($n = 250$), 0.5-mg RBZ ($n = 252$), or sham injection (control group, $n = 257$). In RISE, 377 patients were randomized (127 to sham, 125 to 0.3 mg, and 125 to 0.5 mg). In RIDE, 382 patients were randomized (130 to sham, 125 to 0.3 mg, and 127 to 0.5 mg). The studies began in June, 2007.

Beginning at month 3, all patients were evaluated monthly for the need for macular laser according to protocol-specified criteria: central foveal thickness (CFT) ≥ 250 μm with a <50-μm change from the prior month, with no prior macular laser in the previous 3 months, and an assessment by the evaluating physician that macular laser would be beneficial.

Inclusion Criteria

Adults (≥18 years) with decrease in vision due primarily to DME, central subfield thickness (CST) ≥ 275 μm, study eye BCVA of 20/40 to 20/320, and glycated hemoglobin (HbA1c) ≤ 12% were included in the study. Patients with a history of any of the following were included unless the event occurred within 3 months of day 0:
1. Antiangiogenic drugs in either eye
2. Panretinal photocoagulation
3. Macular laser or intraocular steroids
4. Cerebrovascular accident (CVA) or myocardial infarction (MI).

Study Measures

The primary endpoints were the proportion of patients who gained ≥15 ETDRS letters in BCVA score from baseline at 24 months, mean change from baseline in BCVA, and mean change from baseline in CFT.

Results

- *RISE*: At 24 months, 18.1% of sham patients gained ≥15 letters versus 44.8% of 0.3-mg [$p < 0.0001$; difference vs. sham adjusted for randomization stratification factors, 24.3%; 95% confidence interval (CI), 13.8–34.8] and 39.2% of 0.5-mg RBZ patients ($p < 0.001$; adjusted difference, 20.9%; 95% CI, 10.7–31.1).

- *RIDE*: Significantly, more RBZ-treated patients gained ≥15 letters: 12.3% of sham patients versus 33.6% of 0.3-mg patients ($p < 0.0001$; adjusted difference, 20.8%; 95% CI, 11.4–30.2) and 45.7% of 0.5-mg RBZ patients ($p < 0.0001$; adjusted difference, 33.3%; 95% CI, 23.8–42.8).
- Significant gains in average vision were observed 7 days after the first treatment.
- For all time points comparing 0.3 mg Lucentis to control through month 24, $p < 0.01$.
- Vision improvements observed in patients treated with Lucentis at 24 months were maintained with continued treatment through 36 months.
- A preplanned subgroup analysis reported today indicated that the improvements were generally similar for patients with well-controlled glucose (baseline HbA1c ≤ 8) and poorly controlled glucose (baseline HbA1c > 8).
- Significant improvements in macular edema were noted on OCT, and retinopathy was less likely to worsen and more likely to improve in RBZ-treated patients.
- RBZ-treated patients underwent significantly fewer macular laser procedures (mean of 1.8 and 1.6 laser procedures over 24 months in the sham groups vs. 0.3–0.8 in RBZ groups).
- Ocular safety was consistent with prior RBZ studies; endophthalmitis occurred in four RBZ patients. The total incidence of deaths from vascular or unknown causes, nonfatal myocardial infarctions, and nonfatal cerebrovascular accidents, which are possible effects from systemic VEGF inhibition, was 4.9–5.5% of sham patients and 2.4–8.8% of RBZ patients.

Conclusion

Ranibizumab rapidly and sustainably improved vision, reduced the risk of further vision loss, and improved macular edema in patients with DME, with low rates of ocular and nonocular harm.

SAFETY AND EFFICACY OF RANIBIZUMAB IN DIABETIC MACULAR EDEMA WITH CENTER INVOLVEMENT (RESOLVE)[6]

Purpose

To investigate the safety and efficacy of RBZ in DME involving the foveal center.

Description

RESOLVE was a 12-month, multicenter, randomized, sham-controlled, double-masked study with eyes randomly assigned to intravitreal RBZ (0.3 or

0.5 mg; $n = 51$ each) or sham ($n = 49$). The treatment schedule comprised 3 monthly injections, after which treatment could be stopped/reinitiated with an opportunity for rescue laser photocoagulation (protocol-defined criteria) for 9 months. After month 1, dose-doubling was permitted (protocol-defined criteria, injection volume increased from 0.05 to 0.1 mL and remained at 0.1 mL thereafter). Recruitment was started in October, 2005.

Inclusion Criteria
Patients with age >18 years, type 1 or 2 diabetes, central retinal thickness (CRT) ≥ 300 µm, and BCVA of 73–39 ETDRS letters were included in the study.

Study Measures
Efficacy (BCVA and CRT) and safety were compared between pooled RBZ and sham arms using the full analysis set ($n = 151$, patients receiving ≥1 injection).

Results
At month 12, the mean ± SD BCVA improved from baseline by 10.3 ± 9.1 letters with RBZ and declined by 1.4 ± 14.2 letters with sham ($p < 0.0001$). Mean CRT reduction was 194.2 ± 135.1 µm with RBZ and 48.4 ± 153.4 µm with sham ($p < 0.0001$). Gain of ≥10 letters BCVA from baseline occurred in 60.8% of RBZ and 18.4% of sham eyes ($p < 0.0001$). Safety data were consistent with previous studies of intravitreal RBZ. The mean number of injections administered during 12 months was 10.2 and 8.9 for RBZ and sham, respectively.

Conclusion
Ranibizumab is effective in improving BCVA and is well tolerated in DME. Future clinical trials are required to confirm its long-term efficacy and safety.

RANIBIZUMAB MONOTHERAPY OR COMBINED WITH LASER VERSUS LASER MONOTHERAPY FOR DIABETIC MACULAR EDEMA (RESTORE)[7]

Purpose
To demonstrate the superiority of RBZ 0.5-mg monotherapy or combined with laser over laser alone based on change in BCVA over 12 months in DME.

Description
RESTORE was a 12-month, randomized, double-masked, multicenter, laser-controlled phase III study and included 345 patients enrolled from May, 2008. Patients were randomized to RBZ + sham laser, RBZ + laser or sham injections + laser. RBZ/sham was given for 3 months and then pro re nata (PRN) and laser/sham laser was given at baseline and then PRN (patients

had scheduled monthly visits). Retreatments were given in accordance with ETDRS guidelines at intervals no shorter than 3 months from the previous treatment if considered necessary by the investigator.

Inclusion Criteria
Patients aged >18 years, with type 1 or 2 diabetes mellitus and visual impairment due to DME, were included in the study.

Study Measures
The main outcome measures were mean average change in BCVA from baseline to months 1 through 12 and safety.

Results
- RBZ alone and combined with laser were superior to laser monotherapy in improving the mean average change in BCVA from baseline to months 1 through 12 (+6.1 and +5.9 vs. +0.8; both $p < 0.0001$). At month 12, a significantly greater proportion of patients had a BCVA letter score ≥15 and BCVA letter score level >73 (20/40 Snellen equivalent) with RBZ (22.6% and 53%, respectively) and RBZ + laser (22.9% and 44.9%) versus laser (8.2% and 23.6%).
- Similar results could be found evaluating fluorescein angiography. A significantly larger proportion of patients who underwent RBZ injections alone or RBZ injections associated with laser treatment obtained total resolution of leakage compared with the laser group (19.4% and 13.7% vs. 2.2%).
- The mean CRT was significantly reduced from baseline with RBZ (−118.7 μm) and RBZ + laser (−128.3 μm) versus laser (−61.3 μm; both $p < 0.001$).
- Health-related quality of life, assessed through the National Eye Institute Visual Function Questionnaire 25 (NEI VFQ-25), improved significantly from baseline with RBZ alone and combined with laser ($p < 0.05$ for composite score and vision-related subscales) versus laser.
- Patients received seven (mean) RBZ/sham injections over 12 months. Between months 3 and 11, patients received an average of 4.1 RBZ intravitreal injections in the RBZ arm, 3.8 in the RBZ + laser arm, and 4.5 sham injections in the laser-treated arm.
- No endophthalmitis cases occurred. Increased IOP was reported for one patient each in the RBZ arms. RBZ monotherapy or combined with laser was not associated with an increased risk of cardiovascular or cerebrovascular events in this study.

Conclusion
Ranibizumab monotherapy and combined with laser provided superior visual acuity gain over standard laser in patients with visual impairment due

to DME. Visual acuity gains were associated with significant gains in VFQ-25 scores. At 1 year, no differences were detected between the RBZ and the RBZ + laser arms. RBZ monotherapy and combined with laser had a safety profile in DME similar to that in AMD.

A PROSPECTIVE RANDOMIZED TRIAL OF INTRAVITREAL BEVACIZUMAB OR LASER THERAPY IN THE MANAGEMENT OF DIABETIC MACULAR EDEMA (BOLT)[8,9]

Purpose
To compare repeated IVB and modified ETDRS macular laser therapy (MLT) in patients with persistent clinically significant macular edema (CSME).

Description
BOLT was a prospective, randomized, masked, single-center, 2-year, 2-arm clinical trial in which a total of 80 eyes of 80 patients with center-involving CSME and at least one prior MLT were included. Patients were recruited from 2007 to 2010. Subjects were randomized to either IVB (6 weekly; minimum of three injections and maximum of nine injections in the first 12 months) or MLT (4 monthly; minimum of one treatment and maximum of four treatments in the first 12 months).

Inclusion Criteria
Patients with center-involving CSME, at least one prior MLT and visual acuity of 20/40 to 20/320, were included.

Study Measures
The primary endpoint was the difference in ETDRS BCVA at 12 months between the bevacizumab and laser arms. Secondary outcomes were mean change in BCVA, proportion gaining at least 15 and at least 10 ETDRS letters, losing fewer than 15 and at least 30 letters, change in central macular thickness, ETDRS retinopathy severity, and safety outcomes.

Results
- The baseline mean ETDRS BCVA was 55.7 ± 9.7 (range 34–69) in the bevacizumab group and 54.6 ± 8.6 (range 36–68) in the laser arm. The mean ETDRS BCVA at 12 months was 61.3 ± 10.4 (range 34–79) in the bevacizumab group and 50.0 ± 16.6 (range 8–76) in the laser arm ($p = 0.0006$). Furthermore, the bevacizumab group gained a median of 8 ETDRS letters, whereas the laser group lost a median of 0.5 ETDRS letters ($p = 0.0002$). The odds of gaining ≥10 ETDRS letters over 12 months were 5.1 times greater in the bevacizumab group than in the laser group (adjusted odds ratio, 5.1; 95% CI, 1.3–19.7; $p = 0.019$).

- At 12 months, the central macular thickness decreased from 507 ± 145 μm (range 281–900 μm) at baseline to 378 ± 134 μm (range 167–699 μm) ($p < 0.001$) in the IVB group, whereas it decreased to a lesser extent in the laser group, from 481 ± 121 μm (range 279–844 μm) to 413 ± 135 μm (range 170–708 μm) ($p = 0.02$).
- The median number of injections was nine [interquartile range (IQR) 8–9] in the IVB group, and the median number of laser treatments was three (IQR 2–4) in the MLT group.
- At 2 years, the mean (SD) ETDRS BCVA was 64.4 (13.3) (ETDRS equivalent Snellen fraction: 20/50) in the bevacizumab arm and 54.8 (12.6) (20/80) in the MLT arm ($p = 0.005$). The bevacizumab arm gained a median of 9 ETDRS letters versus 2.5 letters for MLT ($p = 0.005$), with a mean gain of 8.6 letters for bevacizumab versus a mean loss of 0.5 letters for MLT. 49% of patients gained 10 or more letters ($p = 0.001$) and 32% gained at least 15 letters ($p = 0.004$) for bevacizumab versus 7% and 4% for MLT. Percentage who lost fewer than 15 letters in the MLT arm was 86% versus 100% for bevacizumab ($p = 0.03$). The mean reduction in central macular thickness was 146 μm in the bevacizumab arm versus 118 μm in the MLT arm. The median number of treatments over 24 months was 13 for bevacizumab and 4 for MLT.

Conclusion

The study provides evidence to support the use of bevacizumab in patients with center-involving CSME without advanced macular ischemia. Improvements in BCVA and central macular thickness seen with bevacizumab at 1 year were maintained over the second year with a mean of four injections, thus providing evidence supporting longer term use of intravitreous bevacizumab for persistent center-involving CSME.

DME AND VEGF TRAP-EYE: INVESTIGATION OF CLINICAL IMPACT (DA VINCI)[10,11]

Purpose

To compare different doses and dosing regimens of VEGF Trap-Eye with laser photocoagulation in eyes with DME.

Description

DA VINCI was a randomized, double-masked, multicenter, phase 2 clinical trial that included diabetic patients ($n = 221$) with center-involved DME that were enrolled from December, 2008. Participants were assigned randomly to one of five treatment regimens: (1) VEGF Trap-Eye 0.5 mg every 4 weeks (0.5q4), (2) 2 mg every 4 weeks (2q4), (3) 2 mg every 8 weeks after three initial monthly doses (2q8), (4) 2 mg dosing as needed after three initial monthly doses (2PRN), or (5) macular laser photocoagulation. Assessments were completed at baseline and every 4 weeks thereafter.

Inclusion Criteria
Adults 18 years or older with type 1 or 2 diabetes mellitus with clinically significant DME with central involvement and ETDRS BCVA 20/40 to 20/320 (letter score of 73–24) in the study eye were eligible.

Study Measures
These included the change in BCVA at 24 weeks (the primary endpoint) and at 52 weeks, proportion of eyes that gained 15 letters or more in ETDRS BCVA, and mean changes in CRT from baseline.

Results
- Mean improvements in BCVA in the VEGF Trap-Eye groups at week 24 were 8.6, 11.4, 8.5, and 10.3 letters for 0.5q4, 2q4, 2q8, and 2PRN regimens, respectively, versus 2.5 letters for the laser group ($p \leq 0.0085$ vs. laser). Gains from baseline of 0+, 10+, and 15+ letters were seen in up to 93%, 64%, and 34% of VEGF Trap-Eye groups versus up to 68%, 32%, and 21% in the laser group, respectively.
- Mean improvements in BCVA in the VEGF Trap-Eye groups at week 52 were 11.0, 13.1, 9.7, and 12.0 letters for 0.5q4, 2q4, 2q8, and 2PRN regimens, respectively, versus –1.3 letters for the laser group ($p \leq 0.0001$ vs. laser).
- Proportions of eyes with gains in BCVA of 15 or more ETDRS letters at week 52 in the VEGF Trap-Eye groups were 40.9%, 45.5%, 23.8%, and 42.2% versus 11.4% for laser ($p = 0.0031$, 0.0007, 0.1608, and 0.0016, respectively, vs. laser).
- Mean reductions in CRT in the four VEGF Trap-Eye groups at week 24 ranged from –127.3 to –194.5 μm compared with only –67.9 μm in the laser group ($p = 0.0066$ for each VEGF Trap-Eye group vs. laser).
- Mean reductions in CRT in the VEGF Trap-Eye groups at week 52 were –165.4, –227.4, –187.8, and –180.3 μm versus –58.4 μm for laser ($p < 0.0001$ vs. laser).
- VEGF Trap-Eye generally was well-tolerated. The most frequent ocular adverse events with VEGF Trap-Eye were conjunctival hemorrhage, eye pain, ocular hyperemia, and increased IOP, whereas common systemic adverse events included hypertension, nausea, and congestive heart failure.

Conclusion
Intravitreal VEGF Trap-Eye produced a statistically significant and clinically relevant improvement in visual acuity when compared with macular laser

photocoagulation in patients with DME. Significant gains in BCVA from baseline achieved at week 24 were maintained or improved at week 52 in all VEGF Trap-Eye groups. VEGF Trap-Eye warrants further investigation for the treatment of DME.

VEGF TRAP-EYE IN VISION IMPAIRMENT DUE TO DME (VISTA DME)[12]

Purpose
To determine the efficacy of intravitreally administered VEGF Trap-Eye on BCVA assessed by the ETDRS chart in patients with DME with central involvement.

Description
VISTA DME was a double-masked, randomized, active-controlled, phase 3 study that enrolled 872 eyes. In the first arm, patients were treated every month with 2 mg of VEGF Trap-Eye (2q4 group). In the second arm, patients were treated with 2 mg of VEGF Trap-Eye every 2 months after a loading phase of monthly injections (2q8 group). In the third arm, the comparator arm, patients were treated with macular laser photocoagulation. All patients were followed for 3 years.

Inclusion Criteria
Adults ≥ 18 years of age with type 1 or 2 diabetes mellitus with decrease in vision determined to be primarily the result of DME in the study eye and BCVA ETDRS letter score of 73–24 (20/40 to 20/320) in the study eye are eligible.

Study Measures
The primary endpoint was the mean change in visual acuity from baseline as measured by the ETDRS chart at 52 weeks. Secondary outcomes included number of eyes that gained ≥15 letters on ETDRS chart and mean change from baseline CRT.

Results
At 52 weeks
- The mean change in visual acuity from baseline was +12.5, +10.7 and +0.2 in 2q4, 2q8, and laser groups, respectively.
- The mean change in CRT was −185.9, −183.1, and −73.3 in 2q4, 2q8, and laser groups, respectively.
- There was no significant difference in the safety profile of the three groups.

At 100 and 148 weeks
Visual improvement seen at 52 weeks was maintained at 100 and 148 weeks' follow-up results.

Conclusion
Intravitreal AFB shows significantly better anatomical and functional outcomes than laser in patients with center-involving DME with a good safety profile.

FLUOCINOLONE ACETONIDE IN DIABETIC MACULAR EDEMA (FAME)[13,14]

Purpose
To assess the efficacy and safety of intravitreal inserts releasing 0.2 µg/day (low dose) or 0.5 µg/day (high dose) FA in patients with DME.

Description
FAME consisted of two parallel, prospective, randomized, sham injection-controlled, double-masked, multicenter clinical trials conducted in 2011. Subjects with persistent DME despite at least one macular laser treatment were randomized 1:2:2 to sham injection ($n = 185$), low-dose insert ($n = 375$), or high-dose insert ($n = 393$), respectively. Subjects who received study drug or sham injection at baseline and after 6 weeks were eligible for rescue laser. Based on retreatment criteria, additional study drug or sham injections could be given after 1 year.

Study Measures
The primary outcome was the percentage of patients with improvement from baseline BCVA in ETDRS letter score of 15 or more. Secondary outcomes included other parameters of visual function and FTH.

Results
- At month 36, the percentage of patients who gained ≥15 in letter score using the last observation carried forward method was 28.7% (low dose) and 27.8% (high dose) in the FA insert groups compared with 18.9% ($p = 0.018$) in the sham group, and considering only those patients still in the trial at month 36, it was 33.0% (low dose) and 31.9% (high dose) compared with 21.4% in the sham group ($p = 0.030$). Preplanned subgroup analysis demonstrated a doubling of benefit compared with sham injections in patients who reported duration of DME ≥ 3 years at baseline; the percentage who gained ≥15 in letter score at month 36 was 34.0% (low dose; $p < 0.001$) or 28.8% (high dose; $p = 0.002$) compared with

13.4% (sham). An improvement ≥2 steps in the ETDRS retinopathy scale occurred in 13.7% (low dose) and 10.1% (high dose) compared with 8.9% in the sham group.
- At all time points compared with sham, there was significantly more improvement in FTH.
- Almost all phakic patients in the FA insert groups developed cataract, but their visual benefit after cataract surgery was similar to that in pseudophakic patients. The incidence of incisional glaucoma surgery at month 36 was 4.8% in the low-dose group and 8.1% in the high-dose insert group.

Conclusion

Both low- and high-dose FA inserts significantly improved BCVA in patients with DME over 2 years, and the risk-to-benefit ratio was superior for the low-dose insert. This is the first pharmacologic treatment that can be administered by an outpatient injection to provide substantial benefit in patients with DME for at least 2 years. In patients with DME, FA inserts provide substantial visual benefit for up to 3 years and would provide a valuable addition to the options available for patients with DME.

The FDA denied the approval of Alimera's Iluvien fluocinolone insert in November, 2011, citing issues with the risks of adverse reactions, including IOP increases and cataract that were manifest during the 36-month FAME study. The insert, which is designed to deliver drug for up to 3 years, is approved in several European countries.

THREE-YEAR, RANDOMIZED, SHAM-CONTROLLED TRIAL OF DEXAMETHASONE INTRAVITREAL IMPLANT IN PATIENTS WITH DIABETIC MACULAR EDEMA (MEAD STUDY)[15]

Purpose

To evaluate the safety and efficacy of intravitreal dexamethasone implant (OZURDEX—0.35 and 0.7 mg) in treatment of DME.

Background

RISE and RIDE studies paved way for monthly intravitreal RBZ injection for treatment of DME. However, after 2 years of monthly RBZ injections macular edema persisted in nearly 23%, and nearly 40% patients could not achieve BCVA ≥ 20/40 suggesting the need to explore alternatives. Protocol I of DRCR.net reported similar efficacy of intravitreal triamcinolone acetonide or RBZ when used in combination with laser in pseudophakic eyes with DME.

Description

MEAD study comprised of two multicenter phase III randomized controlled trials (2005–2012) including 1,048 patients with previously treated or treatment-naive DME with BCVA between 20/50 and 20/200 and CRT >300 μm on OCT. Patients were randomly assigned to receive 0.7 mg (351 patients), 0.35 mg implant (347 patients), or sham treatment (350 patients). They were followed up for a period of 3 years. Retreatment could be offered after 6 months of any intravitreal injection of implant.

Study Measures

The primary outcome was the number of patients who had greater than 15-letter improvement in visual acuity from baseline at the end of 3 years. The secondary outcome was reduction in mean CRT. Safety parameters such as adverse events and IOP were measured.

Results

- The mean duration of DME before study was 24.9 months. The average number of treatments was 4.1, 4.4, and 3.3 in 0.7-mg, 0.35-mg, and sham group, respectively.
- The percentage of patients having greater than 15-letter improvement at the end of 3 years from baseline was 22.2% in the 0.7-mg implant group, 18.4% in the 0.35-mg implant group, and 12% in the sham group. Patients in both implant groups gained 15-letter improvement significantly earlier than the sham group.
- The mean change in BCVA was 3.5, 3.6, and 2 letters with 0.7 mg, 0.35 mg, and sham groups, respectively, which was significantly greater in both implant groups compared to the sham group.
- The mean reduction in CRT from baseline was –111.6 μm in the 0.7-mg implant group, –107.9 μm in the 0.35-mg implant group, and –41.9 μm in the sham group ($p < 0.001$).
- The rates of cataract-related adverse events in phakic eyes were 67.9% in the 0.7-mg implant group, 64.1 % in the 0.35-mg implant group, and 20.4% in the sham group.
- After cataract surgery, there was no increase in CRT in both dexamethasone implant groups as opposed to sham group which shows protective effect of dexamethasone.
- The percentage of patients with >10 mm Hg increase in IOP was 27.75% in the 0.7-mg implant group, 24.8% in the 0.35-mg implant group, and 3.7% in the sham group. In most patients, IOP was controlled with medication alone. Two patients (one in each dexamethasone implant group) had to undergo trabeculectomy.

- Vitreous hemorrhage was observed in 6.9% in the 0.7-mg implant group, 13.1% in the 0.35-mg implant group, and 7.1% in the sham group which resolved without intervention.

Conclusion

Both dexamethasone implants met the primary efficacy endpoint with an acceptable safety profile.

A RANDOMIZED CLINICAL TRIAL OF INTRAVITREAL BEVACIZUMAB VERSUS INTRAVITREAL DEXAMETHASONE FOR DIABETIC MACULAR EDEMA: THE BEVORDEX STUDY[16]

Purpose

To compare the efficacy of IVB versus intravitreal dexamethasone implant (OZURDEX) in treatment of DME.

Description

The BEVORDEX study was a phase II, prospective, single-masked clinical trial. 88 eyes of 61 patients with center-involving macular edema with BCVA of 20/40 to 20/400 were included in the study (2010–2012). Eyes were included at least 3 months after at least 1 session of laser treatment or treatment-naive eyes where the investigator deemed that laser was unlikely to be beneficial. 42 eyes received 4 weekly IVB injections on PRN basis. 46 eyes received intravitreal dexamethasone implant at 16-week intervals on PRN basis.

Study Measures

The primary outcome was to evaluate the number of eyes that had greater than 10-letter improvement over baseline visual acuity (logMAR scale). The secondary outcomes included mean change in BCVA, central macular thickness, adverse events, and injection frequency. The impact on vision impairment (IVI) questionnaire was used to assess patient-reported outcomes.

Results

At the end of 1 year
- A primary outcome of greater than 10-letter improvement in logMAR visual acuity scale was obtained in 17 out of 42 eyes (40%) in the bevacizumab group and 19 out of 46 eyes (41%) in the dexamethasone implant group.
- Five eyes in the dexamethasone implant group had greater than 10-letter decrease in visual acuity which was attributed to cataract formation. No eye in the bevacizumab group had this outcome.

- The mean reduction in central macular thickness was 122 μm in the bevacizumab group and 187 μm in the dexamethasone implant group ($p = 0.015$).
- The mean number of injections received was 8.6 in the bevacizumab group and 2.7 in the dexamethasone implant group.
- Significant improvement was seen in IVI scores in both groups.

At the end of 2 years
- 20 out of 46 eyes (43%) in the dexamethasone implant group and 19 out of 42 eyes (45%) maintained greater than 10 letter improvement in visual acuity over a period of 2 years.
- The mean visual acuity improved by 6.9 letters in the dexamethasone implant group and 9.6 letters in the RBZ group. In pseudophakic eyes, improvement in visual gain was comparable and less visual gain in the dexamethasone group was attributed to cataract formation.
- The difference in the number of injections required to maintain visual gain significantly decreased over 2 years with the mean number of dexamethasone implant injections being 2.2 and bevacizumab injections being 4.8.

Conclusion

The visual acuity outcome was comparable in both groups with the dexamethasone group achieving better anatomical outcomes with fewer injections. Both treatments were associated with improvement in quality of life.

DEXAMETHASONE IMPLANT FOR DIABETIC MACULAR EDEMA IN NAIVE COMPARED WITH REFRACTORY EYES: THE INTERNATIONAL RETINA GROUP REAL-LIFE 24-MONTH MULTICENTER STUDY. THE IRGREL-DEX STUDY[17]

Purpose

A real-life study for safety and efficacy of repeated dexamethasone implants over 2 years in treatment naive eyes with DME compared to DME eyes refractory to anti-VEGF treatment.

Background

Evidence suggests that the Müller cells may be the first to be affected in DME, showing intracellular edema. Activated Müller cells may cause breakdown of blood retinal barrier, leukocyte recruitment, glial dysfunction, and neuronal cell death. Early treatment with DEX implant is targeted at halting this inflammatory process and preventing irreversible retinal glial cell changes.

Description

This international retrospective multicenter study comprised of 10 study sites and enrolled patients (2011–2017) with DME (naive and refractory) with type 1 or 2 diabetes mellitus with BCVA of 20/32 to 20/200. Refractory DME was defined as worsening of BCVA by 2 ETDRS lines or reduction of <10% of retinal thickness on spectral-domain OCT measured 1 month after at least three anti-VEGF injections that were given at monthly intervals.

Study Measures

BCVA and CST after the first DEX implant were the main outcome measures. For safety data, IOP rise and need for cataract surgery were recorded.

Result

- 130 eyes of 125 patients were included. BCVA and CFT at baseline were similar for naive ($n = 71$) and refractory eyes ($n = 59$). The mean number of previous anti-VEGF injections in the refractory group was 7.4 ± 3.6, and 68% of the refractory cases had 10% reduction in CMT.
- A history of macular laser was present in the naive (6 eyes) and refractory groups (13 eyes) ($p = 0.05$).
- The mean number of DEX implants received over 24 months was 3.5 ± 1.0 (range: 1-4). Only 1% (1/71) of naive eyes received additional treatments during the study period. 25% (15/59) of refractory cases needed further treatment ($p = 0.003$).
- Both groups had significant improvement in vision after 24 months ($p < 0.001$). However, treatment-naive eyes were more likely to gain ≥10 letters and gained significantly more vision than refractory eyes (+11.3 ± 10.0 vs. 7.3 ± 2.7 letters, $p = 0.01$).
- At 6, 12, and 24 months, CST was significantly decreased compared with baseline in both naive and refractory eyes; however, CST was higher in refractory eyes than in naive eyes (CST 279 ± 61 vs. 313 ± 125 μm, $p = 0.10$).
- Of all the phakic patients at baseline, 22 (57.9%) underwent cataract surgery. Nine patients underwent cataract surgery within the first year and 13 within the second year of follow-up. 14% of the studied eyes required topical IOP-lowering treatment after 24 months.

Conclusion

Dexamethasone implants improved vision in DME both in eyes that were treatment naive and in eyes refractory to anti-VEGF treatment; however, improvement was greater in naive eyes.

KESTREL, KITE, and KINGFISHER are phase III clinical trials underway comparing brolucizumab with AFB in patients with DME.

Table 1: Summary of clinical trials on pharmacotherapy in diabetic macular edema.

Title	Purpose	No. of patients	Inclusion criteria	Outcome measure	Result/conclusion
READ-2 (2006)	Compare RBZ with focal/grid laser or combination of both in DME	126	DME with CFT ≥ 250 µm, VA ≤ 20/40 but ≥20/320	Change from baseline in BCVA	• At 6 months, RBZ injections had a better visual outcome than focal/grid laser. • RBZ provided benefit in DME for at least 2 years, and when combined with focal/grid laser, the amount of residual edema was reduced, as were the frequency of injections needed.
RIDE and RISE (2007)	Efficacy and safety of intravitreal RBZ in DME patients	759 (377+382)	Adults with DME with CFT ≥ 275 µm, BCVA of 20/320 to 20/40, and HbA1c ≤ 12%	Proportion of patients who gained ≥15 ETDRS at 24 months, mean change from baseline in BCVA and CFT	RBZ rapidly and sustainably improved vision, reduced the risk of further vision loss, and improved macular edema in patients with DME, with low rates of ocular and nonocular harm.
RESOLVE (2005)	Safety and efficacy of RBZ in DME involving the foveal center	151	Adults, type 1 or 2 diabetes, CFT ≥ 300 µm, and BCVA of 73–39 ETDRS letters	Efficacy in terms of BCVA and CFT and safety at 12 months	RBZ is effective in improving BCVA and is well tolerated in DME.
RESTORE (2008)	Superiority of RBZ 0.5 mg monotherapy or combined with laser over laser alone in DME	345	Adults, type 1 or 2 DM, and visual impairment due to DME	Mean average change in BCVA from baseline to months 1 through 12	RBZ monotherapy and combined with laser provided superior visual acuity over laser in patients with DME.
BOLT (2007)	Bevacizumab versus MLT in CSME	80	Patients with center-involving CSME, at least one prior MLT, BCVA 20/40 to 20/320	Difference in BCVA at 12 months between the bevacizumab and laser arms	The study supports the use of bevacizumab in patients with center-involving CSME without advanced macular ischemia.

Contd...

Title	Purpose	No. of patients	Inclusion criteria	Outcome measure	Result/conclusion
DA VINCI (2008)	VEGF Trap-Eye versus laser in DME	221	Adults >18 years, CSME with central involvement, BCVA 20/40 to 20/320	Change in BCVA at 24 and 52 weeks	VEGF Trap-Eye produced a statistically significant and clinically relevant improvement in BCVA compared with macular laser in DME at 24 and 52 weeks
VISTA DME (2011)	Efficacy of VEGF Trap-Eye on BCVA in DME with central involvement	466	Adults > 18 years, DME, and BCVA 20/40 to 20/320	Mean change in visual acuity from baseline (ETDRS)	VEGF Trap-Eye produced a statistically significant and clinically relevant improvement in BCVA compared with macular laser in DME at 52, 100, and 148 weeks. Results favored 2 monthly dosages of aflibercept due to similar efficacy of monthly and 2 monthly dosages.
FAME (2011)	Low-dose and high-dose fluocinolone acetonide implant (FA) in DME	953	Persistent DME despite at least one macular laser treatment	Percentage of patients with improvement from baseline BCVA in ETDRS letter score of ≥15 at 36 months	• FA inserts improved BCVA over 2 years, and the risk-to-benefit ratio was superior for the low-dose insert. • Almost all phakic patients in the FA groups developed cataract. • The incidence of incisional glaucoma surgery at month 36 was 4.8% in the low-dose group and 8.1% in the high-dose insert group.
MEAD	Safety and efficacy of dexamethasone implant versus sham in treatment of DME	1,048 eyes	Eyes with DME with visual acuity between 20/50 and 20/200 and CRT ≥ 300 μm	Number of patients with ≥15-letter improvement from baseline VA	Eyes that received dexamethasone implant had better VA and greater reduction in CRT over a period of 3 years.

Contd...

Title	Purpose	No. of patients	Inclusion criteria	Outcome measure	Result/conclusion
Bevodex study	Bevacizumab vs dexamethasone implant in treatment of DME	88 eyes of 61 patients	Eyes with center-involving DME	Number of patients with ≥10-letter improvement	Visual acuity outcome was comparable in both groups with dexamethasone group achieving better anatomical outcomes with fewer injections.
The IRGREL-DEX Study	Dexamethasone implant for DME in naive compared with refractory eyes	130 eyes	• Treatment-naive center-involving DME • DME refractory to 3 monthly intravitreal anti-VEGF injection	BCVA and central subfield thickness	• Naive eyes were more likely to gain ≥10 letters and gained significantly more vision than refractory eyes at 24 months. • At 6, 12, and 24 months, CST was significantly decreased compared with baseline in both naive and refractory eyes; however, CST was higher in refractory eyes than in naive eyes.

(BCVA: best corrected visual acuity; CFT: central foveal thickness; CRT: central retinal thickness; CSME: clinically significant macular edema; DM: diabetes mellitus; DME: diabetic macular edema; ETDRS: Early Treatment Diabetic Retinopathy Study; HbA1c: glycated hemoglobin; MLT: macular laser therapy; RBZ: ranibizumab; VA: visual acuity)

REFERENCES

1. READ-2 Study Group; Nguyen QD, Shah SM, Heier JS, Do DV, Lim J, et al. Primary End Point (Six Months) Results of the Ranibizumab for Edema of the mAcula in diabetes (READ-2) study. Ophthalmology 2009; 116: 2175-81.e1.
2. READ-2 Study Group; Nguyen QD, Shah SM, Khwaja AA, Channa R, Hatef E, et al.. Two-year outcomes of the ranibizumab for edema of the mAcula in diabetes (READ-2) study. Ophthalmology. 2010;117:2146-51.
3. READ-2 Study Group; Do DV, Nguyen QD, Khwaja AA, Channa R, Sepah YJ, et al. Ranibizumab for edema of the macula in diabetes study: 3-year outcomes and the need for prolonged frequent treatment. Arch Ophthalmol. 2012;8:1-7.
4. Genetech. Two pivotal Phase III Lucentis studies showed patients with diabetic macular edema experienced significant improvements in vision and fewer developed more advanced retinopathy. https://www.roche.com/investors/updates/inv-update-2011-06-29.htm.
5. RISE and RIDE Research Group; Nguyen QD, Brown DM, Marcus DM, Boyer DS, Patel S, et al. Ranibizumab for DME: Results from 2 phase III randomized trials: RISE and RIDE. Ophthalmology. 2012;119:789-801.
6. Massin P, Bandello F, Garweg J, Hansen LL, Harding SP, Larsen M, et al. Safety and efficacy of ranibizumab in diabetic macular edema (RESOLVE study): a 12-month, randomized, controlled, double masked, multicenter phase II study. Diabetes Care. 2010;33:2399-405.
7. RESTORE study group; Mitchell P, Bandello F, Schmidt-Erfurth U, Lang GE, Massin P. The RESTORE study: ranibizumab monotherapy or combined with laser versus laser monotherapy for diabetic macular edema. Ophthalmology. 2011;118:615-25.
8. Michaelides M, Kaines A, Hamilton RD, Fraser-Bell S, Rajendram R, Quhill F, et al. A prospective randomized trial of intravitreal bevacizumab or laser therapy in the management of diabetic macular edema (BOLT study) 12-month data: report 2. Ophthalmology. 2010;117:1078-86.e2.
9. Rajendram R, Fraser-Bell S, Kaines A, Michaelides M, Hamilton RD, Esposti SD, et al. A 2-year prospective randomized controlled trial of intravitreal bevacizumab or laser therapy (BOLT) in the management of diabetic macular edema: 24-month data: report 3. Arch Ophthalmol. 2012;130:972-9.
10. Do DV, Schmidt-Erfurth U, Gonzalez VH, Gordon CM, Tolentino M, Berliner AJ, et al. The DA VINCI Study: phase 2 primary results of VEGF Trap-Eye in patients with diabetic macular edema. Ophthalmology. 2011;118:1819-26.
11. da Vinci Study Group; Do DV, Nguyen QD, Boyer D, Schmidt-Erfurth U, Brown DM, et al. One-year outcomes of the DA VINCI Study of VEGF Trap-Eye in eyes with diabetic macular edema. Ophthalmology. 2012;119:1658-65.
12. Heier JS, Korobelnik J-F, Brown DM, Schmidt-Erfurth U, Do DV, Midena E, et al. Intravitreal aflibercept for diabetic macular edema: 148-week results from the VISTA and VIVID studies. Ophthalmology. 2016;123(11):2376-85.
13. FAME Study Group; Campochiaro PA, Brown DM, Pearson A, Ciulla T, Boyer D, et al. Long-term benefit of sustained-delivery fluocinolone acetonide vitreous inserts for diabetic macular edema. Ophthalmology. 2011;118:626-35.
14. FAME Study Group; Campochiaro PA, Brown DM, Pearson A, Chen S, Boyer D, et al. Sustained delivery fluocinolone acetonide vitreous inserts provide benefit for at least 3 years in patients with diabetic macular edema. Ophthalmology. 2012;119:2125-32.
15. Boyer DS, Yoon YH, Belfort R, Bandello F, Maturi RK, Augustin AJ, et al. Three-year, randomized, sham-controlled trial of dexamethasone intravitreal implant in patients with diabetic macular edema. Ophthalmology. 2014;121(10):1904-14.
16. Gillies MC, Lim LL, Campain A, Quin GJ, Salem W, Li J, et al. A randomized clinical trial of intravitreal bevacizumab versus intravitreal dexamethasone for diabetic macular edema: the BEVORDEX study. Ophthalmology. 2014;121(12):2473-81.
17. Iglicki M, Busch C, Zur D, Okada M, Mariussi M, Chhablani JK, et al. Dexamethasone implant for diabetic macular edema in naive compared with refractory eyes: The International Retina Group real-life 24-month multicenter study. The IRGREL-DEX study. Retina. 2019;39(1):44-51.

Clinical Trials in Retinal Vascular Occlusions

Neha Goel, Pooja Shah, Vinod Kumar

■ INTRODUCTION

Retinal vein occlusion (RVO) is the second most common retinal vascular disease after diabetic retinopathy. Macular edema leads to vision loss in many patients with either central or branch retinal vein occlusions (CRVO or BRVO). BRVO is the more common of the two presentations, accounting for approximately 80% of RVO.

■ BRANCH VEIN OCCLUSION STUDY (BVOS)[1,2]

Purpose

1. To determine whether scatter argon laser photocoagulation can prevent the development of neovascularization.
2. To determine whether peripheral scatter argon laser photocoagulation can prevent vitreous hemorrhage.
3. To determine whether macular argon laser photocoagulation can improve visual acuity in eyes with macular edema reducing vision to 20/40 or worse.

Background

Many treatments for BRVO were attempted before 1977, but none was proven to be effective. The only treatment that seemed at all promising in preventing visual loss from BRVO was laser photocoagulation.

Description

The BVOS was a multicenter, prospective, randomized, controlled clinical trial supported by the National Eye Institute. Patients seen in six clinics with signs of BRVO were considered for the study. Patient eligibility criteria were as follows:
- *Group I (Eyes at risk for the development of neovascularization)*
  - BRVO occurring 3–18 months earlier (unless entered in group III)
  - An area of 5 disc diameters in diameter of retinal involvement

- Sufficient clearing of intraretinal hemorrhage to permit safe laser photocoagulation.
- *Group II (Eyes at risk for the development of vitreous hemorrhage)*
  - BRVO occurring 3–18 months earlier (unless entered in group I, X, and/or III)
  - Documented disc and/or peripheral retinal neovascularization
  - Sufficient clearing of intraretinal hemorrhage to permit safe laser photocoagulation.
- *Group X (Eyes at high-risk for the development of neovascularization)*
  - BRVO occurring 3–18 months earlier
  - An area of 5 disc diameters in diameter of retinal involvement.
- *Group III (Eyes at risk for vision loss from macular edema)*
  - BRVO occurring 3–18 months earlier
  - Associated macular edema reducing visual acuity to 20/40 or worse.

Approximately 500 patients were enrolled in the study. One-half were randomly assigned to treatment with argon laser photocoagulation; the other one-half remained untreated as controls.

- 319 eyes of 319 patients with BRVO and no retinal neovascularization (group I) and 81 eyes of 81 patients with BRVO and retinal neovascularization (group II) were randomly assigned to *"scatter" laser photocoagulation* or no laser treatment. Scatter treatment of 100–400 laser burns was applied in the drainage area of the occluded vein site 1 burn-width apart, avoiding the fovea (extending no closer than 2 disc diameters from the center of the fovea) and optic disc. Individual laser burns were 200–500 µm in diameter with an exposure time of 0.1–0.2 seconds. The power setting was sufficient to cause a medium-intensity white burn. When performing scatter laser photocoagulation, the following precautions were taken: treatment over the collaterals was not performed, treatment over the retinal hemorrhages was avoided, and treatment was performed at least up to the equator. The patients were followed up to answer questions 1 and 2.
- Recruitment of group X eyes only begun after the minimal sample size required for group I had been reached and so further recruitment terminated. Patients in group X were recruited to maintain a pool of cases that would have a high-risk of developing neovascularization and therefore became eligible for group II. Group X patients were also followed up for *natural history information*.
- 139 eyes of 139 patients with BRVO and macular edema (group III) were randomized either to a *"grid" pattern of photocoagulation* within the involved macular region or to no laser treatment. A fluorescein angiogram < 1 month old had to have been available for each patient. Treatment was performed under topical anesthesia using the argon laser to achieve a grid pattern over the area of capillary leakage identified by fluorescein in the macular region. Burns of 50–100 µm in diameter with an exposure time of 0.05–0.1 seconds were used. Photocoagulation was extended no

closer to the fovea than the edge of the foveal avascular zone and did not extend peripherally beyond the major vascular arcade. Treatment in the papillomacular bundle was not prohibited in the protocol. Repeat treatments were performed as necessary. The information was used to answer question 3.

Inclusion Criteria

Patients with three types of diagnoses were accepted:
1. Major BRVO without neovascularization
2. Major BRVO with neovascularization
3. BRVO with macular edema and reduced vision

All patients must have had onset of signs and/or symptoms of BRVO < 18 months before the initial visit, vision of 5/200 or better, and sufficient clarity of the ocular media to permit confirmation of the condition with fundus photography.

Study Measures

The efficacy of treatment was judged on the basis of visual acuity measurements as well as assessment of the subsequent development of neovascularization and/or vitreous hemorrhage. Stereoscopic color fundus photographs and fundus fluorescein angiograms were evaluated. Patients were followed up for at least 3 years.

The primary outcome in group III was the percentage of patients gaining at least two lines of Snellen acuity from baseline and maintaining this improvement for two consecutive visits.

Results

- In group I, comparing the treated patients with control patients (average follow-up time of 3.74 years), the development of neovascularization was significantly less in laser-treated eyes ($p = 0.009$).
- In group II, it was observed after an average follow-up time of 2.8 years that the development of vitreous hemorrhage was significantly less in treated eyes ($p = 0.005$). Although BVOS was not designed to assess whether peripheral scatter laser photocoagulation should be performed before rather than after the development of neovascularization, it was observed in this study that scatter laser photocoagulation was equally effective after the development of retinal neovascularization as it was before.
- In group III, the average follow-up time was 3.1 years. Comparing the treated patients to control patients in this group, the gain of at least two lines of visual acuity from baseline maintained for two consecutive visits was significantly greater in treated eyes ($p < 0.005$). 63% of the patients in the treated group gained two or more lines of visual acuity (control 36%).

- In this study, it was observed in the natural history of BRVO that 40% of the patients with >5 disc diameters of retinal capillary nonperfusion were at risk of developing retinal neovascularization whereas 60% of these patients will experience vitreous hemorrhage.

Conclusion

- Peripheral scatter argon laser photocoagulation could prevent the development of both neovascularization and vitreous hemorrhage to a significant degree. Peripheral scatter treatment should be applied after, rather than before, the development of neovascularization. The study group recommended laser photocoagulation for patients with BRVO who have developed neovascularization and who meet the eligibility criteria.
- Argon laser photocoagulation improved the visual outcome to a significant degree in eyes with BRVO and visual acuity reduced from macular edema to 6/12 or worse. The study group recommended laser photocoagulation for a patient with macular edema associated with BRVO who meet the eligibility criteria.

CENTRAL VEIN OCCLUSION STUDY (CVOS)[3-7]

Purpose

1. To determine whether early panretinal photocoagulation (PRP) therapy can help prevent iris neovascularization (INV) in eyes with ischemic CRVO.
2. To assess whether grid-pattern photocoagulation therapy will reduce loss of central visual acuity due to macular edema secondary to CRVO.
3. To describe the natural history of eyes with CRVO that have little or no evidence of ischemia (less than 10 disc areas of nonperfusion).
4. To assess whether early PRP is more effective than PRP at the first identification of INV in preventing further ocular morbidity due to progressive neovascular glaucoma in eyes with ischemic CRVO.

Background

Central retinal vein occlusion is a common retinal vascular disorder with potentially blinding complications. The two major complications are reduced central vision caused by macular edema and neovascular glaucoma caused by INV.

Other clinical trials have shown that laser photocoagulation is an effective treatment for complications in diabetic retinopathy and BRVO, which have some features in common with CRVO: neovascularization and reduced visual acuity caused by macular edema occur in all three disorders. Evidence from small-scale studies suggests that a grid pattern of photocoagulation reduces macular edema in CRVO patients, although the associated changes in visual acuity are variable. The CVOS is a detailed investigation of grid pattern photocoagulation in a larger, randomized group of patients.

Description

The CVOS was a multicenter, prospective, randomized, controlled clinical trial supported by the National Eye Institute. 728 eyes of 725 patients seen in nine clinics with signs of CRVO were considered for the study. They were divided into four study groups on the basis of the perfusion status of the retina and the presence of decreased vision associated with macular edema.

Group N

- Duration of CRVO < 1 year
- Intraretinal hemorrhages in all four quadrants
- At least 10 disc areas of retinal nonperfusion
- Study eye iris and angle free of any neovascularization.

181 eyes of 180 patients were included in this group. Eyes were randomly assigned to receive PRP or nontreatment unless INV developed.

Group P

- Duration of CRVO < 1 year
- Intraretinal hemorrhages in all four quadrants
- Retinal nonperfusion, if any, <10 disc areas
- Study eye iris and angle free of any neovascularization.

547 eyes of 546 patients were included in this group. Eyes were followed to provide information about the natural history of the disease. Eyes were entered into group I or N and closed out of group P if sufficiently increased retinal hemorrhage and/or retinal capillary nonperfusion occurred and the eye met the eligibility criteria of the new group.

Group I

- Duration of CRVO < 1 year
- Retinal hemorrhages that prevent measurement of retinal capillary nonperfusion
- Study eye iris and angle free of any neovascularization.

52 eyes of 52 patients were included in this group. Eyes were followed in a natural history study.

Group M

- Duration of CRVO > 3 months
- Macular edema involving fovea

- Visual acuity between 5/200 and 20/50 without any explanation for decreased visual acuity other than CRVO
- Phakic with clear media
- No improvement in visual acuity on consecutive visits.

155 eyes of 155 patients were included in this group. Eyes were randomly assigned to receive grid-pattern photocoagulation or nontreatment.

- Random treatment assignments in groups N and M were made using computer-generated random allocation. Group N eyes were stratified by clinic and group M eyes by both clinic and duration of the CRVO (<1 year or ≥ 1 year).
- Both eyes of the patient could be considered for the study only if they were eligible simultaneously. If both eyes of the patient were eligible for a randomized group, one eye was randomly assigned to PRP treatment and the other to observation. On the assumption that the need to evaluate grid-pattern treatment for macular edema is independent of the treatment status of the periphery of the eye, the protocol allowed eyes in other CVOS groups to be entered into group M as well.
- A green argon laser with a slit-lamp delivery system was used for all treatments. PRP treatment was evenly spaced to or beyond the equator in all quadrants, no closer than 2 disc diameters from the center of the fovea and no closer than 500 μm nasal to the disc. Laser spots were spaced 1/2 to 1 burn-width apart. The grid pattern of laser photocoagulation covered all of the areas of leaking capillaries within 2 disc diameters of the center of the fovea, could not extend beyond 2 disc diameters from the fovea, and could not extend within the foveal avascular zone. Treatment avoided collateral vessels and retinal hemorrhages. 100-μm spots for 0.1 second, to produce medium white burn, with a spacing of about 1/2 to 1 burn-width apart were used.

Inclusion Criteria

Men and women of age 21 years or older and willing to return for follow-up visits for 3 years following assignment into the appropriate group and randomization were included in the study. Each of the four groups had specific eligibility criteria as described above.

In addition, all patients must have visual acuity of light perception or better, intraocular pressure (IOP) <30 mm Hg and sufficient clarity of the ocular media to permit confirmation of the condition with fundus photography and fluorescein angiography. Patients with retinal vascular disease other than that specified in the criteria, such as diabetic retinopathy, BRVO, previous photocoagulation for retinal vascular disease, and vitreous hemorrhage other than breakthrough in the study eye, were ineligible. Patients with macular disease other than that due to CRVO were ineligible for that portion of the study.

Study Measures

Patients in the CVOS were followed up at regular intervals for 3 years. The frequency of follow-up visits varied according to the group to which the CRVO patient was assigned. Patients were initially followed up every 4 months in group P, every month for the first 6 months in group N, every month until the perfusion status of the eye could be determined in group I, and every 4 months in group M. In all these groups, any eye with 2 clock hours of iris new vessels (INV) and/or angle new vessels (ANV) was followed up monthly until the condition stabilized following retinal laser photocoagulation. *It was observed at the first 4 months' follow-up that 16% of the perfused CRVO eyes had developed INV and/or ANV. Therefore, it was decided by the study group to follow-up these patients more closely at 1-month interval at least for the first 6 months after the onset of CRVO.*

Color fundus photographs and fundus fluorescein angiography (FFA) were done at baseline, post-treatment, and at specified follow-up visits for a period of at least 3 years. Standard photographic views were employed. Color stereophotographs of fundus were taken every 4 months (study eye). Iris and color fundus photographs of both eyes and FFA were performed every 12 months. In group M patients, FFA was performed every 4 months and in group I patients, FFA was performed every 2 months. Slit-lamp examination, gonioscopy, and slit-lamp photography were also performed as per the manual of operations. A slit-lamp photograph of the iris with an undilated pupil (study eye) was taken on every visit in all groups.

Visual acuity, the primary outcome factor in the group with macular edema, was measured according to a modified Early Treatment Diabetic Retinopathy Study (ETDRS) protocol at each visit.

Results

- The median visual acuity was 20/63 in group P, 20/400 in group N, 20/400 in group I, and 20/125 in group M. In group M, the visual acuity was low by the design of the study because the patients with CRVO-induced macular edema and visual acuity > 20/50 were excluded from this group.
- 65 (9%) of 722 patients with one eye in study had a prior history of retinal vascular occlusion in fellow eye. Old BRVO was present in 17 eyes, old CRVO in 46 eyes, and old branch retinal artery occlusion (BRAO) in 2 eyes.
- *CVOS group N report*:[6] Four factors associated with the development of anterior segment neovascularization were identified: (1) extensive retinal capillary nonperfusion on fluorescein angiography, (2) large amounts of retinal hemorrhage, (3) short duration of CRVO, and (4) male sex. The strongest predictor of 2 clock hours of iris neovascularization or angle neovascularization (TC-INV/ANV) was the extent of nonperfusion. Eyes with <30 disc diameters of nonperfusion and no other risk factor were at low risk, whereas eyes with 75 disc diameters or more (i.e., eyes

that show virtually no intact capillaries in the posterior pole) are at the highest risk. Prophylactic PRP does not totally prevent TC-INV/ANV, and prompt regression of TC-INV/ANV in response to PRP is more likely to occur in eyes that have not been treated previously. The study group recommended careful observation with frequent follow-up examinations in the early months (including undilated slit-lamp examination of the iris and gonioscopy) and prompt PRP of eyes in which TC-INV/ANV develops.

- *Four-month natural history for eyes in group P:*[3] 16% eyes demonstrated at least 10 disc areas of nonperfusion and/or INV and/or ANV or were transferred to group I at or before the 4-month visit. 22% of these eyes showed INV and/or ANV and required PRP. Eyes with a duration of CRVO of <1 month, visual acuity < 20/200, and presence of 5–9 disc areas of nonperfusion were at a greater risk than eyes with a longer duration.

- *Complete natural history for eyes in group I:* 18% of the eyes developed INV and/or ANV in <1 month after study entry and 58% eyes were eligible for transfer or had developed INV and/or ANV by the 2-month visit. These findings confirm the importance of follow-up examinations in the management of all patients with recent onset of CRVO. Among the remaining patients, 8 of 52 eyes developed good perfusion and were transferred to group P, 22 of 52 eyes developed nonperfusion and were transferred to group N, 16 of 52 eyes developed INV and/or ANV, and in 6 of 52 eyes, the outcome not determined.

- *CVOS group M report:*[7] Macular grid laser photocoagulation had no effect on visual acuity either in patients with CRVO of recent onset (<1 year) or in occlusions of longer duration, during the follow-up period. The initial median visual acuity was 20/160 in treated eyes and 20/125 in control eyes. The final median visual acuity was 20/200 in treated eyes and 20/60 in control eyes. However, treatment clearly reduced the angiographic evidence of macular edema. The results of this study do not support a recommendation for macular grid photocoagulation for the population meeting the CVOS group eligibility criteria. The lack of benefit of macular grid laser photocoagulation in CRVO-induced macular edema is in contrast to its effectiveness in diabetic maculopathy and macular edema due to BRVO. The exact cause of this difference is not clear, but it is probable that diffuse capillary leakage involving the macular area and poor preexisting visual acuity were responsible for the poor outcomes of macular grid laser photocoagulation in CRVO.

Conclusion

- Patients with CRVO are recommended to have frequent follow-up examinations every 1 month for the first 6 months and less frequently thereafter with emphasis on undilated anterior segment examination for prompt detection of INV and/or ANV. Because ANV can rarely occur

even in the absence of INV, careful gonioscopy is important for all patients during follow-up without mydriasis.
- All eyes with CRVO must be evaluated for large areas of capillary nonperfusion.
- Eyes at particular risk are those with recent onset of symptoms (<1 month) and visual acuity worse than 6/60.
- Prophylactic PRP did not prevent the development of INV in eyes with 10 or more disc areas of retinal capillary nonperfusion confirmed by fluorescein angiography. Rather, results of this randomized clinical trial demonstrate that it is safe to wait for the development of early INV and then apply PRP.
- Identification of early INV at the pupillary border is crucial.
- After PRP, monthly follow-up with close scrutiny of the undilated pupil and angle to determine additional PRP or other treatment is required.
- Eyes with such extensive intraretinal hemorrhage that it is not possible to determine the retinal capillary perfusion status act as if they are ischemic or nonperfused.
- Macular grid photocoagulation was effective in reducing the angiographic evidence of macular edema but did not improve visual acuity in eyes with reduced vision due to macular edema from CRVO.

STANDARD CARE VERSUS CORTICOSTEROID FOR RETINAL VEIN OCCLUSION (SCORE) STUDY[8-12]

Purpose

To compare the effectiveness and safety of standard care to intravitreal injection(s) of triamcinolone acetonide for treating macular edema associated with CRVO and BRVO.

Background

Macular edema is a major cause of vision loss in patients with CRVO and BRVO. Currently, there is no effective treatment for macular edema associated with CRVO and standard care treatment is observation. Grid laser photocoagulation may be effective for some patients for macular edema associated with BRVO, but many patients derive limited benefit from this treatment. Therefore, the development of new treatment modalities for macular edema caused by these two conditions is an important research goal.

Over the last several years, many patients with macular edema from CRVO and BRVO have been treated with an intravitreal injection of triamcinolone (a type of steroid). Kenalog, a triamcinolone preparation commonly injected into the eye, is presently Food and Drug Administration (FDA) approved only for its use in muscles and joints. The SCORE study used a formulation of triamcinolone made specifically for the eye.

Description

The SCORE study was a multicenter, randomized, phase III trial conducted from 2004 to 2009 that enrolled 682 participants (271 CRVO participants and 411 BRVO participants). This study, conducted at 84 clinics across the USA, was sponsored by the National Eye Institute. For the purposes of the SCORE study, eyes with hemiretinal vein occlusion (HRVO) were treated as eyes with BRVO and analyzed with the BRVO group. A single eye from each CRVO or BRVO participant was randomized in a 1:1:1 ratio to one of three groups (treatment of neovascular complications as necessary in all three groups):

1. *Standard care group*: Conventional treatment consisting of:
   a. *CRVO*: Observation of macular edema
   b. *BRVO*:
      i. *Study eyes with dense macular hemorrhage*: Immediate observation. Grid laser photocoagulation will be performed if and when clearance of hemorrhage permits grid laser photocoagulation.
      ii. *Study eyes without dense macular hemorrhage*: Immediate grid laser photocoagulation
2. Intravitreal injection(s) of 4 mg of triamcinolone acetonide
3. Intravitreal injection(s) of 1 mg of triamcinolone acetonide

Repeat intravitreal injections of triamcinolone and repeat laser treatment was provided as clinically indicated based on protocol-specific guidelines based on visual acuity, clinical examination, and optical coherence tomography (OCT).

After randomization, participants were examined every 4 months through 3 years to collect ophthalmic information, including visual acuity, IOP, lens examination, OCT, ETDRS protocol 3- and 7-standard field stereoscopic fundus photography and ETDRS protocol fluorescein angiography. Visual acuity testing was done using electronic ETDRS (E-ETDRS) visual acuity testing at 3 m using the Electronic Visual Acuity Tester by a SCORE certified technician. A masked visual acuity examiner with no knowledge of treatment assignments performed visual acuity testing at the 4-, 12-, 24-, and 36-month visits. Fluorescein angiography was performed at 4, 12, and 24 months.

Inclusion Criteria

- Center-involving macular edema secondary to either CRVO or BRVO, with eyes enrolled as early as the time diagnosis of the macular edema, but not longer than 24 months after diagnosis
- Visual acuity score ≥ 19 letters (20/400) and ≤ 73 letters (20/40) by the ETDRS visual acuity protocol in the study eye
- Retinal thickness > 250 μm in the central subfield of the OCT topographic map formed by six radial scans (mean of two measurements)

- No history of laser photocoagulation for macular edema within 4 months prior to randomization. No history of PRP within 4 months prior to randomization or anticipated within the next 4 months following randomization
- No history of intravitreal corticosteroid injection or peribulbar or retrobulbar corticosteroid use for any reason within 6 months prior to randomization
- No vitreoretinal interface disease (vitreomacular traction, epiretinal membrane), foveal atrophy, dense pigmentary changes, or dense subfoveal hard exudates
- Patients with the presence of an ocular condition that, in the opinion of the investigator, might affect macular edema or alter visual acuity during the course of the study were excluded.

Study Measures

The primary outcome was improvement by 15 or more letters from baseline in the best-corrected ETDRS visual acuity score at the 12-month visit. Secondary outcomes included changes from baseline in the best-corrected ETDRS visual acuity score, changes in retinal thickness as assessed by stereoscopic color fundus photography and OCT, and adverse ocular outcomes (injection-related events including infectious endophthalmitis, noninfectious endophthalmitis, retinal detachment, and vitreous hemorrhage; steroid-related toxicities including cataract and elevated IOP).

Results

- The correlation coefficient for the association between baseline OCT-measured center point thickness and best-corrected E-ETDRS visual acuity letter score was –0.27 (95% confidence limit: –0.38 to –0.16) for participants in the CRVO trial and –0.28 (95% confidence limit: –0.37 to –0.19) in the BRVO trial.[8]
- *CRVO trial*: 7%, 27%, and 26% of participants achieved the primary outcome (improvement by 15 or more letters from baseline in the best-corrected ETDRS visual acuity score at the 12-month visit) in the observation, 1-mg, and 4-mg groups, respectively. The odds of achieving the primary outcome were 5.0 times greater in the 1-mg group than the observation group ($p = 0.001$) and 5.0 times greater in the 4-mg group than the observation group ($p = 0.001$); there was no difference identified between the 1- and 4-mg groups ($p = 0.97$). The rates of elevated IOP and cataract were similar for the observation and 1-mg groups but higher in the 4-mg group.[9]
- *BRVO trial*: 29%, 26%, and 27% of participants achieved the primary outcome in the standard care, 1-mg, and 4-mg groups, respectively. None

of the pairwise comparisons between the three groups was statistically significant at month 12. The rates of elevated IOP and cataract were similar for the standard care and 1-mg groups but higher in the 4-mg group.[10]

- For both CRVO and BRVO, younger age was associated with improved visual acuity and central retinal thickness (CRT) outcomes. For CRVO, triamcinolone treatment and less severe anatomic abnormalities of the retina (center point thickness and areas of retinal hemorrhage, thickening, and fluorescein leakage) were predictive of better visual acuity outcomes. For BRVO, no history of coronary artery disease was predictive of improved visual acuity outcomes. For center point thickness outcomes, a shorter duration of macular edema was associated with improvement in both disease entities. For CRVO, a higher baseline visual acuity letter score was predictive of favorable OCT outcomes. For BRVO, a lower baseline visual acuity letter score, presence of dense macular hemorrhage, and no prior grid photocoagulation were predictive of favorable OCT outcomes.[11]

- The cumulative 36-month incidences for CRVO and BRVO eyes, respectively, were 8.5% and 2.4% for neovascularization of the iris (NVI) or neovascular glaucoma (NVG) and 8.8% and 7.6% for neovascularization of the disc/neovascularization elsewhere (NVD/NVE) or preretinal hemorrhage/vitreous hemorrhage. There were no differences in the incidences of neovascular events or risk of nonperfusion when comparing the three treatment groups within diseases. Nonperfusion was the only significant baseline factor for neovascularization in BRVO, with the risk of a neovascular event increasing with greater disc areas of nonperfusion, and the highest risk noted at ≥5.5 disc areas.[12]

Conclusion

- The correlation between OCT-measured center point thickness and visual acuity letter score is modest. The OCT-measured center point thickness represents a useful tool for the detection and monitoring of macular edema in RVO, but it cannot reliably substitute for visual acuity measurements.
- Intravitreal triamcinolone is superior to observation for treating vision loss associated with macular edema secondary to CRVO in patients who have characteristics similar to those in the SCORE-CRVO trial. The 1-mg dose has a safety profile superior to that of the 4-mg dose. Intravitreal triamcinolone in a 1-mg dose, following the retreatment criteria applied in the SCORE study, should be considered for up to 1 year, and possibly 2 years, for patients with characteristics similar to those in the SCORE-CRVO trial.
- There was no difference in visual acuity at 12 months for the standard care group compared with the triamcinolone groups; however, the rates of adverse events (particularly elevated IOP and cataract) were highest

in the 4-mg group. Grid photocoagulation as applied in the SCORE study remains the standard care for patients with vision loss associated with macular edema secondary to BRVO who have characteristics similar to participants in the SCORE-BRVO trial. Grid photocoagulation should remain the benchmark against which other treatments are compared in clinical trials for eyes with vision loss associated with macular edema secondary to BRVO.

- Several factors were predictive of better visual acuity outcomes and more favorable OCT outcomes, including younger age and shorter duration of macular edema, respectively. These factors may assist clinicians in predicting the disease course for patients with CRVO and BRVO.
- Triamcinolone treatment was not associated with lower incidences of neovascular events or nonperfusion status compared with observation or grid photocoagulation. Cumulative 36-month incidences for most neovascular events were significantly higher for nonperfused than perfused eyes. Greater baseline disc areas of nonperfusion increased the risk of neovascularization in BRVO but not CRVO eyes, possibly owing to obscuration of retinal capillary details caused by dense hemorrhage at baseline for CRVO eyes. Increased risk of neovascularization was noted below the historical threshold of 10 disc areas of nonperfusion for RVO.

■ RANIBIZUMAB FOR THE TREATMENT OF MACULAR EDEMA FOLLOWING BRANCH RETINAL VEIN OCCLUSION: EVALUATION OF EFFICACY AND SAFETY (BRAVO)[13]

Purpose

To assess the efficacy and safety of intravitreal injections of 0.3 or 0.5 mg Ranibizumab compared with sham injections in patients with macular edema secondary to BRVO.

Description

This was a phase III, multicenter, prospective, randomized, double-masked, sham injection-controlled study conducted from 2007 to 2009 in which 397 patients with BRVO were enrolled at 93 investigational sites in the United States.

Eligible patients were randomized 1:1:1 to receive monthly intraocular injections of 0.3 or 0.5 mg of ranibizumab or sham injections for 6 months. The study included a treatment period (6 months) and an observation period (6 months). Patients were eligible for laser rescue treatment at 3 months if macular edema showed little or no improvement, visual acuity was 20/40 or worse, and if the central subfield thickness was 250 μm or greater.

Inclusion Criteria

Patients included in the study had macular edema involving the foveal center secondary to BRVO, central subfield macular thickness of 250 μm or greater on OCT, best-corrected visual acuity (BCVA) of 20/40 to 20/400.

Study Measures

The primary efficacy outcome measure was mean change from the baseline BCVA letter score at month 6. Secondary outcomes included other parameters of visual function [such as percentage of patients who gained 3 lines (15 letters) of BCVA at 6 months] and central foveal thickness (CFT).

Results

- The mean [95% confidence interval (CI)] change from the baseline BCVA letter score at month 6 was 16.6 (14.7–18.5) and 18.3 (16.0–20.6) in the 0.3- and 0.5-mg ranibizumab groups, respectively, and 7.3 (5.1–9.5) in the sham group ($p < 0.0001$ for each ranibizumab group vs. sham group).
- Improvement in BCVA was evident as early as 1 week, with patients achieving a mean gain of 7.6, 7.4, and 1.9 letters in the 0.3- and 0.5-mg ranibizumab and sham groups at 1 week, respectively.
- The percentage of patients who gained ≥ 15 letters in BCVA at month 6 was 55.2% (0.3 mg) and 61.1% (0.5 mg) in the ranibizumab groups and 28.8% in the sham group ($p < 0.0001$ for each ranibizumab group vs. sham group).
- At month 6, significantly more ranibizumab-treated patients (0.3 mg, 67.9%; 0.5 mg, 64.9%) had BCVA of ≥ 20/40 compared with sham patients (41.7%; $p < 0.0001$ for each ranibizumab group vs. sham group).
- At month 6, the CFT had decreased by a mean of 337 μm (0.3 mg) and 345 μm (0.5 mg) in the ranibizumab groups and 158 μm in the sham group ($p < 0.0001$ for each ranibizumab group vs. sham group). The median percent reduction in excess foveal thickness at month 6 was 97.0% and 97.6% in 0.3- and 0.5-mg groups and 27.9% in the sham group.
- More patients in the sham group (54.5%) received a rescue grid laser compared with the 0.3-mg (18.7%) and 0.5-mg (19.8%) ranibizumab groups.
- The safety profile was consistent with previous phase III ranibizumab trials, and no new safety events were identified in patients with BRVO.

Conclusion

Intraocular injections of 0.3 or 0.5 mg ranibizumab provided rapid, effective treatment for macular edema following BRVO with low rates of ocular and nonocular safety events.

CENTRAL RETINAL VEIN OCCLUSION STUDY: EVALUATION OF EFFICACY AND SAFETY (CRUISE)[14]

Purpose
To assess the efficacy and safety of intravitreal injections of 0.3- or 0.5-mg ranibizumab compared with sham injections in patients with macular edema secondary to CRVO.

Description
CRUISE was a phase III, multicenter, prospective, randomized, double-masked, sham injection-controlled study conducted from 2007 to 2009 in which 392 patients with CRVO were enrolled at 95 investigational sites in the United States.

Eligible patients were randomized 1:1:1 to receive monthly intraocular injections of 0.3 or 0.5 mg of ranibizumab or sham injections for 6 months. The study included a treatment period (6 months) and an observation period (6 months).

Inclusion Criteria
Patients included in the study had macular edema involving the foveal center secondary to CRVO, a central subfield macular thickness of 250 μm or greater on OCT, and a BCVA of 20/40 to 20/320.

Study Measures
The primary efficacy outcome measure was a mean change from the baseline BCVA letter score at month 6. Secondary outcomes included other parameters of visual function [such as percentage of patients who gained 3 lines (15 letters) of BCVA at 6 months] and CFT.

Results
- The mean (95% CI) change from the baseline BCVA letter score at month 6 was 12.7 (9.9–15.4) and 14.9 (12.6–17.2) in the 0.3- and 0.5-mg ranibizumab groups, respectively, and 0.8 (−2.0 to 3.6) in the sham group ($p < 0.0001$ for each ranibizumab group vs. sham group).
- Gain in BCVA was seen as early as 1 week, with patients achieving mean gains of 8.8, 9.3, and 1.1 letters in the 0.3- and 0.5-mg ranibizumab and sham groups at 1 week, respectively.
- The percentage of patients who gained ≥ 15 letters in BCVA at month 6 was 46.2% (0.3 mg) and 47.7% (0.5 mg) in the ranibizumab groups and 16.9% in the sham group ($p < 0.0001$ for each ranibizumab group vs. sham group).

- At month 6, significantly more ranibizumab-treated patients (0.3 mg = 43.9%; 0.5 mg = 46.9%) had BCVA of ≥ 20/40 compared with sham patients (20.8%; $p < 0.0001$ for each ranibizumab group vs. sham group).
- At month 6, the CFT had decreased by a mean of 434 µm (0.3 mg) and 452 µm (0.5 mg) in the ranibizumab groups and 168 µm in the sham group ($p < 0.0001$ for each ranibizumab group vs. sham group).
- The median percentage reduction in excess foveal thickness at month 6 was 94.0% and 97.3% in the 0.3- and 0.5-mg groups, respectively, and 23.9% in the sham group.
- The safety profile was consistent with previous phase III ranibizumab trials, and no new safety events were identified in patients with CRVO.

Conclusion

Intraocular injections of 0.3- or 0.5-mg ranibizumab provided rapid improvement in 6-month visual acuity and macular edema following CRVO, with low rates of ocular and nonocular safety events.

Following the BRAVO and CRUISE trials, the US FDA approved the use of ranibizumab for the treatment of macular edema due to retinal venous occlusions.

GLOBAL EVALUATION OF IMPLANTABLE DEXAMETHASONE IN RETINAL VEIN OCCLUSION WITH MACULAR EDEMA (GENEVA)[15,16]

Purpose

To evaluate the safety and efficacy of one or two treatments with dexamethasone intravitreal implant (DEX implant; OZURDEX, Allergan, Inc., Irvine, CA) compared with sham in eyes with vision loss due to macular edema associated with BRVO or CRVO.

Background

Macular edema is a common cause of vision loss in both BRVO and CRVO. The pathogenesis of macular edema in RVO involves hydrostatic effects from increased venous pressure, the presence of inflammatory cytokines (e.g., prostaglandins and interleukin-6), the dysregulation of endothelial tight junction proteins, or increased amounts of vascular permeability factors, such as vascular endothelial growth factor (VEGF). Corticosteroids can help reduce many of these processes; they have potent anti-inflammatory effects, can reduce vascular permeability, inhibit fibrin deposition and leukocyte movement, suppress homing and migration of inflammatory cells, stabilize endothelial cell tight junctions, and inhibit the synthesis of VEGF, prostaglandins, and other cytokines. Dexamethasone is a potent, water-soluble corticosteroid that can be delivered to the vitreous cavity by the DEX implant, which is composed of a biodegradable copolymer of lactic acid and glycolic acid containing micronized dexamethasone. The drug-copolymer complex gradually releases the total dose of dexamethasone over a series of months after insertion into the eye through a small pars plana puncture using a customized applicator system.

The US FDA approved OZURDEX™ (DEX implant) 0.7 mg as the first drug therapy indicated for the treatment of macular edema following BRVO or CRVO in 2009.

Description

GENEVA consisted of two identical, multicenter, prospective studies including a randomized, 6-month, double-masked, sham-controlled phase followed by a 6-month open-label extension (each of which included patients with BRVO and patients with CRVO). A total of 1,256 patients with vision loss due to macular edema associated with BRVO or CRVO were included.

At baseline, patients received DEX implant 0.7 mg ($n = 421$), DEX implant 0.35 mg ($n = 412$), or sham ($n = 423$) in the study eye. At day 180, patients could receive DEX implant 0.7 mg if the BCVA was <84 letters or retinal thickness was >250 μm.

Inclusion Criteria

Patients who were at least 18 years of age and had decreased visual acuity as a result of clinically detectable macular edema associated with either CRVO or BRVO were recruited. The duration of macular edema (defined as the time since the initial diagnosis of macular edema) was required to be between 6 weeks and 9 months in patients with CRVO and between 6 weeks and 12 months in patients with BRVO. Eligible patients had to have BCVA of between 34 letters (20/200) and 68 letters (20/50) in the study eye and better than 34 letters in the nonstudy eye. The retinal thickness in the central subfield (as measured by OCT) had to be ≥300 μm in the study eye.

Patients with clinically significant epiretinal membrane, active retinal/disc/INV, glaucoma, and ocular hypertension needing more than one medication were excluded, as were those with lens opacities including cataract.

Study Measures

The primary outcome measure for the pooled data from the two studies was the time to achieve a ≥15-letter improvement in BCVA. Secondary end points included BCVA, CRT, and safety. The primary outcome for the open-label extension was safety; BCVA was also evaluated.

Results

- About 66% of patients had BRVO and 36% had CRVO. The mean visual acuity at baseline was 54 letters. 10% had previous laser treatment (as expected, nearly all of these had BRVO).
- After a single administration, the time to achieve a ≥15-letter improvement in BCVA was significantly less in both DEX implant groups compared with sham ($p < 0.001$). The percentage of eyes with a ≥15-letter improvement in BCVA was significantly higher in both DEX implant groups compared with sham at days 30–90 ($p < 0.001$). The percentage of eyes with a ≥15-letter loss in BCVA was significantly lower in the DEX implant 0.7-mg group compared with sham at all follow-up visits ($p ≤ 0.036$). Improvement in mean BCVA was greater in both DEX implant groups compared with sham at all follow-up visits ($p ≤ 0.006$). Improvements in BCVA with DEX implant were seen in patients with BRVO and in patients with CRVO, although the patterns of response differed. The percentage of DEX implant-treated eyes with an IOP of ≥25 mm Hg peaked at 16% at day 60 (both doses) and was not different from sham by day 180. There was no significant interd-group difference in the occurrence of cataract or cataract surgery.[14]
- At day 180, 997 patients received open-label DEX implant. Except for cataract, the incidence of ocular adverse events was similar in patients who received their first or second DEX implant. Over 12 months, cataract progression occurred in 90 of 302 phakic eyes (29.8%) that received two DEX implant 0.7-mg injections versus 5 of 88 sham-treated phakic eyes (5.7%); cataract surgery was performed in 4 of 302 (1.3%) and 1 of 88 (1.1%) eyes, respectively. In the group receiving two 0.7-mg DEX implants ($n = 341$), a ≥ 10-mm Hg IOP increase from baseline was observed in (12.6% after the first treatment and 15.4% after the second). The IOP increases were usually transient and controlled with medication or observation; an additional 10.3% of patients initiated IOP-lowering medications after the second treatment. A ≥15-letter improvement in BCVA from baseline was achieved by 30% and 32% of patients 60 days after the first and second DEX implant, respectively.[15]

Conclusion

Among patients with macular edema owing to BRVO or CRVO, single and repeated treatment with DEX implant had a favorable safety profile over 12 months. DEX implant can both reduce the risk of vision loss and improve the speed and incidence of visual improvement in eyes with macular edema secondary to BRVO or CRVO and may be a useful therapeutic option for eyes with these conditions. In patients who qualified for and received two DEX implant injections, the efficacy and safety of the two implants were similar with the exception of cataract progression.

CONTROLLED PHASE 3 EVALUATION OF REPEATED INTRAVITREAL ADMINISTRATION OF VEGF TRAP-EYE IN CENTRAL RETINAL VEIN OCCLUSION: UTILITY AND SAFETY (COPERNICUS)[17,18,19]

Purpose

To assess the efficacy and safety of intravitreal VEGF Trap-Eye (VTE; also known as aflibercept, EYLEA) in eyes with macular edema secondary to CRVO.

Background

VTE is a fully human recombinant fusion protein, consisting of soluble extracellular domains of VEGF receptors 1 and 2 fused to the Fc portion of human immunoglobulin 1 (IgG1), which binds all forms of VEGF-A along with the related placental growth factor (PlGF). VTE is a specific and highly potent blocker of these growth factors. VTE is specially purified and contains iso-osmotic buffer concentrations, allowing for intravitreal injection.

Bayer HealthCare and Regeneron are collaborating on the global development of VTE for the treatment of the neovascular age-related macular degeneration (wet AMD), CRVO, diabetic macular edema (DME), and other ocular disorders. In September, 2012, the US FDA approved EYLEA® (aflibercept) injection for the treatment of macular edema following CRVO. This approval of EYLEA® was based on 24-week data from the phase 3 COPERNICUS and GALILEO studies. Results from weeks 24 through 52 of the COPERNICUS and GALILEO studies have not yet been reviewed by the FDA.

Description

COPERNICUS was a multicenter, randomized, prospective, controlled trial that included 189 patients (1 eye/patient) with macular edema secondary to CRVO. Eyes were randomized 3:2 to receive VTE 2 mg or sham injection monthly for 6 months (115 patients received VTE and 74 were randomized to the control arm). At the end of the initial 6 months, all patients randomized to VTE were dosed on a PRN (as needed) basis for another 6 months, guided by anatomic and visual acuity monitoring. Patients randomized to sham injections in the first 6 months were eligible for cross over to VTE PRN dosing in the second 6 months. During the second 6 months of the studies, all patients were eligible for rescue laser treatment.

From weeks 52 to 100, patients were evaluated quarterly to receive intravitreal aflibercept injection (IAI) PRN. If needed, patients could receive IAI as frequently as every 4 weeks.

Study Measures

The proportion of eyes with a ≥15-letter gain (ETDRS) or more in BCVA at week 24 was the primary efficacy end point. Mean changes in BCVA and CRT, proportion of eyes progressing to neovascularization of the anterior segment, optic disc, or elsewhere in the retina and quality-of-life National Eye Institute Visual Function Questionnaire 25 (NEI VFQ-25) outcomes were other measures.

Results

At week 24, 56.1% of VTE-treated eyes gained 15 letters or more from baseline versus 12.3% of sham-treated eyes ($p < 0.001$). The VTE-treated eyes gained a mean of 17.3 letters versus sham-treated eyes, which lost 4.0 letters ($p < 0.001$). CRT decreased by 457.2 μm in eyes treated with VTE versus 144.8 μm in sham-treated eyes ($p < 0.001$), and progression to any neovascularization occurred in 0 and 5 (6.8%) of VTE-treated eyes and sham-treated eyes, respectively ($p = 0.006$). Conjunctival hemorrhage, reduced visual acuity, and eye pain were the most common adverse events. Serious ocular adverse events were reported by 3.5% of VTE-treated patients and 13.5% of sham patients. Incidences of nonocular serious adverse events generally were well balanced between both groups.

At week 52, 55.3% of patients receiving VTE dosed monthly for 24 weeks, and then on a PRN basis over the next 28 weeks, gained at least 15 letters compared to 30.1% of patients who received sham injections for the first 24 weeks followed by VTE PRN from week 24 to week 52 ($p = 0.0006$). In terms of gain in visual acuity from baseline to week 52, patients receiving VTE gained, on average, 16.2 letters of vision compared to a mean gain of 3.8 letters for *patients* who switched from sham to VTE PRN ($p < 0.0001$). The most common adverse events for both groups were conjunctival hemorrhage, eye pain, reduced visual acuity, and increased IOP.

At 100 weeks, the proportion of patients who gained ≥15 letters was 49.1% versus 23.3% ($p < 0.01$) in the VTE group and sham-VTE groups, respectively. The mean BCVA change from baseline was +13.0 versus +1.5 letters at week 100 in the VTE group and sham-VTE groups. The mean CRT reduction from baseline was 390.0 versus 343.3 μm at week 100 in the VTE group and sham-VTE groups. The mean (SD) number of PRN IAIs was 6.0 (3.4) versus 7.1 (3.4) from week 24 to 100 in the VTE group and sham-VTE groups, respectively.

Conclusion

Monthly injections of 2-mg intravitreal aflibercept for patients with macular edema secondary to CRVO resulted in a statistically significant improvement in visual acuity at week 24, which was largely maintained through week 52 with intravitreal aflibercept PRN dosing. IAI was generally well tolerated.

GENERAL ASSESSMENT LIMITING INFILTRATION OF EXUDATES IN CENTRAL RETINAL VEIN OCCLUSION WITH VEGF TRAP-EYE (GALILEO)[20]

Purpose
To evaluate intravitreal VTE in patients with macular edema secondary to CRVO.

Description
In this double-masked study, 177 patients were randomized (3:2 ratio) to intravitreal injections of VTE 2 mg or sham procedure every month for 6 months (104 patients were randomized and treated with VTE and 68 randomized and treated in the control arm). BCVA was evaluated using the ETDRS chart and the CRT was measured with OCT. After 6 monthly injections, patients continued to receive VTE treatment during weeks 24 to 52 only if they met prespecified retreatment criteria (PRN), except for patients in the sham control group who continued to receive sham injections through week 52.

Results
From baseline until week 24, more patients receiving VTE (60.2%) gained ≥15 letters compared with those receiving sham injections (22.1%) ($p < 0.0001$). VTE patients gained a mean of 18.0 letters compared with 3.3 letters with sham injections ($p < 0.0001$). Mean CRT decreased by 448.6 and 169.3 μm in the VTE and sham groups, respectively ($p < 0.0001$). The most frequent ocular adverse events in the VTE arm were typically associated with the injection procedure or the underlying disease, and included eye pain (11.5%), increased IOP (9.6%), and conjunctival hemorrhage (8.7%).

The 1-year GALILEO results showed that the proportion of subjects that gained at least 15 letters of vision from baseline to week 52 was 60.2% of patients receiving VTE, compared to 32.4% of patients receiving sham injections (exploratory tertiary endpoint; $p = 0.0004$). In terms of gain in visual acuity from baseline until week 52, patients receiving VTE gained, on an average, 16.9 letters of vision compared to a mean gain of 3.8 letters for patients receiving sham injections (exploratory tertiary endpoint; $p < 0.0001$).

Conclusion
VTE 2 mg every 4 weeks was efficacious in CRVO with an acceptable safety profile. Vision gains with VTE were significantly higher than with observation/PRP if needed. Based on these data, VTE may provide a new treatment option for CRVO.

STUDY OF COMPARATIVE TREATMENTS FOR RETINAL VEIN OCCLUSION 2 (SCORE 2)[21-24]

Purpose
To study if bevacizumab is noninferior to aflibercept for macular edema secondary to CRVO or HRVO.

Background
Bevacizumab has been widely used for the treatment of macular edema due to venous occlusions. However, there has been no study to compare it with aflibercept which has shown efficacy in various studies.

Description
- SCORE2 is a multicenter (including private practice), randomized noninferiority clinical trial in the United States and included 362 patients with macular edema due to CRVO or HRVO. Eyes were randomized to receive intravitreal bevacizumab (n = 182) or aflibercept (n = 180) every 4 weeks till 6 months.
- After a good response at month 6, the eyes received either monthly injections or treat-and-extend (TAE) regimens of aflibercept or bevacizumab. 293 eyes were involved in this sub-group.
- After poor response to aflibercept or bevacizumab treatment at month 6, eyes receiving monthly aflibercept were switched to a dexamethasone implant at month 6 and, if needed, at months 9, 10, or 11. Eyes receiving monthly bevacizumab were switched to aflibercept at months 6, 7, and 8 and then to a TAE aflibercept regimen until month 12. 49 eyes were a part of this protocol.

Study Measures
The primary outcome was a mean change in ETDRS BCVA at 6 months. The noninferiority margin was 5 letters.

Results
At 6 months, the mean visual acuity was 69.3 letters (mean increase of 18.6 from baseline) in the bevacizumab group and 69.3 (mean increase of 18.9 from baseline) in the aflibercept group, meeting the criteria for noninferiority. Macular thickness also reduced similarly in both the groups. Ocular adverse events were similar in two groups.

At 12 months:
- The treatment group difference (the change in visual acuity letter score in the monthly group minus the change in the TAE group) from month 6 to month 12 was 1.88 for aflibercept and 1.98 for bevacizumab.

- In the aflibercept arm, the mean number of injections between months 6 and 11 was 5.8 in the monthly injection group and 3.8 in the TAE group: in the bevacizumab arm, the mean number of injections was 5.8 in the monthly group and 4.5 in the TAE group.
- Of the 49 eyes, aflibercept and bevacizumab treatment had failed in 14 and 35 patients, respectively.
- In eyes with switch from aflibercept to dexamethasone, the mean BCVA change from month 6 to 12 was 2.63 and 46.0 µm for central subfield thickness. In eyes with switch from bevacizumab to aflibercept, the mean BCVA change from month 6 to 12 was 10.27 and −125.4 µm for central subfield thickness.

Conclusions

- Bevacizumab was noninferior to aflibercept in patients with macular edema due to CRVO or HRVO in terms of visual acuity at 6 months after treatment.
- From 6 to 12 months, TAE was associated with one to two fewer injections than the monthly group. However, the authors recommended caution while interpreting the two approaches as equal since there was a wide variation in CIs.
- Eyes treated with aflibercept after a poor response to bevacizumab had improvement in BCVA and macular thickness. Few eyes had a poor response to aflibercept and were switched to dexamethasone.
- No differences in BCVA and macular thickness were identified at 12 months when participants originally assigned to aflibercept were compared with those assigned to bevacizumab.

■ STUDY TO ASSESS THE CLINICAL EFFICACY AND SAFETY OF INTRAVITREAL AFLIBERCEPT INJECTION IN PATIENTS WITH BRANCH RETINAL VEIN OCCLUSION (VIBRANT)[25,26]

Purpose
To compare IAI with macular grid laser photocoagulation for the treatment of macular edema in BRVO.

Background
After the introduction of anti-VEGFs, laser photocoagulation as the treatment of macular edema due to BRVO has declined which was the earlier gold standard. This study was aimed to compare aflibercept with laser photocoagulation.

Description

VIBRANT was a double-masked, active-controlled, randomized, phase III trial conducted at multiple centers (58) in USA and Japan.
- Treatment-naive eyes with macular edema due to BRVO (not more than 1-year old) with BCVA of 20/40 to 20/320 were randomized to either IAI 2 mg every 4 weeks ($n = 91$) from baseline to week 20 or grid laser ($n = 92$) at baseline with a single grid laser rescue treatment, if needed, from weeks 12 to 20.
- In the aflibercept group after the initial 6 monthly injections, injection was given every 8 weeks through week 48 with rescue grid laser, if needed, at week 36. In the grid laser group, IAI was added every 8 weeks after 3 monthly doses from week 24 onward.
- Exclusion criteria included a history of vitreoretinal surgery within 12 months or any intraocular surgery within the last 3 months; reductions in visual acuity from causes other than BRVO; and presence of DME or retinopathy, ocular inflammation, or uncontrolled glaucoma.

Study Measures

The primary outcome measure was the number of eyes that gained ≥15 ETDRS letters from baseline at 24 weeks. Secondary end points included mean change from baseline BCVA and central macular thickness (CMT) at 24 weeks. All outcome measures at week 52 were exploratory, and p values were considered nominal.

Results

At week 24, 52.7% eyes in the IAI group and 26.7% in the laser group gained ≥15 ETDRS letters at 24 weeks ($p = 0.0003$). The mean BCVA improvement at 24 weeks was 17.0 letters in the IAI group and 6.9 letters in the laser group ($p < 0.0001$). The mean reduction in CMT at 24 weeks was 280.5 μm in the IAI group and 128.0 μm in the laser group ($p < 0.0001$).

At week 52, 57.1% eyes in the IAI group and 41.1% in the laser group gained ≥15 ETDRS letters ($p = 0.0296$). The mean BCVA improvement at 52 weeks was 17.1 letters in the IAI group and 12.2 letters in the laser group ($p = 0.0035$). The mean reduction in CMT at 52 weeks was 283.9 μm in the IAI group and 249.3 μm in the laser group ($p < 0.0218$). 10.6% of eyes received rescue laser at week 36 in the aflibercept group. 80.7% received rescue IAI from week 24 to 48.

Conclusion

Six monthly aflibercept injections provided significantly greater visual benefit and reduction in CMT at 24 weeks than grid laser photocoagulation in eyes with macular edema due to BRVO.

After 6 monthly IAI, injections every 8 weeks maintained control of macular edema and visual benefits till 52 weeks. In the laser group, rescue IAI from week 24 through 52 resulted in substantial visual improvements.

■ HEAD-TO-HEAD COMPARISON OF RANIBIZUMAB PRN VERSUS SINGLE-DOSE DEXAMETHASONE FOR BRANCH RETINAL VEIN OCCLUSION (COMRADE-B)[27]

Purpose
To compare the efficacy and safety of ranibizumab 0.5 mg versus dexamethasone 0.7 mg in macular edema secondary to BRVO at 6 months.

Description
COMRADE-B was a 6-month, phase IIIb, multicenter, randomized, double-masked study that enrolled 244 patients with macular edema due to BRVO, at maximum 6 months prior to screening with ETDRS visual acuity of 20/40 to 20/400, from 74 sites across the European union (2011–2013). Patients with anti-VEGF treatment in the study eye or the fellow eye within 3 months prior to baseline, panretinal scatter photocoagulation or sectoral laser photocoagulation performed within 3 months before baseline or anticipated to be performed in the 4 months following randomization, use of intraocular corticosteroid within 6 months before baseline, and glaucoma were excluded. Patients were randomized 1:1; the ranibizumab group ($n = 126$) received consecutive monthly 0.5-mg IVR for 3 months followed by PRN regimen while the dexamethasone group ($n = 118$) received single sustained-release intravitreal 0.7-mg DEX implant followed by sham injections monthly until month 3 followed by a PRN regimen.

Study Measures
These included mean average change in BCVA, CMT, time to achieve a significant improvement in BCVA, defined as ≥15 letters, and rate of IOP rise.

Results
- The gain in BCVA was similar between the two groups for the first 3 months followed by a decline in the dexamethasone group. At month 6, the difference in BCVA gains from baseline was +17.3 letters in the ranibizumab group versus +9.2 letters in the dexamethasone group.
- Patients in the ranibizumab group received a mean of 2.94 loading injections and 1.74 PRN retreatment injections, while those in the dexamethasone group received a single loading injection. Elevated IOP and adverse events were more frequent with dexamethasone than with ranibizumab treatment.

Conclusion

Ranibizumab PRN resulted in greater visual acuity gains in macular edema following BRVO compared with single-dose dexamethasone implant over a 6-month study period, observed from month 3. In clinical practice, retreatment with dexamethasone may be required prior to this point.

◼ CLINICAL EFFICACY AND SAFETY OF RANIBIZUMAB VERSUS DEXAMETHASONE FOR CENTRAL RETINAL VEIN OCCLUSION (COMRADE-C): A EUROPEAN LABEL STUDY[28]

Purpose

To compare the efficacy and safety of ranibizumab 0.5 mg versus dexamethasone 0.7 mg in macular edema secondary to CRVO at 6 months.

Description

COMRADE-C was a 6-month, phase IIIb, multicenter, randomized, double-masked study that enrolled 243 patients with macular edema due to CRVO. Patients were randomized (1:1) to receive either monthly ranibizumab followed by PRN treatment ($n = 124$) or a single sustained-release dexamethasone implant followed by PRN sham injections ($n = 119$).

Study Measures

Main outcomes were mean average change in BCVA from baseline to month 1 through month 6, mean change in BCVA, and adverse events.

Results

185 patients completed study.
- The gain in BCVA was similar between the two groups for the first 2 months followed by decline in the dexamethasone group. At month 6, the BCVA gains from baseline were +12.86 letters in the ranibizumab versus +2.96 letters in the dexamethasone group, significantly favoring ranibizumab.
- The mean injection number of ranibizumab was 4.52. Ocular adverse events were reported in more patients in the dexamethasone group than in the ranibizumab group (86.6% vs. 55.6%).

Conclusion

Ranibizumab PRN resulted in greater visual acuity gains in macular edema following CRVO compared with the single-dose dexamethasone implant over a 6-month study period, observed from month 2. In clinical practice, retreatment with dexamethasone may be required prior to this point.

COMPARISON OF RANIBIZUMAB VERSUS DEXAMETHASONE FOR MACULAR EDEMA FOLLOWING RETINAL VEIN OCCLUSION: 1-YEAR RESULTS OF THE COMRADE EXTENSION STUDY[29]

Purpose
The COMRADE extension trial was designed to provide additional 6-month data of patients who completed the core studies.

Description
In this open-label, phase IV study, 92 BRVO patients (ranibizumab 52, DEX 40) and 83 CRVO patients (ranibizumab 61, DEX 22) who completed the COMRADE core studies were prospectively enrolled, monitored monthly, and received either 0.5 mg ranibizumab or a 0.7-mg DEX implant as needed according to the original study group.

Results
94.6% of BRVO patients and 97.6% of CRVO patients completed the extension study.
- The mean average change in BCVA in BRVO patients was significantly better for ranibizumab than DEX ($p = 0.0249$). The CRVO results were consistent with BRVOs, although not significant ($p = 0.1119$).
- Over the course of the extension, more adverse events were reported. In BRVO patients, adverse events were reported more in the dexamethasone group (62.5%) compared with ranibizumab (55.8%). Among CRVO patients, 65.5% in the ranibizumab group and 59.1% in the DEX group developed adverse events. The overall rise in IOP was more with the dexamethasone implant.

Conclusion
Ranibizumab revealed a better ocular safety profile and produced greater average BCVA gains than the dexamethasone implant. By the end of the additional 6-month study period, this difference in BCVA was more pronounced in BRVO than in CRVO patients.

The main limitation of the COMRADE studies was that DEX patients received only a single intravitreal treatment during the first 6 months, which is presumably not adequate. However, frequent DEX implants could lead to more steroid-related side effects, especially to an increased IOP.

Table 1: Summary of clinical trials in retinal vascular occlusions.

Title	Purpose	No. of patients	Inclusion criteria	Outcome measure	Result/conclusion
BVOS (1984)	Scatter argon photocoagulation for prevention of NV and vitreous hemorrhage and improving visual acuity in eyes with macular edema reducing vision to 20/40 or worse	539	• Major BRVO without NV • Major BRVO with NV • BRVO with macular edema and reduced vision	Visual acuity and development of NV or vitreous hemorrhage	• Scatter argon photocoagulation prevents the development of NV and vitreous hemorrhage but should be applied after the development of NV • Argon laser improved visual outcome in eyes with BRVO and visual acuity reduced from macular edema to 6/12 or worse
CVOS (1988)	• Early PRP for prevention of INV in ischemic CRVO • Early PRP versus PRP at first identification of INV • Grid-pattern photocoagulation for loss of central visual acuity due to macular edema	725	Patients of CRVO, age 21 or older, visual acuity of light perception or better, IOP <30 mm Hg and sufficient clarity of the ocular media	Visual acuity, fundus evaluation, fluorescein angiography, and INV	• Prophylactic PRP did not prevent the development of INV. It is safe to wait for the development of early INV and then apply PRP • Macular grid photocoagulation was effective in reducing angiographic evidence of macular edema but did not improve visual acuity • Patients with CRVO are recommended to have frequent follow-up examination every 1 month for the first 6 months to look for NVI

Contd...

Clinical Trials in Retinal Vascular Occlusions

Contd...

Title	Purpose	No. of patients	Inclusion criteria	Outcome measure	Result/conclusion
SCORE (2004)	Standard care versus intravitreal injection(s) of triamcinolone acetonide for macular edema of CRVO and BRVO	682	Center-involving macular edema secondary to either CRVO or BRVO, <24-month old, VA ≥ 19 letters and ≤73 letters, retinal thickness > 250 μm in the central subfield	Improvement by 15 or more letters from baseline in best-corrected ETDRS visual acuity score at the 12-month visit	• Intravitreal triamcinolone is superior to observation for treating vision loss associated with macular edema secondary to CRVO but not in BRVO • 1-mg dose has a safety profile superior to that of the 4-mg dose
BRAVO (2007)	Intravitreal ranibizumab versus sham injections in patients with macular edema due to BRVO	397	Macular edema involving foveal center due to BRVO, CFT ≥ 250 μm on OCT and BCVA of 20/40 to 20/400	Mean change in BCVA letter score at month 6 from baseline	Ranibizumab provided rapid and effective treatment for macular edema following BRVO with low rates of ocular and nonocular safety events
CRUISE (2007)	Intravitreal ranibizumab versus sham injections in patients with macular edema due to CRVO	392	Macular edema involving foveal center due to CRVO, CFT ≥ 250 μm on OCT, and BCVA of 20/40 to 20/320	Mean change in BCVA letter score at month 6 from baseline	Ranibizumab provided rapid improvement in 6-month visual acuity and macular edema following CRVO, with low rates of ocular and nonocular safety events

Contd...

Title	Purpose	No. of patients	Inclusion criteria	Outcome measure	Result/conclusion
GENEVA (2004)	Dexamethasone intravitreal implant versus sham in vision loss due to macular edema due to BRVO or CRVO	1,256	Decreased VA due to ME associated with either CRVO or BRVO, BCVA of between 34 and 68 letters, central subfield ≥ 300 μm on OCT	Time to achieve a ≥15-letter improvement in BCVA	Dexamethasone intravitreal implant can both reduce the risk of vision loss and improve the speed and incidence of visual improvement in eyes with ME secondary to BRVO or CRVO
COPERNICUS	Intravitreal VEGF Trap-Eye in eyes with macular edema secondary to CRVO	189	Center-involved macular edema secondary to CRVO for no longer than 9 months, central subfield thickness ≥ 250 μm, BCVA of 20/40 to 20/320	Proportion of eyes with a ≥15-letter gain BCVA at week 24	Intravitreal VEGF Trap-Eye for macular edema secondary to CRVO resulted in a significant improvement in visual acuity
GALILEO	Intravitreal VEGF Trap-Eye in patients with macular edema secondary to CRVO	177	Center-involved macular edema secondary to CRVO for no longer than 9 months, central subfield thickness ≥ 250 μm, BCVA of 20/40 to 20/320	Percentage of eyes which gained ≥15 letters at week 24	Intravitreal VEGF Trap-Eye was efficacious in CRVO with an acceptable safety profile

Contd...

Title	Purpose	No. of patients	Inclusion criteria	Outcome measure	Result/conclusion
SCORE2	To study if bevacizumab is noninferior to aflibercept for macular edema secondary to central retinal or hemiretinal vein occlusion	362	Patients with macular edema due to central retinal or hemiretinal vein occlusion	Mean change ETDRS BCVA at 6 and 12 months	• At 6 months, bevacizumab was noninferior to aflibercept in terms of visual acuity at 6 months • No differences in BCVA and macular thickness were identified at 12 months when participants originally assigned to aflibercept were compared with those assigned to bevacizumab. Eyes treated with aflibercept after a poor response to bevacizumab had improvement in BCVA and macular thickness. Few eyes had a poor response to aflibercept and were switched to dexamethasone
VIBRANT	To compare intravitreal aflibercept with macular grid laser photocoagulation for the treatment of macular edema in BRVO	183	Treatment-naive eyes with macular edema due to BRVO (not more than 1-year old)	Number of eyes that gained ≥15 ETDRS letters from baseline at 24 weeks. Outcome measures at week 52 were exploratory.	• At week 24, 52.7% eyes in the IAI group and 26.7% in the laser group gained ≥15 ETDRS letters ($p = 0.0003$) • The mean reduction in CMT at 24 weeks was 280.5 μm in the IAI group and 128.0 μm in the laser group ($p < 0.0001$) • At week 52, 57.1% eyes in the IAI group and 41.1% in the laser group gained ≥15 ETDRS letters at 52 weeks ($p = 0.0296$)

(BCVA: best-corrected visual acuity; BRVO: branch retinal vein occlusion; CFT: central foveal thickness; CRVO: central retinal vein occlusion; ME: macular edema; PRP: panretinal photocoagulation; INV: iris neovascularization; IOP: intraocular pressure; NV: neovascularization; NVI: neovascularization of the iris; OCT: optical coherence tomography; VA: visual acuity; VEGF: vascular endothelial growth factor)

REFERENCES

1. Branch Vein Occlusion Study Group. Argon laser scatter photocoagulation for prevention of neovascularization and vitreous hemorrhage in branch vein occlusion. Arch Ophthalmol. 1986;104:34-41.
2. Branch Vein Occlusion Study Group. Argon laser photocoagulation for macular edema in branch vein occlusion. Am J Ophthalmol. 1984;98:271-82.
3. The Central Vein Occlusion Study Group. Baseline and early natural history report. Arch Ophthalmol. 1993;111:1087-95.
4. The Central Vein Occlusion Study Group. Natural history and clinical management of central retinal vein occlusion. Arch Ophthalmol. 1997;115:486-91.
5. Clarkson JG, Central Vein Occlusion Study Group. Central vein occlusion study: Photographic protocol and early natural history. Trans Am Ophthalmol Soc. 1994;92:203-15.
6. The Central Vein Occlusion Study Group. A randomized clinical trial of early panretinal photocoagulation for ischemic central vein occlusion. The CVOS Group N Report. Ophthalmology. 1995;102:1434-44.
7. The Central Vein Occlusion Study Group. Evaluation of grid pattern photocoagulation for macular edema in central vein occlusion. The CVOS Group M Report. Ophthalmology. 1995;102:1425-33.
8. SCORE Study Investigator Group. SCORE Study report 1: baseline associations between central retinal thickness and visual acuity in patients with retinal vein occlusion. Ophthalmology 2009;116:504-12.
9. SCORE Study Research Group. SCORE Study report 5: A randomized trial comparing the efficacy and safety of intravitreal triamcinolone with observation to treat vision loss associated with macular edema secondary to central retinal vein occlusion. Arch Ophthalmol. 2009;127:1101-14.
10. SCORE Study Research Group. SCORE Study report 6: A randomized trial comparing the efficacy and safety of intravitreal triamcinolone with standard care to treat vision loss associated with macular edema secondary to branch retinal vein occlusion. Arch Ophthalmol. 2009;127:1115-28.
11. SCORE Study Investigator Group. SCORE Study report 10: Baseline predictors of visual acuity and retinal thickness outcomes in patients with retinal vein occlusion. Ophthalmology. 2011;118:345-52.
12. SCORE Study Investigator Group. SCORE Study report 11: Incidences of neovascular events in eyes with retinal vein occlusion. Ophthalmology. 2011;118:1364-72.
13. BRAVO Investigators. Ranibizumab for macular edema following branch retinal vein occlusion: six-month primary end point results of a phase III study. Ophthalmology. 2010;117:1102-12.e1.
14. CRUISE Investigators. Ranibizumab for macular edema following central retinal vein occlusion: six-month primary end point results of a phase III study. Ophthalmology. 2010;117:1124-33.e1.
15. Ozurdex GENEVA Study Group. Randomized, sham-controlled trial of dexamethasone intravitreal implant in patients with macular edema due to retinal vein occlusion. Ophthalmology. 2010;117:1134-46.e3.
16. Ozurdex GENEVA Study Group, Li J. Dexamethasone intravitreal implant in patients with macular edema related to branch or central retinal vein occlusion twelve-month study results. Ophthalmology. 2011;118:2453-60.
17. Boyer D, Heier J, Brown DM, Clark WL, Vitti R, Berliner AJ, et al. Vascular endothelial growth factor Trap-Eye for macular edema secondary to central retinal vein occlusion: six-month results of the phase 3 COPERNICUS study. Ophthalmology 2012; 119:1024-1032.
18. Brown DM, Heier JS, Clark WL, Boyer DS, Vitti R, Berliner AJ, et al. Intravitreal aflibercept injection for macular edema secondary to central retinal vein occlusion:

1-year results from the phase 3 COPERNICUS study. Am J Ophthalmol. 2013;155:429-37.e7.
19. Clark WL. Two-year results of the COPERNICUS study evaluating intravitreal aflibercept injection (IAI) for macular edema secondary to central retinal vein occlusion (CRVO). Invest Ophthalmol Vis Sci. 2013;54(15):4515.
20. Holz FG, Roider J, Ogura Y, Korobelnik JF, Simader C, Groetzbach G, et al. VEGF Trap-Eye for macular oedema secondary to central retinal vein occlusion: 6-month results of the phase III GALILEO study. Br J Ophthalmol. 2013;97:278-84.
21. Scott IU, Van Veldhuisen PC, Ip MS, Blodi BA, Oden NL, Awh CC, et al. Effect of bevacizumab vs aflibercept on visual acuity among patients with macular edema due to central retinal vein occlusion: the SCORE2 randomized clinical trial. JAMA. 2017;317(20):2072-87.
22. Scott IU, Van Veldhuisen PC, Ip MS, Blodi BA, Oden NL, Altaweel M, et al. Comparison of monthly vs treat-and-extend regimens for individuals with macular edema who respond well to anti-vascular endothelial growth factor medications: secondary outcomes from the SCORE2 randomized clinical trial. JAMA Ophthalmol. 2018;136(4):337-45.
23. Ip MS, Oden NL, Scott IU, Van Veldhuisen PC, Blodi BA, Ghuman T, et al. Month 12 outcomes after treatment change at month 6 among poor responders to aflibercept or bevacizumab in eyes with macular edema secondary to central or hemiretinal vein occlusion: A secondary analysis of the SCORE2 study. JAMA Ophthalmol. 2019;137(3):281-7.
24. Scott IU, Oden NL, Van Veldhuisen PC, Ip MS, Blodi BA, Chan CK. Month 24 outcomes after treatment initiation with anti-vascular endothelial growth factor therapy for macular edema due to central retinal or hemiretinal vein occlusion: SCORE2 Report 10: A secondary analysis of the SCORE2 randomized clinical trial. JAMA Ophthalmol. 2019;137(12):1389-98.
25. Campochiaro PA, Clark WL, Boyer DS, Heier JS, Brown DM, Vitti R, et al. Intravitreal aflibercept for macular edema following branch retinal vein occlusion: the 24-week results of the VIBRANT study. Ophthalmology. 2015;122(3):538-44.
26. Clark WL, Boyer DS, Heier JS, Brown DM, Haller JA, Vitti R, et al. Intravitreal aflibercept for macular edema following branch retinal vein occlusion: 52-week results of the VIBRANT study. Ophthalmology. 2016;123(2):330-6.
27. Hattenbach LO, Feltgen N, Bertelmann T, Schmitz-Valckenberg S, Berk H, Eter N, et al. Head-to-head comparison of ranibizumab PRN versus single-dose dexamethasone for branch retinal vein occlusion (COMRADE-B). Acta Ophthalmol. 2018;96(1):e10-8.
28. Hoerauf H, Feltgen N, Weiss C, Paulus EM, Schmitz-Valckenberg S, Pielen A, et al. Clinical efficacy and safety of ranibizumab versus dexamethasone for central retinal vein occlusion (COMRADE C): A European label study. Am J Ophthalmol. 2016;169:258-67.
29. Feltgen N, Hattenbach LO, Bertelmann T, Callizo J, Rehak M, Wolf A, et al. Comparison of ranibizumab versus dexamethasone for macular oedema following retinal vein occlusion: 1-year results of the COMRADE extension study. Acta Ophthalmol. 2018;96(8):e933-41.

Clinical Trials in Age-related Macular Degeneration-I

Neha Goel, Vinod Kumar

■ INTRODUCTION

Age-related macular degeneration (AMD) is the leading cause of blindness among elderly patients in developed countries. Choroidal neovascularization (CNV), the hallmark of "wet" or "neovascular" AMD, is responsible for approximately 90% of cases of severe vision loss due to AMD.

■ LASER PHOTOCOAGULATION

Macular Photocoagulation Study (MPS)[1-7]

Purpose

To evaluate laser treatment of CNV through randomized, controlled clinical trials. The MPS consisted of three sets of randomized, controlled clinical trials:

1. *Argon Study*: To determine whether argon blue-green laser photocoagulation of leaking abnormal blood vessels in choroidal neovascular membranes outside the fovea [200–2,500 µm from the center of the foveal avascular zone (FAZ)] is of benefit in preventing or delaying loss of central vision in patients with AMD, presumed ocular histoplasmosis (POH), and idiopathic neovascular membranes (INVM). A separate trial was conducted for each of the three underlying conditions.
2. *Krypton Study*: To determine whether krypton red laser photocoagulation of choroidal neovascular lesions with the posterior border 1–199 µm from the center of the FAZ is of benefit in preventing or delaying large losses of visual acuity in patients with AMD, POH, and INVM. A separate trial was conducted for each of the three underlying conditions.
3. *Foveal Study*: To determine whether laser photocoagulation is of benefit in preventing or delaying further visual acuity loss in patients with new (never treated) or recurrent (previously treated with laser photocoagulation) CNV due to AMD, under the center of the FAZ. Two separate trials, one for each type of lesion, were carried out.

Description

MPS was an interventional, randomized, multicenter, controlled phase 3 trial that began in February, 1979, and was funded by the National Eye Institute. In each randomized trial conducted by the MPS Group, focal laser photocoagulation was compared to observation without treatment. Patients were assigned to laser treatment or to observation with equal probability.

- The first set of MPS randomized trials, the Argon Study, focused on the effectiveness of photocoagulation with the argon blue-green laser in eyes with discrete extrafoveal CNV. Recruitment was terminated in 1,982 (*AMD*—236 eyes) and 1,983 (*POH*—262 eyes and *INVM*—67 eyes) patients because of demonstrated short-term treatment benefit, and some eyes in the "no-treatment" groups were treated later in their clinical course as a result of the evidence of early benefit. Follow-up was to continue for 5 years so that treatment effectiveness over a 5-year period can be assessed.
- After the initiation of the Argon Study, a new krypton red laser became available. The new wavelength offered theoretical advantages over the argon laser for treating CNV that extended inside the FAZ of the macula. The Krypton Study design was analogous to the Argon Study, with the investigation of three underlying conditions, except that CNV was closer to the FAZ center. For patients with *AMD*, recruitment ended in December, 1987, after 247 patients had been assigned to photocoagulation and 249 patients had been assigned to no treatment. Recruitment of patients with *POH* was stopped after 143 had been assigned to photocoagulation and 145 to observation only because more untreated eyes than treated eyes had experienced severe visual acuity loss. In eyes with *INVM*, 24 were assigned to laser photocoagulation and 25 to laser treatment.
- The third set of MPS clinical trials, the Foveal Study, was designed to determine whether laser photocoagulation was effective for delaying or preventing further visual acuity loss in *AMD* patients who have subfoveal CNV. Visual acuities of treated and untreated eyes were compared 4 years after enrolment, in the *Subfoveal New CNV Study* (eyes without prior laser treatment), and 3 years after enrolment, in the *Subfoveal Recurrent CNV Study* (eyes with subfoveal recurrent CNV at the periphery of an earlier laser treatment scar). Among patients assigned to laser treatment in the Foveal Study, argon laser treatment was compared with krypton red laser treatment of these lesions.

Inclusion Criteria

To be eligible, men and women must have been experiencing visual symptoms attributable to the macular lesion and must have had visible, well-demarcated hyperfluorescence characteristic of classic CNV on fluorescein angiography.

Age-related macular degeneration patients were 50 years of age or older and had drusen visible in the macula of at least one eye. POH patients were at least 18 years old and had at least one characteristic histo spot in one or both eyes. INVM patients were at least 18 years old and had no evidence of AMD, POH, angioid streaks, high myopia, diabetic retinopathy, or any other condition that could be the cause of the neovascularization. In particular, INVM patients had neither drusen greater than MPS Standard Photograph No. 1.1 nor histo spots in either eye.

Additional patient eligibility criteria were as follows:
- *Argon Study*: Discrete CNV outside the fovea (200–2,500 μm from the center of the FAZ) and visual acuity of 20/100 or better in the study eye
- *Krypton Study*: A neovascular lesion consisting of neovascularization and possibly blood and/or pigment that extended into the FAZ. The posterior border of CNV could extend as close as 1 μm to the FAZ center. The visual acuity of the study eye was 20/400 or better.
- *Foveal Study*: Only patients with AMD were eligible for this study. Fluorescein angiography of the eligible eye had to show evidence of a leaking choroidal neovascular membrane, some part of which extended under the center of the FAZ, or a neovascular lesion consisting of an old laser treatment scar and contiguous leaking neovascularization within 150 μm of the center of the FAZ. New, never-treated subfoveal lesions were less than 4 disc areas in size. Recurrent lesions were <6 disc areas in size, including the old treatment scar and new neovascularization. The best-corrected visual acuity was no better than 20/40 and no worse than 20/320.

Study Measures

A change in the best-corrected visual acuity from the baseline was the primary outcome for all MPS trials.

Results

- *Argon Study:* Argon laser treatment, as applied in the study, dramatically reduced severe visual acuity loss in these conditions. Laser treatment of such lesions is beneficial in preventing or delaying large losses of visual acuity for at least 5 years. In eyes with AMD as the underlying cause, the relative risk (RR) of losing 6 or more lines of visual acuity from the baseline level among untreated eyes ($n = 117$) compared with laser-treated eyes ($n = 119$) was 1.5 from 6 months through 5 years after entry ($p = 0.001$). In addition, after 5 years, untreated eyes had lost a mean of 7.1 lines of visual acuity, while laser-treated eyes had lost 5.2 lines. Recurrent neovascularization had been observed in 54% of laser-treated eyes by the end of the 5-year follow-up period. Among eyes with POH, untreated eyes

(n = 130) had 3.6 times the risk of losing 6 or more lines of visual acuity compared to laser-treated eyes (n = 132) (p < 0.0001). Also, untreated eyes had lost a mean of 4.4 lines of visual acuity after 5 years, compared with only 0.9 lines lost by laser-treated eyes. Among laser-treated eyes, recurrent neovascularization had been observed in 26% by 5 years after enrolment.[1,2]

- *Krypton Study*: There was a beneficial effect of krypton red laser treatment in eyes with AMD. The estimated RR of a loss of 6 or more lines of visual acuity from baseline to any examination from 6 months through 5 years after enrolment for untreated eyes in comparison with treated eyes was 1.20 (p = 0.04). Normotensive patients with AMD realized the greatest benefit from laser treatment (RR, 1.82) and hypertensive patients experienced little or no benefit (RR, 0.93). Untreated eyes with POH were at a much greater risk of a 6-line decrease in visual acuity from the 1-year through the 5-year examination than were treated eyes (unadjusted RR, 2.60; RR, 4.26 after adjustment for visual acuity and hypertension at baseline; p < 0.001 for both). The treatment effect for eyes with INVM was between the effects for eyes with AMD and eyes with POH.[3-6]

- *Foveal Study*: Patients treated with laser had larger losses of visual acuity from baseline than untreated eyes. Laser treatment was particularly effective for subfoveal recurrent CNV. Overall, eyes receiving direct laser treatment to the fovea for new CNV immediately lost more visual acuity than observed eyes. However, the amount of visual acuity loss in observed eyes increased to the level of loss in treated eyes at 12 months and exceeded the level thereafter. 4 years after enrolment in the Subfoveal New CNV Study, 39 (47%) of 83 untreated eyes and 17 (22%) of 77 laser-treated eyes had lost 6 or more lines of visual acuity from baseline levels (p = 0.002). At the 3-year examination in the Subfoveal Recurrent CNV Study, 21 (36%) of 58 untreated eyes and 6 (12%) of 49 treated eyes had lost 6 or more lines of visual acuity from baseline levels (p = 0.009).[7]

Conclusion

- For patients with any of the above three conditions, eyes with well-demarcated areas of classic CNV, as defined by fluorescein angiography, had a better visual prognosis when treated with laser photocoagulation, performed according to MPS guidelines, than when managed by observation. These outcome data apply to all three conditions when the position of the neovascularization is extrafoveal or juxtafoveal, i.e., when the CNV does not involve the center of the fovea. The early beneficial effects of laser treatment on visual acuity persisted for at least 5 years.
- Eyes with AMD and subfoveal CNV benefited more from laser treatment than from observation when MPS eligibility guidelines and treatment

protocol were observed. Eyes with smaller lesions and worse initial visual acuity had greater and earlier benefits of laser treatment. Eyes with large subfoveal neovascular lesions and good initial visual acuity are not good candidates for focal laser photocoagulation. The benefits of laser treatment have persisted through at least 4 years of follow-up in the Subfoveal New CNV Study and 3 years of follow-up in the Subfoveal Recurrent CNV Study.

■ VERTEPORFIN PHOTODYNAMIC THERAPY

Following the MPS, it was realized that only an estimated 13–26% of patients who have CNV meet the strict criteria used to select patients who would benefit from treatment. Laser photocoagulation for CNV itself causes thermal injury to the overlying retina and can cause a subsequent absolute scotoma. Consequently, most patients who have subfoveal lesions are not treated, because they might experience an immediate and permanent decline in central vision equivalent to the decline experienced in untreated patients. Unfortunately, most patients have a lesion that extends under the center of the retina. Moreover, even for patients receiving laser photocoagulation to lesions that do not extend under the foveal center, there is a high incidence (at least 50%) of recurrence of CNV through the foveal center within 1–3 years, which could result in further vision loss.

Verteporfin [a benzoporphyrin derivative monoacid (BPD-MA); Visudyne, Novartis AG] is a light-activated drug. The application of photodynamic therapy (PDT) with verteporfin involves two main steps: (1) intravenous infusion of the light-activated drug and (2) activation of the drug by light at a specific wavelength (689 nm) corresponding to an absorption peak of the drug with a low-power, nonthermal laser. The drug can be taken up by neovasculature and light-activation induces a photochemical reaction in the target area that causes immunologic and cellular damage, including endothelial damage of new vessels. Endothelial damage and the resulting platelet adhesion, degranulation, and subsequent thrombosis and occlusion of the vasculature might be the predominant mechanism by which light-activated drugs work.

The significance of PDT lies in its dual selectivity. Only rapidly dividing cells as seen in CNV will have receptor-mediated uptake of the photosensitizing drug, and only the area of CNV irradiated by the laser light will be activated to the triplet state. Thus, collateral damage to the adjacent normal choriocapillaris, retinal pigment epithelium (RPE), and neurosensory retina is minimized. The goal is to avoid the absolute scotoma caused by laser photocoagulation and permit the treatment of a broader range of subfoveal CNV with respect to lesion size and initial visual acuity.

Currently, verteporfin is the only US Food and Drug Administration (FDA)-approved photosensitizer used in PDT.

Treatment of Age-related Macular Degeneration with Photodynamic Therapy (TAP)[8-10]

Purpose
To evaluate the effect of PDT with verteporfin in patients with subfoveal CNV caused by AMD.

Description
The TAP study consisted of two multicenter, double-masked, placebo-controlled, randomized clinical trials that were conducted at 22 ophthalmology practices in Europe and North America from 1998. 609 patients with AMD and subfoveal classic CNV underwent a 2:1 randomization between treatment and control (sham treatment); 402 were assigned to verteporfin and 207 to placebo. Patients were randomly assigned to verteporfin (6 mg/m^2 of the body surface area) or placebo (5% dextrose in water) administered via intravenous infusion of 30 mL over 10 minutes. 15 minutes after the start of the infusion, a laser light at 689 nm delivered 50 J/cm^2 at an intensity of 600 mW/cm^2 over 83 seconds using a spot size with a diameter 1,000 μm larger than the greatest linear dimension of the CNV lesion. At follow-up examinations every 3 months, retreatment with the same regimen was applied if angiography showed persistent or new leakage.

Patients who completed the 2-year randomized, placebo-controlled portion of the TAP investigation could participate in the open-label extension study for an additional 3 years. Patients in the study extension received open-label verteporfin therapy in the study eye, fellow eye, or both eyes, irrespective of original treatment assignment to placebo or verteporfin, if leakage from CNV was evident on fluorescein angiography. Follow-up visits occurred at 3-month intervals through to month 48, with a final follow-up visit at month 60.

Inclusion Criteria
Patients with subfoveal classic CNV lesions caused by AMD measuring 5,400 μm or less in greatest linear dimension and best-corrected visual acuity of 20/40 to 20/200 were included in the study.

Study Measures
The primary outcome was the proportion of eyes with fewer than 15 letters (approximately 3 lines) of visual acuity loss at the month 24 examination, adhering to an intent-to-treat analysis.

Results

At 1 year

Visual acuity, contrast sensitivity, and fluorescein angiographic outcomes were better in the verteporfin-treated eyes than in the placebo-treated eyes at every follow-up examination through the month 12 examination.

- 246 (61%) of 402 eyes assigned to verteporfin compared with 96 (46%) of 207 eyes assigned to placebo had lost fewer than 15 letters of visual acuity from baseline ($p < 0.001$).
- In subgroup analyses, the visual acuity benefit (<15 letters lost) of verteporfin therapy was clearly demonstrated (67% vs. 39%; $p < 0.001$) when the area of classic CNV occupied 50% or more of the area of the entire lesion (termed *predominantly classic CNV lesions*), especially when there was no occult CNV. No statistically significant differences in visual acuity were noted when the area of classic CNV was >0% but <50% of the area of the entire lesion (termed *minimally classic CNV lesions*).
- Few ocular or other systemic adverse events were associated with verteporfin treatment, compared with placebo, including transient visual disturbances (18% vs. 12%), injection-site adverse events (13% vs. 3%), transient photosensitivity reactions (3% vs. 0%), and infusion-related low back pain (2% vs. 0%).

At 2 years

351 (87%) of 402 patients in the verteporfin group compared with 178 (86%) of 207 patients in the placebo group completed the month 24 examination. Beneficial outcomes with respect to visual acuity and contrast sensitivity noted at the month 12 examination in verteporfin-treated patients were sustained through the month 24 examination.

- 213 (53%) of 402 verteporfin-treated patients compared with 78 (38%) of 207 placebo-treated patients lost fewer than 15 letters ($p < 0.001$).
- In subgroup analyses for predominantly classic lesions at baseline, 94 (59%) of 159 verteporfin-treated patients compared with 26 (31%) of 83 placebo-treated patients lost fewer than 15 letters at the month 24 examination ($p < 0.001$). For minimally classic lesions at baseline, no statistically significant differences in visual acuity were noted.

At 5 years

Of the 402 verteporfin-treated patients in the randomized trials, 320 (80%) enrolled in the extension study; 193 (60%) of these completed the extension study up to 5 years. Patients received an average of approximately two treatments during the 3 years of the extension study. 77 (62%) of the 124 verteporfin-treated patients with predominantly classic lesions at baseline who enrolled in the extension completed the month 60 examination. 26 (34%) of these 77 patients had lost 3 or more lines of visual acuity by month 24 and 27 (35%) had lost this amount of vision by month 60; the mean change in visual acuity from baseline was also similar at the month 24 and month 60 examinations (−1.5 and −1.6 lines, respectively). When visual acuity results were examined for all extension patients who received verteporfin at baseline, regardless of baseline lesion composition and extension study completion status, a similar pattern of visual acuity stabilization was evident. Few additional instances of infusion-related back pain or photosensitivity reactions were reported from months 24 to 60. No additional safety issues were noted after bilateral treatment.

Conclusion

- The visual acuity benefits of verteporfin therapy for AMD patients with predominantly classic CNV subfoveal lesions were safely sustained for 2 years, providing compelling evidence to use verteporfin therapy for these cases. For AMD patients with subfoveal lesions that are minimally classic, there was insufficient evidence to warrant routine use of verteporfin therapy.
- Vision outcomes for verteporfin-treated patients with predominantly classic lesions at baseline remained relatively stable from months 24 to 36, although only approximately one-third of the verteporfin-treated patients originally enrolled with this lesion composition had a month 36 examination. Vision outcomes remained relatively stable from months 24 to 60 even though the treatment rate was low during this period. The TAP Study Group identified no new safety concerns to preclude repeating verteporfin therapy as described in this study through 5 years.

Verteporfin in Photodynamic Therapy (VIP)[11-14]

Purpose

1. To determine if PDT with verteporfin can improve the chance of stabilizing or improving vision (<8 letter loss) safely in patients with subfoveal CNV caused by pathologic myopia.
2. To determine if PDT with verteporfin can safely reduce the risk of vision loss compared with a placebo in patients with subfoveal CNV caused by AMD who were identified with a lesion composed of occult with no classic CNV or with presumed early onset classic CNV with a good visual acuity letter score.

Background

The VIP study evaluated patients who were not originally eligible for the TAP study.

Description

The VIP study was a multicenter, double-masked, placebo-controlled, randomized clinical trial conducted at 28 ophthalmology practices in Europe and North America from 1998. 120 patients with subfoveal CNV caused by pathologic myopia were recruited in the first part. 339 patients with AMD, with subfoveal CNV lesions with either occult with no classic CNV or evidence of classic CNV, were recruited in the second part. The treatment protocol was the same as used in the TAP.

Inclusion Criteria

Myopic CNV
Patients with subfoveal CNV caused by pathologic myopia with a greatest linear dimension no >5,400 μm and best-corrected visual acuity (Snellen equivalent) of approximately 20/100 or better were recruited in the first part.

CNV in AMD
Patients with AMD, with subfoveal CNV lesions measuring no >5,400 μm in greatest linear dimension with either:
- Occult with no classic CNV, best-corrected visual acuity score of at least 50 (Snellen equivalent approximately 20/100), and evidence of hemorrhage or recent disease progression or
- Evidence of classic CNV with a best-corrected visual acuity score of at least 70 (better than a Snellen equivalent of approximately 20/40) were recruited in the second part.

Study Measures

Myopic CNV
The primary outcome was the proportion of eyes at the follow-up examination 12 months after study entry with fewer than 8 letters (approximately 1.5 lines) of visual acuity lost, adhering to an intent-to-treat analysis.

CNV in AMD
The main outcome measure was at least moderate vision loss, i.e. a loss of at least 15 letters (approximately 3 lines), adhering to an intent-to-treat analysis with the last observation carried forward to impute for missing data.

Results

Myopic CNV
79 of the 81 verteporfin-treated patients (98%) compared with 36 of the 39 placebo-treated patients (92%) completed the *month 12* examination. At baseline, >90% of each group had evidence of classic CNV. Visual acuity, contrast sensitivity, and fluorescein angiographic outcomes were better in the verteporfin-treated eyes than in the placebo-treated eyes at every follow-up examination through the month 12 examination. At the month 12 examination, 72% of the verteporfin-treated patients compared with 44% of the placebo-treated patients lost fewer than eight letters

($p < 0.01$) including 26 (32%) versus 6 (15%) improving at least five letters (≥1 line). 70 (86%) of the verteporfin-treated patients compared with 26 (67%) of the placebo-treated patients lost fewer than 15 letters ($p = 0.01$). Few ocular or other systemic adverse events were associated with verteporfin therapy compared with placebo treatment.[11]

77 of 81 patients (95%) in the verteporfin group, compared with 36 of 39 patients (92%) in the placebo group, completed the *month 24* examination. At this time point, 29 of 81 verteporfin-treated patients (36%) compared with 20 of 39 placebo-treated patients (51%) lost at least 8 letters ($p = 0.11$). The distribution of change in visual acuity at the month 24 examination was in favor of a benefit for the cases assigned to verteporfin ($p = 0.05$). This included improvement by at least 5 letters (equivalent to at least 1 line) in 32 verteporfin-treated cases (40%) versus 5 placebo-treated cases (13%) and improvement by at least 15 letters (equivalent to at least 3 lines) in 10 verteporfin-treated cases (12%) versus zero placebo-treated cases. No additional photosensitivity adverse reactions or injection site adverse events were associated with verteporfin therapy in the second year of follow-up.[13]

CNV in AMD[12,14]

210 (93%) and 193 (86%) of the 225 patients in the verteporfin group compared with 104 (91%) and 99 (87%) of the 114 patients in the placebo group completed the month 12 and 24 examinations, respectively. On average, verteporfin-treated patients received five treatments over the 24 months of follow-up.

1. The primary outcome was similar for the verteporfin-treated and the placebo-treated eyes through the month 12 examination, although a number of secondary visual and angiographic outcomes significantly favored the verteporfin-treated group.
2. Between the month 12 and 24 examinations, the treatment benefit grew so that by the month 24 examination, the verteporfin-treated eyes were less likely to have moderate or severe vision loss. Of the 225 verteporfin-treated patients, 121 (54%) compared with 76 (67%) of 114 placebo-treated patients lost at least 15 letters ($p = 0.023$). Likewise, 67 of the verteporfin-treated patients (30%) compared with 54 of the placebo-treated patients (47%) lost at least 30 letters ($p = 0.001$).
3. Statistically significant results favoring verteporfin therapy at the month 24 examination were consistent between the total population and the subgroup of patients with a baseline lesion composition identified as occult CNV with no classic CNV. This subgroup included 166 of the 225 verteporfin-treated patients (74%) and 92 of the 114 placebo-treated patients (81%). In these patients, 91 of the verteporfin-treated group (55%) compared with 63 of the placebo-treated group (68%) lost at least 15 letters ($p = 0.032$), whereas 48 of the verteporfin-treated group (29%) and 43 of the placebo-treated group (47%) lost at least 30 letters ($p = 0.004$).

4. Other secondary outcomes, including visual acuity letter score worse than 34 (approximate Snellen equivalent of 20/200 or worse), mean change in visual acuity letter score, development of classic CNV, progression of classic CNV, and size of lesion, favored the verteporfin-treated group at both the month 12 and month 24 examinations for both the entire study group and the subgroup of cases with occult with no classic CNV at baseline.
5. Subgroup analyses of lesions composed of occult with no classic CNV at baseline suggested that the treatment benefit was greater for patients with either smaller lesions (4 disc areas or less) or lower levels of visual acuity [letter score < 65, an approximate Snellen equivalent of 20/50(–1) or worse] at baseline. Continued monitoring is recommended for patients with occult with no classic lesions, similar to those patients enrolled in the VIP trial who did not initially receive treatment when they had relatively large lesions with good visual acuity. In these cases, if visual acuity decreases or predominantly classic features develop, PDT with verteporfin may be considered.

Conclusion

- Verteporfin therapy for subfoveal CNV caused by pathologic myopia safely maintained a visual benefit compared with a placebo therapy through 2 years of follow-up. Although the primary outcome was not statistically significantly in favor of verteporfin therapy at 2 years as it had been at 1 year of follow-up, the distribution of change in visual acuity at the month 24 examination was in favor of the verteporfin-treated group and showed that this group was more likely to have improved visual acuity through the month 24 examination. The VIP Study Group recommends verteporfin therapy for subfoveal CNV resulting from pathologic myopia based on both the 1- and the 2-year results of this randomized clinical trial.
- PDT with verteporfin should be considered for the treatment of patients with AMD with subfoveal lesions composed of occult with no classic CNV who are presumed to have recent disease progression. Patients to be treated should be aware of a small (4%) risk of acute, severe vision decrease.

Visudyne in Minimally Classic Choroidal Neovascularization (VIM)[15]

Purpose

To compare the treatment effect and safety of PDT with verteporfin using a standard (SF) or reduced (RF) light fluence rate with that of placebo therapy in patients with subfoveal minimally classic CNV with AMD.

Description

VIM was a phase 2, multicenter, double-masked, placebo-controlled, randomized clinical trial conducted in 19 ophthalmology practices in North America and Europe. Patients were recruited from 2001 to 2002. 117 patients were randomly assigned (1:1:1) to verteporfin infusion (6 mg/m^2) and light application with an RF rate (300 mW/cm^2) for 83 seconds (light dose of 25 J/cm^2) or an SF rate of 600 mW/cm^2 for 83 seconds (light dose of 50 J/cm^2) or to placebo infusion with RF or SF. Treatment was repeated every 3 months if the treating physician noted fluorescein leakage from CNV on angiography. Patients in whom a predominantly classic lesion developed could receive open-label standard verteporfin treatment.

The best-corrected visual acuity was measured every 3 months, and angiographic changes were assessed by the Photograph Reading Center through the 3-month examination unless an ocular adverse event or conversion to a predominantly classic lesion was identified by an investigator. Safety was assessed throughout the study. All outcomes were on an intent-to-treat basis.

Inclusion Criteria

Patients with the initial best-corrected visual acuity of at least 20/250 and a lesion size of no >6 MPS disc areas were eligible.

Results

103 (88%) of 117 patients completed the 24-month examination. 12 (30%) of 40 patients assigned to placebo received open-label standard verteporfin treatment after confirmation of the presence of predominantly classic CNV. At month 12, a loss of at least 3 lines of visual acuity occurred in 5 (14%) of 36 eyes assigned to RF and 10 (28%) of 36 eyes assigned to SF, compared with 18 (47%) of 38 eyes assigned to placebo (RF, $p = 0.002$; SF, $p = 0.08$; RF + SF, $p = 0.004$). At month 24, this loss occurred in 9 (26%) of 34 eyes assigned to RF and 17 (53%) of 32 eyes assigned to SF, compared with 23 (62%) of 37 eyes assigned to placebo (RF, $p = 0.003$; SF, $p = 0.45$; RF + SF, $p = 0.03$). Progression to predominantly classic CNV by 24 months was more common in the placebo group [11 (28%) of 39 patients compared with 2 (5%) of 38 in the RF group ($p = 0.007$) and 1 (3%) of 37 in the SF group ($p = 0.002$)]. No unexpected ocular or systemic adverse events were identified. Treatment-related, usually transient visual disturbances were 13% with SF, 10% with placebo, and 5% with RF.

Conclusion

Verteporfin therapy safely reduced the risks of losing at least 15 letters (≥3 lines) of visual acuity and progression to predominantly classic CNV for at least 2 years in individuals with subfoveal minimally classic lesions due to AMD measuring 6 MPS disc areas or less. Based on the overall evidence available on verteporfin therapy for these lesions, the VIM Study Group would consider recommending verteporfin therapy for relatively small minimally classic lesions similar to those enrolled in the VIM trial.

Submacular Surgery Trials (SST)[16-19]

Purpose

1. To determine whether surgical removal of subfoveal CNV and associated hemorrhage in patients with AMD, ocular histoplasmosis syndrome (OHS), or idiopathic CNV stabilizes or improves vision more often than observation.
2. To determine how surgical removal compared to observation of subfoveal CNV due to AMD, OHS, or idiopathic causes changes the patient's perception of health- and vision-related "quality of life," as measured by a telephone interview using the Medical Outcomes Survey Short Form-36 (MOS SF-36) instrument, the Hospital Anxiety and Depression Scale, and the National Eye Institute Visual Function Questionnaire 25 (NEI VFQ-25).
3. To determine whether randomized trials of surgery are warranted for patients with subfoveal CNV associated with AMD not suitable for laser treatment.

Background

The MPS group demonstrated that laser treatment is effective for recurrent subfoveal CNV after laser treatment and for selected patients with subfoveal CNV who had no prior treatment. More recently, PDT with verteporfin was shown to reduce the risk of moderate and severe loss of vision in selected patients with subfoveal CNV associated with AMD.

Recently, alternative therapies to laser photocoagulation and PDT have been proposed for the management of CNV and are intended to increase the chance of stabilizing or improving vision at a greater rate than with observation. The most promising of these alternatives at this time is surgical removal of the neovascular lesion, i.e., submacular surgery. The rationale for this surgical approach is that removal of the CNV may halt enlargement of the visual defect, spare photoreceptors in the central macula, and allow adjacent ocular structures to function normally. Data regarding the effectiveness of this approach is limited to reports of case series which suffer from the absence of untreated controls, limited number of cases evaluated, or lack of long-term follow-up to assess the impact of recurrent CNV, delayed atrophy of the outer retina, and adverse outcomes such as cataract and retinal detachment, requiring additional treatment.

Description

The Submacular Surgery Trials comprise a set of multicenter, randomized clinical trials. A total of 19 clinical centers collaborated in conducting a clinical trial for patients with neovascular POH and INVM (Group H protocol). A total of 29 clinical centers collaborated in conducting two additional clinical trials for patients with neovascular AMD (Group B and Group N protocol). A total of 1,015 participants were enrolled in all three trials from May, 1997, till September, 2001.

Vision data collected at baseline include a protocol refraction, best-corrected logMAR visual acuity (ETDRS charts), contrast threshold (Pelli–Robson charts), and reading speed (enlarged text). Other baseline data recorded include stereoscopic color fundus photographs, fluorescein angiograms, and lens photographs as well as health- and vision-related quality-of-life interview data (by telephone).

Eligible patients who gave a signed, informed consent were randomly assigned to surgery (within 8 days of randomization) or observation. Patients, assigned to surgery, are seen 1-month postsurgery for an examination and photographs. All participants are examined at 3, 6, 12, 24, 36, and 48 months after randomization to collect vision data (collected in a masked fashion at 24 and 48 months after randomization) and to repeat photography. Quality-of-life telephone interviews are repeated at 6, 12, 24, 36, and 48 months after randomization.

Inclusion Criteria

Group H (histoplasmosis/idiopathic CNV): Patients with evidence of CNV due to OHS or idiopathic cause, with visual acuity (SST protocol) of 20/50 to 20/800, fluorescein angiographic evidence of subfoveal CNV lesion (new or recurrent after laser photocoagulation) which is < 9 MPS disc areas.

Group B (blood): Patients with evidence of large hemorrhages from subfoveal neovascular AMD lesions (new or recurrent after laser photocoagulation), visual acuity (SST protocol) of 20/100 to light perception, with the area of hemorrhage larger than the area of fluorescein angiographically visible CNV, with any visible CNV < 9 MPS disc areas.

Group N (new CNV): Patients with new CNV (no prior laser) due to AMD, visual acuity (SST protocol) of 20/100 to 20/800, fluorescein angiographic evidence of subfoveal CNV lesion which is < 9 MPS disc areas, with poorly demarcated boundaries.

Study Measures

The primary outcome was improvement in visual acuity from baseline to the 2-year examination or retention of baseline visual acuity through the 2-year examination. Secondary outcomes included change in quality of life from baseline to the 2- and 4-year examinations, change in visual acuity over

4 years, large losses of visual acuity, and adverse ocular outcomes (e.g., those requiring additional treatment such as cataract, retinal detachment, or recurrent CNV).

Results

All evaluated surgically excised CNV specimens consisted of fibrovascular tissue, fibrocellular tissue, or hemorrhage. Surgically excised CNV associated with AMD in this series was larger and often was located beneath the RPE compared with non-AMD CNV, although fewer than half of all the specimens could be oriented by topographic relationship to the RPE.

SST Group H trial

Among 225 patients enrolled, 113 study eyes were assigned to observation and 112 to surgery.

- 46% of the eyes in the observation arm and 55% in the surgery arm had a successful outcome (success ratio, 1.18; 95% confidence interval, 0.89–1.56). The median visual acuity at the 24-month examination was 20/250 among eyes in the observation arm and 20/160 for eyes in the surgery arm. The prespecified subgroup of eyes with visual acuity worse than 20/100 at baseline ($n = 92$) had more successes with surgery: 31 (76%) of 41 eyes in the surgery arm versus 20 (50%) of 40 eyes in the observation arm examined at 24 months (success ratio, 1.53; 95% confidence interval, 1.08–2.16). Recurrent CNV developed by the 24-month examination in 58% of surgically treated eyes.
- 5 (4%) of 111 eyes in the surgery arm subsequently had a rhegmatogenous retinal detachment. 27 (24%) of 112 initially phakic eyes in the surgery arm (none in the observation arm) had cataract surgery during follow-up, all among patients older than 50 years of age.
- Vision-targeted quality of life improved more after submacular surgery than with observation, supporting a possible small overall benefit of surgery suggested by the ophthalmic outcomes.

SST Group B trial

Of 336 patients enrolled, 168 were assigned to each treatment arm.

- Loss of ≥2 lines (≥8 letters) of VA occurred in 56% of surgery eyes versus 59% of observation eyes examined at 24 months. Although severe loss of VA was not the primary outcome of interest, surgery more often prevented such loss: 36% in the observation arm versus 21% in the surgery arm at the 24-month examination ($\chi^2\ p = 0.004$).
- Of initially phakic eyes, the cumulative percentage that had undergone cataract surgery by 24 months was 44% in the surgery arm compared with 6% in the observation arm. 27 eyes (16%) in the surgical arm, compared with 3 eyes (2%) in the observation arm, had a rhegmatogenous retinal detachment.

- No difference was detected with respect to vision-targeted quality-of-life outcomes for patients randomized to surgery or observation.

SST Group N trial

Of 454 patients enrolled, 228 study eyes were assigned to observation and 226 to surgery.
- The percentages of eyes that had successful outcomes were similar in the two arms: 44% assigned to observation and 41% assigned to surgery. Median VA losses from baseline to the 24-month examination were 2.1 lines (10.5 letters) in the observation arm and 2.0 lines (10 letters) in the surgery arm. Median VA declined from 20/100 at baseline to 20/400 at 24 months in both arms. No subgroup of patients was identified in which submacular surgery led to better VA outcomes.
- In the surgery arm, 55 (39%) of 142 initially phakic eyes had cataract surgery by the 24-month examination, compared with 6 (5%) of 133 eyes in the observation arm. Rhegmatogenous retinal detachment occurred in 12 surgery eyes (5%) and 1 observation eye.
- Although health-related quality-of-life outcomes were better in the submacular surgery arm than in the observation arm, surgery (per protocol) is not recommended because VA outcomes were similar in the treatment arms.

Conclusion
- Overall, findings supported no benefit or a smaller benefit to surgery than the trial was designed to detect. Findings support consideration of surgery for eyes with subfoveal CNV and best-corrected visual acuity worse than 20/100 that meet other eligibility criteria for the SST Group H Trial. Other factors that may influence the treatment decision include the risks of retinal detachment, cataract among older patients, and recurrent CNV and the possibility that additional treatment will be required after submacular surgery.
- Submacular surgery, as performed in the SST Group B Trial, did not increase the chance of stable or improved VA (the primary outcome of interest) and was associated with a high-risk of rhegmatogenous RD but did reduce the risk of severe VA loss in comparison with observation.
- Submacular surgery, as performed in the SST Group N Trial, did not improve or preserve VA for 24 months in more eyes than observation and is not recommended for patients with similar lesions.

Table 1: Laser photocoagulation in CNV.

Title	Purpose	Inclusion criteria	No. of patients	Outcome measure	Follow-up	Results	Conclusion
MPS—Argon study 1979	To evaluate laser treatment of CNV (well-demarcated classic)	Extrafoveal CNV in AMD, POH, INVM with VA ≥ 20/100	236, 262, 67	Change in BCVA from baseline	5 years	Relative risk of losing ≥ 6 lines—untreated versus treated—1.5 (AMD), 3.6 (POH)	Laser is beneficial in extrafoveal and juxtafoveal well-demarcated classic CNV
MPS—Krypton study 1979		Juxtafoveal CNV in AMD, POH, INVM with VA ≥ 20/400	496, 288, 49		5 years	Relative risk—1.2 (AMD), 2.6 (POH). Benefit in normotensive AMD patients	
MPS—Foveal study 1979		Subfoveal new (<4 disc areas) or recurrent (<6 disc areas) CNV in AMD with VA 20/320 to 20/40	160 new, 107 recurrent		New—4 years, recurrent—3 years	Effect in recurrent > new	Laser is beneficial in subfoveal classic CNV if small and worse initial VA

(AMD: age-related macular degeneration; BCVA: best-corrected visual acuity; CNV: choroidal neovascularization; INVM: idiopathic neovascular membranes; PDT: photodynamic therapy; POH: presumed ocular histoplasmosis; BA: visual acuity; VA: visual acuity)

Table 2: Photodynamic therapy in choroidal neovascularization.

Title	Purpose	Inclusion criteria	No. of patients	Outcome measure	Follow-up	Results	Conclusion
TAP 1998	PDT in subfoveal CNV in AMD	Subfoveal classic CNV, size ≤ 5,400 μm, VA ≥ 20/100	609—2:1 (402 PDT, 207 placebo)	Eyes with <15 letters VA loss at 2 years	3 monthly for 2 years, retreatment if leakage, extension—5 years	53% of treated versus 38% sham lost <15 letters. Statistically significant in pred classic, not minimally classic	PDT is beneficial in pred classic subfoveal CNV
VIP—myopic CNV 1998	PDT in subfoveal CNV in myopia	Subfoveal CNV, size ≤ 5,400 μm, VA ≥ 20/100	120—2:1	Eyes with < 8 letters VA loss	3 monthly for 2 years, retreatment if leakage	At 1 year, 72% of treated versus 44% sham lost <8 letters. At 2 years, 36% treated versus 51% untreated lost 8 letters	PDT is beneficial in subfoveal CNV in myopia
VIP—CNV in AMD 1998	PDT in subfoveal CNV in AMD, occult or classic with good VA	Subfoveal CNV, size ≤ 5,400 μm, occult—VA ≥ 20/100 with recent progression; classic—VA >20/40	339—2:1	Loss of 15 letters, i.e., moderate vision loss	3 monthly for 2 years, retreatment if leakage	54% of treated versus 67% of untreated lost 15 letters	Occult CNV should be treated with PDT if <4 disc areas, VA < 20/50 or if classic features develop
VIM 2001	SF/RF PDT in subfoveal minimally classic CNV in AMD	Subfoveal, minimally classic, VA ≥ 20/250, lesion size < 6 MPS disc areas	117—1:1:1	Loss of 15 letters	3 monthly for 2 years, retreatment if leakage	Loss of 15 letters occurred in 26% of RF and 53% of SF, compared with 62% of placebo	PDT is beneficial in small subfoveal minimally classic CNV in AMD

Table 3: Submacular surgery trials.

Title	Purpose	Inclusion criteria	No. of patients	Outcome measure	Follow-up	Results	Conclusion
SST-H 1997	Surgical removal of subfoveal CNV in OHS or INVM versus observation	Subfoveal CNV (new or recurrent after laser), < 9 MPS disc areas, VA 20/50 to 20/800	225	Improvement in VA or retention of VA	4 years	46% of the eyes in the observation arm and 55% in the surgery arm had a successful outcome at 2 years	Findings supported no benefit or a smaller benefit to surgery than the trial was designed to detect
SST-B 1997	Surgical removal of subfoveal CNV in AMD versus observation	Large hemorrhages from subfoveal CNV (area of hemorrhage >CNV on FA), VA of 20/100 to light perception	336		2 years	Loss of ≥2 lines (≥8 letters) of VA occurred in 56% of surgery eyes versus 59% of observation eyes examined at 24 months	Submacular surgery did not increase or stabilize VA, high risk of RD, but reduced the risk of severe VA loss compared to observation
SST-N 1997	Surgical removal of subfoveal CNV in AMD versus observation	New subfoveal CNV due to AMD, <9 MPS disc areas, with poorly demarcated boundaries, VA of 20/100 to 20/800	454		2 years	Percentages of eyes that had successful outcomes were similar in the two arms	Submacular surgery that did not improve or preserve VA is not recommended

REFERENCES

1. Macular Photocoagulation Study Group. Argon laser photocoagulation for neovascular maculopathy. Three-year results from randomized clinical trials. Arch Ophthalmol. 1986;104:694-701.
2. Macular Photocoagulation Study Group. Argon laser photocoagulation for neovascular maculopathy. Five-year results from randomized clinical trials. Arch Ophthalmol. 1991;109:1109-14.
3. Macular Photocoagulation Study Group. Krypton laser photocoagulation for neovascular lesions of age-related macular degeneration. Results of a randomized clinical trial. Arch Ophthalmol. 1990;108:816-24.
4. Macular Photocoagulation Study Group. Krypton laser photocoagulation for neovascular lesions of ocular histoplasmosis. Results of a randomized clinical trial. Arch Ophthalmol. 1987;105:1499-507.
5. Macular Photocoagulation Study Group. Krypton laser photocoagulation for idiopathic neovascular lesions. Results of a randomized clinical trial. Arch Ophthalmol. 1990;108:832-37.
6. Macular Photocoagulation Study Group. Laser photocoagulation for juxtafoveal choroidal neovascularization. Five-year results from randomized clinical trials. Arch Ophthalmol. 1994;112:500-9.
7. Macular Photocoagulation Study Group. Laser photocoagulation of subfoveal neovascular lesions of age-related macular degeneration. Updated findings from two clinical trials. Arch Ophthalmol. 1993;111:1200-9.
8. TAP Study Group. Photodynamic therapy of subfoveal choroidal neovascularization in age-related macular degeneration with verteporfin: one-year results of 2 randomized clinical trials—TAP report. Arch Ophthalmol. 1999;117:1329-45.
9. Bressler NM; TAP Study Group. Photodynamic therapy of subfoveal choroidal neovascularization in age-related macular degeneration with verteporfin: two-year results of 2 randomized clinical trials—TAP report 2. Arch Ophthalmol. 2001;119:198-207.
10. Kaiser PK; TAP Study Group: Verteporfin therapy of subfoveal choroidal neovascularization in age-related macular degeneration: 5-year results of two randomized clinical trials with an open-label extension: TAP report no. 8. Graefes Arch Clin Exp Ophthalmol. 2006;244:1132-42.
11. Verteporfin in Photodynamic Therapy Study Group. Photodynamic therapy of subfoveal choroidal neovascularization in pathologic myopia with verteporfin. 1-year results of a randomized clinical trial—VIP report no. 1. Ophthalmology. 2001;108:841-52.
12. Verteporfin in Photodynamic Therapy Study Group. Verteporfin therapy of subfoveal choroidal neovascularization in age-related macular degeneration: two-year results of a randomized clinical trial including lesions with occult with no classic choroidal neovascularization—verteporfin in photodynamic therapy report 2. Am J Ophthalmol. 2001;131:541-60.
13. Blinder KJ, Blumenkranz MS, Bressler NM, Bressler SB, Donato G, Lewis H, et al. Verteporfin therapy of subfoveal choroidal neovascularization in pathologic myopia: 2-year results of a randomized clinical trial—VIP report no. 3. Ophthalmology. 2003;110:667-73.
14. Pieramici DJ, Bressler SB, Koester JM, Bressler NM. Occult with no classic subfoveal choroidal neovascular lesions in age-related macular degeneration: clinically relevant natural history information in larger lesions with good vision from the Verteporfin in Photodynamic Therapy (VIP) Trial: VIP Report No. 4. Arch Ophthalmol. 2006;124:660-4.

15. Visudyne in Minimally Classic Choroidal Neovascularization Study Group; Azab M, Boyer DS, Bressler NM, Cihelkova I, Hao Y, et al. Verteporfin therapy of subfoveal minimally classic choroidal neovascularization in age-related macular degeneration: 2-year results of a randomized clinical trial. Arch Ophthalmol. 2005;123:448-57.
16. Hawkins BS, Bressler NM, Bressler SB, Davidorf FH, Hoskins JC, Marsh MJ, et al. Surgical removal vs observation for subfoveal choroidal neovascularization, either associated with the ocular histoplasmosis syndrome or idiopathic: I. Ophthalmic findings from a randomized clinical trial: Submacular Surgery Trials (SST) Group H Trial: SST Report No. 9. Arch Ophthalmol. 2004;122:1597-611.
17. Submacular Surgery Trials (SST) Research Group; Bressler NM, Bressler SB, Childs AL, Haller JA, Hawkins BS, et al. Surgery for hemorrhagic choroidal neovascular lesions of age-related macular degeneration: ophthalmic findings: SST report no. 13. Ophthalmology. 2004;111:1993-2006.
18. Submacular Surgery Trials (SST) Research Group; Hawkins BS, Bressler NM, Miskala PH, Bressler SB, Holekamp NM, et al. Surgery for subfoveal choroidal neovascularization in age-related macular degeneration: ophthalmic findings: SST report no. 11. Ophthalmology. 2004;111:1967-80.
19. Grossniklaus HE, Green WR. Histopathologic and ultrastructural findings of surgically excised choroidal neovascularization. Submacular Surgery Trials Research Group. Arch Ophthalmol. 1998;116:745-9.

Clinical Trials in Age-related Macular Degeneration –II

Neha Goel, Arpit Sharma, Rohan Chawla

■ INTRODUCTION

Neovascular age-related macular degeneration (AMD) is associated with increased vascular permeability and the development of choroidal neovascularization (CNV). This increase in vascular permeability leads to abnormal intraretinal or subretinal fluid, foveal involvement results in serious visual impairment. Vascular endothelial growth factor (VEGF)-A is a major regulator of angiogenesis and vascular permeability and has been shown to be involved in the development of neovascular AMD.

Therapy targeted against VEGF and its isoforms has revolutionized the treatment of neovascular AMD. In 2004, the US Food and Drug Administration (FDA) approved pegaptanib sodium injection (Macugen, Eyetech), the first anti-VEGF agent to target CNV. In 2006, ranibizumab (Lucentis, Genentech), a humanized monoclonal antibody fragment targeting VEGF-A, was approved by the FDA for the treatment of neovascular AMD. While awaiting FDA approval of ranibizumab, ophthalmologists began treating neovascular AMD with off-label use of bevacizumab, which was approved in 2004 for intravenous treatment of metastatic colon cancer in combination with chemotherapy. Both ranibizumab and bevacizumab were derived from the same murine antibody to VEGF; however, ranibizumab is an anti-VEGF antibody fragment while bevacizumab is a humanized full-length anti-VEGF antibody. On November 18, 2011, VEGF Trap-Eye (aflibercept, EYLEA) was approved by the FDA for the treatment of neovascular AMD. In addition to inhibiting VEGF, aflibercept also blocks the formation of abnormal blood vessels by inhibiting placental growth factor. On October 8, 2019 Brolucizumab (RTH258, Beovu by Novartis), a 26 kD single chain antibody fragment was approved by US FDA for neovascular AMD with every 3 month dosing after 3 monthly injection as loading dose. It inhibits activation of VEGF receptors through prevention of the ligand-receptor interaction.

■ PEGAPTANIB SODIUM (MACUGEN)

VEGF Inhibition Study in Ocular Neovascularization (VISION)[1-3]

Purpose

To assess the vision benefit of treating early subfoveal CNV secondary to AMD with pegaptanib sodium.

Background

Pegaptanib sodium (Macugen) is a pegylated anti-VEGF aptamer. Aptamers are oligonucleotide ligands that are selected for high-affinity binding to molecular targets. Pegaptanib sodium is an RNA aptamer directed against VEGF165, the VEGF isoform primarily responsible for pathologic ocular neovascularization and vascular permeability.

Methods

The VISION study included two concurrent, prospective, randomized, double-masked, multicenter, dose-ranging, controlled phase III clinical trials. 1,186 patients were randomized to sham (0 mg), 0.3 mg, 1.0 mg, or 3.0 mg of the drug. Intravitreal injections were given in one eye per patient every 6 weeks over a period of 48 weeks.

1,053 patients (out of 1,186) continued in the VISION study for a second year. At week 54, those initially assigned to pegaptanib were rerandomized (1:1) to continue or discontinue therapy for 48 more weeks (8 injections). Those initially assigned to sham were rerandomized (1:1:1:1:1) to continue sham, discontinue sham, or receive 1 of 3 pegaptanib doses.

At 102 weeks, subjects receiving pegaptanib 0.3 mg or 1 mg in years 1 or 2 continued (941 out of 1053); those receiving pegaptanib 3 mg or who did not receive treatment in years 1 and 2 were rerandomized to 0.3 mg or 1 mg for year 3.

Inclusion Criteria

Patients with all angiographic choroidal neovascularization lesion compositions of AMD were eligible.

Study Measures

The primary endpoint was proportion of patients avoiding 3 lines of vision loss at 1 year. The secondary endpoints were visual gain (>15 letters) of vision and mean change from baseline visual acuity.

In the second year, mean change in visual acuity (VA) over time and mean change in the standardized area under the curve of VA and proportions of patients experiencing a loss of ≥15 letters from week 54 to week 102; losing <15 letters (responders) from baseline to week 102; gaining ≥0, ≥1, ≥2, and ≥3 lines of VA; and progressing to legal blindness (20/200 or worse) were the outcome measures.

Results

In year 1, 1,190 subjects received at least one study treatment (0.3 mg, $n = 295$; 1 mg, $n = 301$; 3 mg, $n = 296$; sham, $n = 298$); 7,545 intravitreous injections of pegaptanib were administered. In year 2, 425 subjects (0.3 mg, $n = 128$; 1 mg, $n = 126$; 3 mg, $n = 120$; sham, $n = 51$) continued the same masked treatment as in year 1 and received at least one study treatment in year 2; 2,663 intravitreous injections of pegaptanib were administered in these subjects.

At 1 year:
- Efficacy was demonstrated, without a dose-response relationship, for all three doses of pegaptanib ($p <0.001$ for the comparison of 0.3 mg with sham injection; $p <0.001$ for the comparison of 1.0 mg with sham injection; and $p = 0.03$ for the comparison of 3.0 mg with sham injection).
- 70% of treated (0.3 mg) vs. 55% of controls achieved the primary endpoint ($p <0.001$).
- The risk of severe loss of visual acuity (loss of 30 letters or more) was reduced from 22% in the sham-injection group to 10% in the group receiving 0.3 mg of pegaptanib ($p <0.001$).
- More patients receiving pegaptanib (0.3 mg), as compared with sham injection, maintained their visual acuity or gained acuity (33% vs. 23%; $p = 0.003$).
- As early as 6 weeks after beginning therapy with the study drug, and at all subsequent points, the mean visual acuity among patients receiving 0.3 mg of pegaptanib was better than in those receiving sham injections ($p <0.002$).
- Among the adverse events that occurred, endophthalmitis (in 1.3% of patients), traumatic injury to the lens (in 0.7%), and retinal detachment (in 0.6%) were the most serious and required vigilance. These events were associated with a severe loss of visual acuity in 0.1% of patients.

At 2 years:
In combined analysis, mean VA was maintained in patients continuing with 0.3-mg pegaptanib compared with those discontinuing therapy or receiving usual care.
- In patients who continued pegaptanib, the proportion who lost >15 letters from baseline in the period from week 54 to week 102 was half (7%) that of patients who discontinued pegaptanib or remained on usual care (14% for each). Kaplan-Meier analysis showed that patients continuing 0.3-mg pegaptanib for a second year were less likely to lose ≥15 letters than those rerandomized to discontinue after 1 year ($p <0.05$).

- The proportion of patients gaining vision was higher for those assigned to 2 years of 0.3-mg pegaptanib than receiving usual care.
- Progression to legal blindness was reduced for patients continuing 0.3-mg pegaptanib for 2 years.
- In patients receiving pegaptanib for >1 year, there were no reports of endophthalmitis or traumatic cataract in year 2; retinal detachment was reported in 4 patients (all rhegmatogenous, 0.15%/injection).

At 3 years:

As in years 1 and 2, pegaptanib was well-tolerated in year 3. Adverse events were mainly ocular in nature, mild, transient, and injection-related. Serious adverse events were rare. No evidence of systemic safety signals attributed to vascular endothelial growth factor inhibition arose in year 3. There were no findings in relation to vital signs or electrocardiogram results suggesting a relationship to pegaptanib treatment.

Conclusion

Continuing visual benefit was observed in patients who were randomized to receive therapy with pegaptanib in year 2 of the VISION trials when compared with 2 years' usual care or cessation of therapy at year 1. The 3 year safety profile of pegaptanib sodium was favorable in patients with neovascular AMD.

RANIBIZUMAB (LUCENTIS)

Anti-VEGF Antibody for the Treatment of Predominantly Classic Choroidal Neovascularization in AMD (ANCHOR)[4-6]

Purpose

To compare ranibizumab (RBZ) with photodynamic therapy (PDT) with Verteporfin in the treatment of predominantly classic neovascular AMD.

Background

Ranibizumab (Lucentis; Genentech, South San Francisco, California) is a recombinant, humanized, monoclonal antibody antigen-binding fragment that neutralizes all VEGF-A isoforms. In phase 1 and 2 clinical studies, RBZ demonstrated encouraging signs of biologic activity, with acceptable safety, when administered intravitreally for up to 6 months in patients with neovascular AMD.

Description

It was a multicenter, randomized, double-blind, active-treatment–controlled study. Patients were randomly assigned into one of three groups:
1. PDT with verteporfin every 3 months as needed plus a monthly sham intravitreal injection ($n = 143$);

2. 0.3 mg intravitreal RBZ with sham PDT (saline) as needed every 3 months (*n* = 140); or
3. 0.5 mg with sham PDT (saline) as needed every 3 months (*n* = 140).

In the group that received PDT with verteporfin, intravenous administration of verteporfin was followed by laser irradiation of the macula, according to instructions provided in the product package insert. In the RBZ groups, sham verteporfin therapy was achieved by an intravenous infusion of saline rather than verteporfin, followed by laser irradiation of the macula identical to that in the active verteporfin-therapy group.

Ranibizumab was injected into the study eye at a monthly interval (ranging from 23 to 37 days, for a total of 12 injections, excluding the injection at month 12) in the first year, beginning on day 0. The PDT therapy or sham PDT therapy was administered at Study Day 0 and then quarterly as needed based on the investigator's evaluation of fluorescein angiography (FA) every 3 months. A subset (*n* = 61) had optical coherence tomography (OCT) assessments.

Inclusion Criteria

Patients with predominantly classic, subfoveal CNV not previously treated with PDT or anti-angiogenic drugs were eligible. Patients had to be more than 50 years of age; have a lesion whose total size was no more than 5,400 μm in greatest linear dimension; have BCVA of 20/40 to 20/320 (Snellen equivalent); have no permanent structural damage to the central fovea; and have had no previous treatment. No patients were excluded because of preexisting cardiovascular, cerebrovascular, or peripheral vascular conditions.

Study Measures

The primary, intent-to-treat efficacy analysis was at 12 months, with continued measurements to month 24. Key measures included the percentage losing <15 letters from baseline visual acuity (VA) score (month 12 primary efficacy outcome measure), percentage gaining ≥15 letters from baseline, and mean change over time in VA score and FA-assessed lesion characteristics. Adverse events were monitored.

Results

- Of the 423 patients enrolled (143 PDT, 140 each in the 2 RBZ groups), 94.3% of those given 0.3 mg of RBZ and 96.4% of those given 0.5 mg lost fewer than 15 letters, as compared with 64.3% of those in the verteporfin group (p <0.001 for each comparison). Visual acuity improved by 15 letters or more in 35.7% of the 0.3-mg group and 40.3% of the 0.5-mg group, as compared with 5.6% of the verteporfin group (p <0.001 for each comparison). Mean visual acuity increased by 8.5 letters in the

0.3-mg group and 11.3 letters in the 0.5-mg group, as compared with a decrease of 9.5 letters in the verteporfin group ($p <0.001$ for each comparison). Among 140 patients treated with 0.5 mg of RBZ, presumed endophthalmitis occurred in 2 patients (1.4%) and serious uveitis in 1 (0.7%).
- Of 423 patients, the majority completed the 2-year study. Consistent with results at month 12, at month 24 the VA benefit from RBZ was statistically significant and clinically meaningful: 89.9–90.0% of RBZ-treated patients had lost <15 letters from baseline (vs. 65.7% of PDT patients); 34–41.0% had gained ≥15 letters (vs. 6.3% of PDT group); and, on average, VA was improved from baseline by 8.1–10.7 letters (vs. a mean decline of 9.8 letters in PDT group). Changes in lesion anatomic characteristics on FA also favored RBZ (all comparisons $p <0.0001$ vs. PDT). Overall, there was no imbalance among groups in rates of serious ocular and nonocular adverse events. In the pooled RBZ groups, 3 of 277 (1.1%) patients developed presumed endophthalmitis in the study eye. The rate of presumed endophthalmitis in the study eye per injection was 3 of 5,921 injections (0.05%) in the RBZ groups.
- At months 12 and 24, RBZ was superior to PDT ($p <0.0001$) for mean changes from baseline in total area of lesion, CNV area, and total area CNV leakage. Month 12 OCT showed greater center point thickness decrease from baseline with RBZ than with PDT ($p = 0.0003$). RBZ benefits over PDT were evident by 3 months (fluorescein angiography) and 7 days (OCT).
- Lower baseline VA score, smaller baseline CNV lesion size, and younger baseline age were associated with greater gain of letters with RBZ treatment and less loss of letters with PDT.

Conclusion

Ranibizumab administered as monthly intravitreal injections of 0.3 mg or 0.5 mg over a 24-month period was effective, and superior to PDT treatment, in maintaining or improving VA and lesion characteristics inpatients with new onset, predominantly classic subfoveal neovascular AMD. Rates of serious adverse events were low.

Minimally Classic/Occult Trial of the Anti-VEGF Antibody Ranibizumab in the Treatment of Neovascular ARMD (MARINA)[7-9]

Purpose

To evaluate the role of RBZ in the treatment of minimally classic/occult neovascular ARMD.

Background

While the ANCHOR trial investigated efficacy of RBZ only in predominantly classic CNV, its sister study, MARINA, evaluated the efficacy of RBZ in nonclassic (minimally classic and occult) CNV.

Description

At 96 sites in the United States, 716 patients were enrolled in this 2-year, prospective, randomized, double-blind, sham-controlled study of the safety and efficacy of repeated intravitreal injections of RBZ in minimally classic or occult CNV in AMD. Eligible patients were randomly assigned in a 1:1:1 ratio to receive monthly:
- Sham ($n = 238$)
- 0.3 mg RBZ ($n = 238$)
- 0.5 mg RBZ ($n = 240$)

Injections in the study eye for 24 months. Verteporfin PDT was allowed if the CNV in the study eye became predominantly classic.

Stereoscopic fundus photography and FA were done at baseline and months 3, 6, 12, and 24. OCT was performed at a subset of investigative sites (46 patients) at baseline, day 7, and months 1 and 12.

Inclusion Criteria

Patients with age >50 years old; BCVA 20/40 to 20/320; primary or recurrent CNV associated with AMD, involving the foveal center; minimally classic or occult with no classic CNV; maximum lesion size of 12 optic-disc areas, and presumed recent progression of disease were eligible. There were no exclusion criteria regarding preexisting cardiovascular, cerebrovascular, or peripheral vascular conditions.

Study Measures

The primary efficacy analysis was at 12 months, with continued measurements to month 24. The main outcome measures included the percentage losing <15 letters from baseline VA score (month 12 primary efficacy outcome measure), percentage gaining ≥15 letters from baseline and mean change over time in VA score.

Results

716 patients were enrolled in the study.
- At 12 months, 94.5% of the group given 0.3 mg of RBZ and 94.6% of those given 0.5 mg lost fewer than 15 letters, as compared with 62.2% of patients receiving sham injections. At 24 months, 90.0% of patients in the 0.5 mg RBZ group and 52.9% of those in the sham injection group met the primary goal ($p < 0.0001$).

- Visual acuity improved by 15 or more letters in 24.8% of the 0.3-mg group and 33.8% of the 0.5-mg group, as compared with 5.0% of the sham-injection group. The benefit in visual acuity was maintained at 24 months.
- At 12 months, mean increases in visual acuity were 6.5 letters in the 0.3-mg group and 7.2 letters in the 0.5-mg group, as compared with a decrease of 10.4 letters in the sham-injection group ($p < 0.001$ for both comparisons). At 24 months, patients in the 0.5 mg RBZ group gained 6.6 letters, compared with a mean loss of 14.9 letters in the sham injection group ($p < 0.001$).
- At 12 and 24 months, statistically significant benefits of RBZ over sham treatment were observed for mean change from baseline in the areas of CNV lesion, total CNV, leakage from CNV, SSRD, and disciform scar/subretinal fibrosis. At 12 months (final OCT), the mean change in foveal center point thickness on OCT was a significant decrease in the RBZ group compared with the sham group.
- During 24 months, presumed endophthalmitis was identified in five patients (1.0%) and serious uveitis in six patients (1.3%) given RBZ.
- The most important predictors of VA outcomes were, in decreasing order of importance, baseline VA score, CNV lesion size, and age.

Conclusion

The MARINA trial demonstrated that patients treated with RBZ for nonclassic neovascular AMD had substantially better VA outcomes than those who received sham injections. In addition, patients treated with RBZ showed stabilization of lesion size in contrast to increases in the sham group. These efficacy outcomes were achieved with a low rate of serious ocular adverse events and with no clear difference from the sham-treated group in the rate of nonocular adverse events.

Phase IIIb, Multicenter, Randomized, Double-masked, Sham Injection-controlled Study of Efficacy and Safety of Ranibizumab in Subjects with Subfoveal CNV with or without Classic CNV Secondary to AMD (PIER)[10,11]

Purpose

To evaluate the efficacy and safety of RBZ administered monthly for 3 months and then quarterly in patients with subfoveal CNV secondary to AMD.

Background

MARINA and ANCHOR collectively showed the efficacy of RBZ in both classic and nonclassic neovascular AMD. Both studies relied on monthly injections over a 24-month period. The most significant visual gain occurred in the first

3 months with stabilization over the next 21 months. Following the MARINA and ANCHOR trials, several studies looked at ways to decrease the treatment burden while maintaining similar visual gains. These trials include PIER, EXCITE, PrONTO, SUSTAIN, and HORIZON.

Description

It was a Phase IIIb, multicenter, randomized, double-masked, sham injection-controlled trial in patients with predominantly or minimally classic or occult with no classic CNV lesions. A total of 184 patients were randomized 1:1:1 to 0.3 mg RBZ ($n = 60$), 0.5 mg RBZ ($n = 61$), or sham ($n = 63$) treatment groups. During study year 2, eligible sham-group patients crossed over to 0.5 mg RBZ quarterly. Later in year 2, all eligible randomized patients rolled over to 0.5 mg RBZ monthly.

Inclusion Criteria

All lesion types were eligible for the PIER study if the active CNV accounted for at least 50% of the total lesion.

Study Measures

The primary efficacy endpoint was mean change from baseline VA at month 12. Key visual outcomes at month 24 were mean change from baseline VA, proportion of patients who lost <15 VA letters from baseline, proportion of patients who gained ≥15 VA letters from baseline, and mean change from baseline of total area of CNV.

Results

At month 12, mean changes from baseline VA at 12 months were -16.3, -1.6, and -0.2 letters for the sham, 0.3 mg, and 0.5 mg groups, respectively ($p \geq 0.0001$, each RBZ dose vs. sham). RBZ arrested CNV growth and reduced leakage from CNV. However, the treatment effect declined in the RBZ groups during quarterly dosing (e.g., at 3 months the mean changes from baseline VA had been gains of 2.9 and 4.3 letters for the 0.3 mg and 0.5 mg doses, respectively). Results of subgroups analyses of mean change from baseline VA at 12 months by baseline age, VA, and lesion characteristics were consistent with the overall results. Few serious ocular or nonocular adverse events occurred in any group.

At month 24, visual acuity had decreased an average of 21.4, 2.2, and 2.3 letters from baseline in the sham, 0.3 mg, and 0.5 mg groups ($p <0.0001$ for each RBZ group vs. sham). 78.2% patients in the 0.3 mg group and 82.0% in the 0.5 mg group had lost <15 letters from baseline VA compared with 41.3% sham-injection patients ($p <0.0001$). VA of sham patients who crossed over (and subsequently rolled over) to RBZ decreased across time, with an average loss of 3.5 letters 10 months after crossover. VA of 0.3 mg and 0.5 mg group patients who rolled over to monthly RBZ increased for an average gain of 2.2 and 4.1 letters, respectively, 4 months after rollover. The ocular safety profile of RBZ was favorable and consistent with previous reports.

Conclusion

Ranibizumab administered monthly for 3 months and then quarterly, provided significant VA benefit to patients with AMD-related subfoveal CNV and was well-tolerated. However, with the quarterly dosing, there was a steady decline in VA during months 4 through 24 in PIER compared to the VA stabilization achieved in ANCHOR and MARINA with monthly RBZ injections. RBZ appeared to provide additional VA benefit to treated patients who rolled over to monthly dosing, but not to patients who began receiving RBZ after >14 months of sham injections. The incidence of serious ocular or nonocular adverse events was low.

Efficacy and Safety of Ranibizumab in Patients with Subfoveal CNV Secondary to AMD (EXCITE)[12]

Purpose

To demonstrate noninferiority of a quarterly treatment regimen to a monthly regimen of RBZ in patients with subfoveal CNV secondary to AMD.

Description

It was a 12-month, multicenter, randomized, double-masked, active-controlled, phase IIIb study. A total of 353 patients were enrolled in the study and randomized 1:1:1, comparing the PIER quarterly regimen [0.3 mg (n = 120) and 0.5 mg (n = 118)] with the ANCHOR/MARINA monthly injections of 0.3 mg RBZ (n = 115) for classic and nonclassic subfoveal neovascular AMD. Treatment comprised of a loading phase (3 consecutive monthly injections) followed by a 9-month maintenance phase (either monthly or quarterly injection).

Study Measures

Mean change in BCVA measured by ETDRS charts and central retinal thickness (CRT) from baseline to month 12 and the incidence of adverse events (AEs) were evaluated.

Results

- There was a prompt increase in vision with the initial 3 monthly injections in all three arms. At 3 months the 0.3 mg monthly arm had a +7.5 ETDRS letter gain. The 0.3 mg and 0.5 mg quarterly injection arms had a +6.8 and

+6.6 ETDRS letter gains, respectively. As seen previously in ANCHOR/MARINA, the monthly injection arm maintained its visual gain over the 12-month period with a final visual gain of +8.3 ETDRS letters at 12 months. In the quarterly injection arm the visual gain declined over the 12-month period with a final VA gain of +4.9 letters and +3.8 letters in the 0.3 mg and 0.5 mg quarterly RBZ, respectively.
- In the per-protocol population (293 patients), BCVA, increased from baseline to month 12 by 4.9, 3.8, and 8.3 letters in the 0.3 mg quarterly (104 patients), 0.5 mg quarterly (88 patients), and 0.3 mg monthly (101 patients) dosing groups, respectively. Similar results were observed in the intent-to-treat (ITT) population (353 patients).
- The mean decrease in CRT from baseline to month 12 in the ITT population was -96.0 µm in 0.3 mg quarterly, -105.6 µm in 0.5 mg quarterly, and -105.3 µm in 0.3 mg monthly group.
- The most frequent ocular AEs were conjunctival hemorrhage (17.6%, pooled quarterly groups; 10.4%, monthly group) and eye pain (15.1%, pooled quarterly groups; 20.9%, monthly group). There were 9 ocular serious AEs and 3 deaths; 1 death was suspected to be study-related (cerebral hemorrhage; 0.5 mg quarterly group). The incidences of key arterial thromboembolic events were low.

Conclusion

After 3 initial monthly RBZ injections, both monthly (0.3 mg) and quarterly (0.3 mg/0.5 mg) RBZ treatments maintained BCVA in patients with CNV secondary to AMD. At month 12, BCVA gain in the monthly regimen was higher than that of the quarterly regimens. The noninferiority of a quarterly regimen was not achieved with reference to 5.0 letters. The safety profile was similar to that reported in prior RBZ studies. The three arms of EXCITE validated the results of ANCHOR, MARINA, and PIER trials with RBZ monthly intravitreal injections demonstrating the best VA outcomes.

Prospective Optical Coherence Tomography Imaging of Patients with Neovascular AMD Treated with Intraocular Ranibizumab (PrONTO)[13,14]

Purpose

To evaluate an OCT-guided, variable-dosing regimen with intravitreal RBZ for the treatment of patients with neovascular AMD.

Description

It was a 2-year, open-label, prospective, single-center, uncontrolled, nonrandomized, investigator-sponsored clinical study. A total of 40 patients, age 50 years and older, with subfoveal CNV and a central retinal thickness

(CRT) of at least 300 μm as measured by OCT were enrolled and 37 completed the 2-year study. Patients received three consecutive monthly intravitreal injections of 0.5 mg RBZ. After the first three monthly injections, retreatment with RBZ was performed at each subsequent monthly visit if any of the five different retreatment criteria was met:
1. VA loss of at least five letters with OCT evidence of fluid in the macula
2. An increase in OCT CRT of at least 100 μm
3. New macular hemorrhage
4. New area of classic CNV
5. Evidence of persistent fluid on OCT 1 month after the previous injection.

During the second year, the retreatment criteria were amended to include retreatment if any qualitative increase in the amount of fluid was detected using OCT.

Inclusion Criteria

The study included AMD patients with subfoveal CNV and a CRT of at least 300 μm as measured by OCT.

Study Measures

The major 2-year outcome measurements in the PrONTO study were the change in VA scores and OCT measurements from baseline, OCT-CRT measurements, and the total number of injections received by a patient during 2 years.

Results

At month 12, the mean visual acuity improved by 9.3 letters ($p < 0.001$) and the mean OCT CRT decreased by 178 μm ($p < 0.001$). Visual acuity improved 15 or more letters in 35% of patients. These visual acuity and OCT outcomes were achieved with an average of 5.6 injections over 12 months. After a fluid-free macula was achieved, the mean injection-free interval was 4.5 months before another reinjection was necessary.

At month 24, the mean VA improved by 11.1 letters ($p < 0.0001$) and the OCT-CRT decreased by 212 μm ($p < 0.0001$). These outcomes were achieved with a mean number of injections of 5.6 over the course of 1 year and 9.9 injections over 2 years. The most common reason for retreatment was loss of ≥5 letters of VA with evidence of fluid detected on macular OCT. After 12 months, VA improved at least three lines in 35% of patients and in 43% of patients by month 24. During the 2-year study period, a total of 386 injections were performed with no episodes of endophthalmitis or uveitis. There were no ATEs or deaths attributable to the injection of RBZ.

Conclusion

The PrONTO study was designed to minimize the number of retreatments but not the number of visits. The use of an OCT-guided variable-dosing regimen with RBZ resulted in VA outcomes similar to results from the Phase III MARINA and ANCHOR studies while averaging 59% less (9.9 vs. 24) injections over 2 years. Without a control group, it is unknown whether the eyes in PrONTO study would have done even better with monthly dosing.

Study of Ranibizumab in Patients with Subfoveal CNV Secondary to AMD (SUSTAIN)[15]

Purpose
To evaluate the safety and efficacy of individualized RBZ treatment (PRN regime) in patients with neovascular AMD.

Description
It was a 12-month; prospective, phase III, multicenter, open-label, single-arm study. A total of 513 RBZ-naïve patients were included. Three initial monthly injections of RBZ (0.3 mg) and thereafter pro re nata (PRN) retreatment for 9 months were administered if either of the following two retreatment criteria are met:
1. More than 5-letter loss in VA from the previous highest VA score during the first 3 months; or
2. 100 μm increase in CRT from the previous lowest measurement during the first 3 months.
   Patients switched to 0.5 mg RBZ after approval in Europe.

Study Measures
Frequency of adverse events, monthly change of best-corrected visual acuity (BCVA) and central retinal thickness (CRT) from baseline, the time to first retreatment, and the number of treatments were assessed.

Results
- A total of 249 patients (48.5%) reported ocular AEs, and 8 (1.5%) deaths, 5 (1.2%) patients with ocular serious AEs of the study eye (retinal hemorrhage, cataract, retinal pigment epithelial tear, reduced visual acuity, vitreous hemorrhage), and 19 (3.7%) patients with arteriothromboembolic events were observed. Most frequent AEs in the study eye were reduced VA (18.5%), retinal hemorrhage (7.2%), increased intraocular pressure (7.0%), and conjunctival hemorrhage (5.5%).
- The average number of retreatments from months 3 to 11 was 2.7.
- Mean BCVA increased steadily from baseline to month 3 to reach +5.8 letters, decreased slightly from month 3 to 6, and remained stable from month 6 to 12, reaching +3.6 at month 12.
- Mean change in CRT was -101.1 μm from baseline to month 3 and -91.5 μm from baseline to month 12.

Conclusion

Like PrONTO, early results from the SUSTAIN trial have shown a rapid increase in VA in the first 3 months, which deteriorates slightly, but not nearly as much as in PIER, over the 9 months of PRN dosing. Visual acuity in SUSTAIN patients with individualized retreatment based on VA/OCT assessment reached on average a maximum after the first 3 monthly injections, decreased slightly under PRN during the next 2–3 months, and was then sustained throughout the treatment period. The safety results were comparable to the favorable tolerability profile of RBZ observed in previous pivotal clinical studies; individualized treatment with less than monthly retreatments showed a similar safety profile as observed in previous randomized clinical trials with monthly RBZ treatment. Efficacy outcomes were achieved with a low average number of retreatments.

PHase III, Double-masked, Multicenter, Randomized, Active Treatment-controlled Study of the Efficacy and Safety of 0.5 mg and 2.0 mg Ranibizumab Administered Monthly or on an As-needed Basis (PRN) in Patients with Subfoveal neOvasculaR Age-related Macular Degeneration (HARBOR)[16]

Purpose

To evaluate the 12-month efficacy and safety of intravitreal RBZ 0.5 mg and 2.0 mg administered monthly and on an as-needed (PRN) basis in treatment-naïve patients with subfoveal neovascular AMD.

Description

It was a 24-month, phase III, randomized, multicenter, double-masked, dose-response study of patients aged ≥50 years with subfoveal wet AMD (2009–2012). 1,098 patients were randomized to receive RBZ 0.5 mg or 2.0 mg intravitreal injections administered monthly or on a PRN basis after 3 monthly loading doses.

Inclusion Criteria

Men and women aged 50 years or more with CNV lesions <12 disc areas and BCVA 20/40–20/320 (Snellen equivalent) were eligible.

Study Measures

The primary efficacy end point was the mean change from baseline in BCVA at month 12. Key secondary end points included the mean number of RBZ injections, the mean change from baseline in central foveal thickness (CFT) over time, and the proportion of patients who gained ≥15 letters of BCVA. Unless otherwise specified, end point analyses were performed using the last-observation-carried-forward method to impute missing data.

Results

At month 12, the mean change from baseline in BCVA for the 4 groups was +10.1 letters (0.5 mg monthly), +8.2 letters (0.5 mg PRN), +9.2 letters (2.0 mg monthly), and +8.6 letters (2.0 mg PRN). The proportion of patients who gained ≥15 letters from baseline at month 12 in the 4 groups was 34.5%, 30.2%, 36.1%, and 33.0%, respectively. The mean change from baseline in CFT at month 12 in the 4 groups was -172.0 μm, -161.2 μm, -163.3 μm, and -172.4 μm, respectively. The mean number of injections was 7.7 and 6.9 for the 0.5-mg PRN and 2.0-mg PRN groups, respectively. Ocular and systemic safety profiles were consistent with previous RBZ trials in AMD and comparable between groups.

Conclusions At month 12, the RBZ 2.0-mg monthly group did not meet the prespecified superiority comparison and the RBZ 0.5-mg and 2.0-mg PRN groups did not meet the prespecified noninferiority (NI) comparison. However, all treatment groups demonstrated clinically meaningful visual improvement (+8.2 to +10.1 letters) and improved anatomic outcomes, with the PRN groups requiring approximately 4 fewer injections (6.9-7.7) than the monthly groups (11.2-11.3). No new safety events were observed despite a 4-fold dose escalation in the study. The HARBOR study confirmed that RBZ 0.5 mg dosed monthly provides optimum results in patients with wet AMD. There is no additional benefit from the high dose (2.0 mg) in treatment-naïve wet AMD patients.

Safety Assessment of Intravitreal Lucentis for AMD (SAILOR)[17,18]

Purpose

To evaluate the safety and efficacy of intravitreal RBZ in a large population of subjects with neovascular AMD.

Description

It was a 12-month randomized (cohort 1) or open-label (cohort 2) multicenter, phase IIIb clinical trial. A total of 4,300 subjects with angiographically determined subfoveal CNV secondary to AMD were included.

Cohort 1 subjects were randomized 1:1 to receive 0.3 mg (n = 1,169) or 0.5 mg (n = 1,209) intravitreal RBZ for 3 monthly loading doses. Dose groups were stratified by AMD treatment history (treatment-naïve vs. previously treated). Cohort 1 subjects were retreated on the basis of OCT or visual acuity (VA) criteria. Cohort 2 subjects (n = 1,922) received an initial intravitreal dose of 0.5 mg RBZ and were retreated at physician discretion. Safety was evaluated at all visits.

Study Measures

Safety outcomes included the incidence of ocular and nonocular adverse events and serious adverse events (SAEs). Efficacy outcomes included changes in BCVA over time.

Results

81.7% of cohort 1 subjects and 49.9% of cohort 2 subjects completed the 12-month study. The average total number of RBZ injections was 4.9 for cohort 1 and 3.6 for cohort 2.

- The rates of individual key ocular SAEs, which included endophthalmitis or presumed endophthalmitis, were similar in both cohorts (<1%).
- The rates of key nonocular SAEs and ATEs were similar across cohort 1 dose groups, but were generally lower in cohort 2. Nonvascular death, stroke, and hemorrhage rates were numerically higher in the 0.5 mg group. The incidence of nonocular AEs potentially related to anti-VEGF therapy was low and similar across cohorts and dose groups.
- The incidence of vascular and nonvascular deaths during the 12-month study was 0.9% and 0.7% in the cohort 1 0.3 mg group, 0.8% and 1.5% in the cohort 1 0.5 mg group, and 0.7% and 0.9% in cohort 2, respectively. The incidence of death due to unknown cause was 0.1% in both cohort 1 dose groups and cohort 2. The number of vascular deaths and deaths due to unknown cause did not differ across cohorts or dose groups.
- Stroke rates were 0.7%, 1.2%, and 0.6% in the 0.3 mg and 0.5 mg groups and cohort 2, respectively. A prior history of stroke, arrhythmia, and congestive heart failure was a significant risk factor for stroke.
- At month 12, cohort 1 treatment-naïve subjects had gained an average of 0.5 (0.3 mg) and 2.3 (0.5 mg) VA letters and previously treated subjects had gained 1.7 (0.3 mg) and 2.3 (0.5 mg) VA letters.

Conclusion

Intravitreal RBZ was safe and well-tolerated in a large population of subjects with neovascular AMD. SAILOR was able to demonstrate that the incidence of cerebrovascular and cardiovascular adverse events was similar to that observed in previous RBZ studies. RBZ had a beneficial effect on VA. Unfortunately, SAILOR did not have a sham control arm. The safety results do not differentiate between the inherent risks of intravitreal RBZ versus an elderly control subject population. Although the risks of arterial thromboembolic events related to RBZ are low, ophthalmologists should be aware of these risks to appropriately educate and treat patients with neovascular AMD. Future investigations will seek to establish optimal dosing regimens for persons with neovascular AMD.

Extension Trial of Ranibizumab for Neovascular Age-related Macular Degeneration (HORIZON)[19]

Purpose
To evaluate the long-term safety and efficacy of multiple intravitreal RBZ injections administered at the investigator's discretion in patients with CNV secondary to AMD.

Description
The HORIZON Study is an open-label, multicenter, 2-year extension study investigating the safety and efficacy of RBZ in neovascular AMD for patients who completed either the ANCHOR, MARINA, or FOCUS trials. The 853 patients enrolled in HORIZON could receive additional 0.5 mg RBZ injection in the same study eye as in the initial study at intervals no more frequently than every 30 days, up to a maximum of 12 injections per year. The frequency of the injections was at the discretion of investigators. The patients were categorized into three groups:
1. Patients treated with RBZ in the initial study (RBZ treated-initial; $n = 600$);
2. Patients randomized to control who crossed over to receive RBZ (RBZ treated-XO; $n = 190$)
3. RBZ-naïve patients (RBZ untreated; $n = 63$).

Inclusion Criteria
Patients who completed the controlled treatment phase of 1 of 3 prospective, randomized, 2-year clinical trials of RBZ were eligible for enrollment.

Study Measures
The primary outcome measure was the incidence and severity of ocular and nonocular adverse events. The secondary outcome measure was BCVA assessed every 3 months.

Results
In the initial-RBZ-treated group, 69% received additional injections with mean of 3.6 injections over a 2-year period.
- There was 1 occurrence of mild endophthalmitis per 3,552 HORIZON injections in the RBZ treated-initial/RBZ treated-XO groups.
- There were no serious AE reports of lens damage, retinal tears, or rhegmatogenous retinal detachments in the study eyes.
- The proportion of patients with any single post dose intraocular pressure ≥30 mm Hg was 9.2%, 6.6%, and 0%, and the proportion of patients with glaucoma was 3.2%, 4.2%, and 3.2% in the RBZ treated-initial, RBZ treated-XO, and RBZ untreated groups, respectively.
- Cataract AEs were less frequent in the RBZ untreated group: 6.3% versus 12.5% and 12.1% in the RBZ treated-initial and RBZ treated-XO groups, respectively.

- The proportion of patients with arterial thromboembolic events as defined by the Antiplatelet Trialists' Collaboration was 5.3% in the RBZ treated-initial and RBZ treated-XO groups, and 3.2% in the RBZ untreated group.
- 24-month VA results were available on 384 of 600 initially treated patients. These 384 patients experienced a three line Snellen VA improvement (20/100 to 20/50), in the original trials. With 2 years of PRN dosing in HORIZON, VA decreased two lines from a baseline of 20/50 to 20/80.
- At month 48 (2 years of HORIZON), the mean change in BCVA (ETDRS letters) relative to the initial study baseline was 2.0 in the RBZ treated-initial group versus -11.8 in the pooled RBZ treated-XO and RBZ untreated groups.

Conclusion

Multiple RBZ injections were well-tolerated for ≥4 years. The incidence of serious ocular and nonocular AEs during the 2-year study period of HORIZON trial were low and consistent with those observed during the 24 months of treatment in the prior Phase III trials. With less frequent follow-up leading to less treatment, there was an incremental decline of the VA gains achieved with monthly treatment.

Seven-year Outcomes in Ranibizumab-treated Patients in ANCHOR, MARINA, and HORIZON: A Multicenter Cohort Study[20,21]

Purpose

Seven years outcomes in Ranibizumab-treated patients in ANCHOR, MARINA and HORIZON trials (Seven Up study)

Description

The participants in ANCHOR and MARINA trials were among the earliest patients to receive ranibizumab therapy. Upon completion, these subjects were also eligible to enter the HORIZON extension study. This accounted for a unique AMD patient cohort providing longest ranibizumab treatment period within a clinical trial protocol (4 years) and the longest duration of follow-up available at that time (7–8 years).

7–8 years after being enrolled in the ANCHOR or MARINA trials, 65 patients with exudative AMD were recalled for evaluation. This group had received 2 years of monthly ranibizumab treatment, followed by an additional 2 years of as-needed ranibizumab treatment in the HORIZON protocol.

It was a multicenter, cross-sectional 7 year update of this unique cohort.

Study Measures

The primary end point was percentage with best-corrected visual acuity (BCVA) of 20/70 or better; secondary outcomes included mean change in letter score compared with previous time points and anatomic results on fluorescein angiography, spectral-domain ocular coherence tomography (OCT), and fundus autofluorescence (FAF).

Results
At a mean of 7 years after entry into ANCHOR or MARINA, 37% of study eyes had 20/70 or better BCVA (23% had BCVA of 20/40 or better).
- 37% of study eyes had BCVA of 20/200 or worse.
- 43% of study eyes had a stable or improved letter score compared with ANCHOR or MARINA baseline measurements, whereas 34% declined by 15 letters or more, with overall a mean decline of 8.6 letters ($p < 0.005$).
- Since exit from the HORIZON study, study eyes received a mean of 6.8 VEGF injections during the mean 3.4-year interval; a subgroup of patients who received 11 or more anti-VEGF injections had a significantly better mean gain in letter score since HORIZON exit ($p < 0.05$).
- Active exudative disease was detected by spectral-domain OCT in 68% of study eyes, and 46% were receiving ongoing ocular anti-VEGF treatments.
- Macular atrophy was detected by FAF in 98% of eyes, with a mean area of 9.4 mm^2; the area of atrophy correlated significantly with poor visual outcome ($p < 0.0001$).

Conclusions
Approximately 7 years after ranibizumab therapy in the ANCHOR or MARINA trials, one-third of patients demonstrated good visual outcomes, whereas another third had poor outcomes. Compared with baseline, almost half of eyes were stable, whereas one third declined by 15 letters or more. More alarming, macular atrophy was detected by FAF in 98% of all studied eyes, with the area of atrophy mainly localized in the fovea and significantly correlated with a poor visual outcome. Even at this late stage in the therapeutic course, exudative AMD patients remain at risk for substantial visual decline.

Comment
This study further raises question of whether pan-VEGF suppression is linked with macular atrophy. However, direct cause-effect relation cannot be concluded.

The Port Delivery System with Ranibizumab for Neovascular Age-related Macular Degeneration: Results from the Randomized Phase 2 Ladder Clinical Trial[22]

Purpose
To evaluate the safety and efficacy of the Port Delivery System with ranibizumab (PDS) for neovascular age-related macular degeneration (nAMD) treatment.

Background

Though monthly anti-VEGF injections have provided 1-2 lines of improvement in vision in nAMD patients in clinical trials the same has not been translated to the real-world scenario. A major problem may be the frequent requirement of patient visits and injections.

The PDS is a novel, long-acting drug delivery system that contains a refillable implant. It is surgically implanted through a small incision in the pars plana. Drug can be replenishment through a self-sealing septum without the need to remove the implant. Ranibizumab moves by diffusion down a concentration gradient through a porous control into the vitreous cavity.

Description

This was a phase 2, multicenter, randomized, active treatment controlled, dose-ranging trial and was conducted at 49 sites in the United States.

Inclusion Criteria

- Newly diagnosed with wet AMD within 9 months of diagnosis
- Participant must have received at least 2 prior anti-VEGF (any) injections. However, the last anti-VEGF injection must have been ranibizumab and must have occurred at least 7 days prior to the screening visit
- Demonstrated response to anti-VEGF treatment
- BCVA of 20/20–20/200 Snellen equivalent.

Exclusion Criteria

- History of laser photocoagulation, vPDT, intravitreal corticosteroid injection, vitrectomy surgery, submacular surgery, device implantation, or other surgical intervention for AMD in the study eye
- Subretinal hemorrhage involving the center of the fovea
- Subfoveal fibrosis, or atrophy in the study eye
- Uncontrolled ocular hypertension or glaucoma in the study eye.

Study Measures

The primary end point was the time to first implant refill assessed when the last enrolled patient completed the month 9 visit. Secondary efficacy outcomes included change in visual function and changes in CM.

Results

- Median time to first implant refill was 8.7, 13.0, and 15.0 months in the PDS 10-mg/mL, 40-mg/mL, and 100-mg/mL arms, respectively.
- Mean BCVA change from baseline to 9 months was -3.2, -0.5, +5.0, and +3.9 ETDRS letters in the PDS 10-mg/mL, 40-mg/mL, 100-mg/mL, and monthly ranibizumab arms, respectively.

- Mean CMT change from baseline was similar in the PDS 100-mg/mL and monthly ranibizumab arms.
- Postoperative vitreous hemorrhage rate was 4.5% in PDS arms.

Conclusion

The PDS 100-mg/mL arm showed visual and anatomic outcomes comparable with monthly intravitreal ranibizumab 0.5-mg injections but with a reduced total number of ranibizumab treatments.

Currently phase 3 trial of PDS comparing it with monthly dosing of ranibizumab is underway and has completed the enrollment.

BEVACIZUMAB (AVASTIN)

Systemic Bevacizumab (Avastin®) Therapy for Neovascular Age-related Macular Degeneration (SANA)[23,24]

Purpose

To evaluate the safety, efficacy, and durability of bevacizumab for the treatment of subfoveal CNV in patients with neovascular AMD.

Description

It was an open-label, single-center, uncontrolled clinical study. Patients (n = 18) were treated at baseline with an intravenous infusion of bevacizumab (5 mg/kg) followed by 1 or 2 additional doses given at 2-week intervals. Retreatment with bevacizumab was performed if there was evidence of recurrent CNV.

Patients were examined every week for the first 6 weeks, every 2 weeks for the next 6 weeks, and every 4 weeks thereafter for a total of 24 weeks. Safety assessments were performed at all visits. Ophthalmologic evaluations included protocol VA measurements, ocular examinations, and optical coherence tomography (OCT) imaging at each visit.

Inclusion Criteria

Patients with AMD with subfoveal CNV, BCVA letter scores of 70 to 20 (approximate Snellen equivalent, 20/40–20/400) and a central retinal thickness of 300 µm were included.

Study Measures

Safety assessments were performed, along with assessments of changes from baseline in VA scores, OCT measurements, and angiographic lesion characteristics.

Results

- No serious ocular or systemic adverse events were identified through 24 weeks. The only adverse event identified was a mild elevation of mean systolic and diastolic blood pressure measurements (+11 mm Hg, $p = 0.004$; +8 mm Hg, $p <0.001$) evident by 3 weeks and easily controlled with antihypertensive medications. By 24 weeks, the systolic and diastolic mean blood pressures were at or below baseline measurements.
- Visual acuity in the study eyes improved within the first 2 weeks, and by 24 weeks, the mean VA letter score increased by 14 letters in the study eyes ($p <0.001$), and the mean OCT central retinal thickness measurement decreased by 112 μm ($p <0.001$). By 24 weeks, retreatment was needed for only 6 of the 18 study eyes, and after retreatment, the recurrent leakage was eliminated, with restoration of any lost VA.

Conclusions

Systemic bevacizumab therapy for neovascular AMD was well-tolerated and effective for all 18 patients through 24 weeks, with an improvement in VA, OCT, and angiographic outcomes. By 6 months, most patients did not require any additional treatment beyond the initial 2 or 3 infusions. Despite these impressive results, it is unlikely that systemic bevacizumab will be studied in a large clinical trial because of the potential risks associated with systemic anti-VEGF therapy and the perception that intravitreal therapy is safer.

Avastin® (Bevacizumab) for Choroidal Neovascularization (ABC) Trial[25-27]

Purpose

To evaluate the efficacy and safety of intravitreal bevacizumab injections for the treatment of neovascular AMD.

Background

Bevacizumab, derived from the same parent molecule as RBZ, is a humanized anti-VEGF-A antibody that also binds all VEGF-A isoforms and their biologically active degradation products. Given its substantially lower cost than RBZ, bevacizumab has gained increasing popularity as an off-label AMD treatment. Although bevacizumab is FDA approved only for intravenous use in combination with chemotherapy for the treatment of colorectal, breast, lung and renal cell cancers, clinical experience with intravitreal bevacizumab has shown that this agent is well-tolerated and associated with improved vision and decreased retinal thickness in patients with exudative AMD. Most of the evidence supporting the use of bevacizumab for neovascular AMD has come from interventional case series and this clinical trial was initiated because of the increasing and widespread use of this agent in the treatment of neovascular AMD (an off-label indication) despite a lack of definitive unbiased safety and efficacy data. The ABC Trial was the first double-masked randomized control trial to investigate the efficacy and safety of intravitreal bevacizumab in the treatment of neovascular AMD.

Description

It was a prospective, double-masked, multicenter, randomized controlled trial comparing intravitreal bevacizumab injections to standard therapy in the treatment of neovascular AMD, conducted at three ophthalmology centers in the United Kingdom. 131 patients with neovascular AMD randomized 1:1 to intervention or control. Intravitreous bevacizumab (1.25 mg, three loading injections at 6 week intervals followed by further treatment if required at 6 week intervals) or standard treatment available at the start of the trial (PDT with verteporfin for predominantly classic type neovascular AMD, or intravitreal pegaptanib or sham treatment for occult or minimally classic type neovascular AMD). RBZ treatment was not included in the control arm as it had not been licensed for use at the start of recruitment for this trial. This trial completed recruitment in November 2007. Contrast sensitivity was determined during the study using a Pelli-Robson chart.

Study Measures

The primary outcome was the proportion of patients gaining ≥ 15 letters of visual acuity at 1 year and secondary outcomes included the proportion of patients with stable vision and mean visual acuity change.

Results

Of the 131 patients enrolled in the trial, five patients did not complete the study because of adverse events, loss to follow-up, or death.
- In the bevacizumab group, 21 (32%) patients gained 15 or more letters from baseline visual acuity compared with two (3%) in the standard care group ($p < 0.001$); the estimated adjusted odds ratio was 18.1 (95% CI 3.6–91.2) and the number needed to treat was 4 (3–6).
- In addition, the proportion of patients who lost fewer than 15 letters of visual acuity from baseline was significantly greater among those receiving bevacizumab treatment [91% (59) v 67% (44) in standard care group; $p < 0.001$].
- Mean visual acuity increased by 7.0 letters in the bevacizumab group with a median of seven injections compared with a decrease of 9.4 letters in the standard care group ($p < 0.001$), and the initial improvement at week 18 (plus 6.6 letters) was sustained to week 54.
- All end points with respect to visual acuity in the study eye at 54 weeks favored bevacizumab treatment over standard care.

- At the week-54 examination, bevacizumab-treated patients were more likely to gain at least 6 letters or more of contrast sensitivity than the patients receiving standard care [23 (35.4%) versus 10 (15.2%), $p = 0.009$]. In addition the bevacizumab-treated patients were less likely to lose 6 or more letters with a better mean letter change at week 54 than the patients receiving standard care [3 (4.6%) versus 14 (21.2%), and +4.0 versus -0.7 letters; $p < 0.05$ for both comparisons].
- Among 65 patients treated with bevacizumab, there were no cases of endophthalmitis or serious uveitis related to the intervention.
- 380 retreatment decisions were made after 3 fixed injections for 64 patients randomized to bevacizumab that completed 1-year follow-up. The most common criterion for retreatment was persistent intraretinal fluid on OCT imaging, and fluorescein angiography did not drive any retreatment decision. The mean (median) change in visual acuity and OCT central macular thickness after the 3 loading treatments to week 54 was +0.4 (+1.0) letters and +2.0 (+1.0) μm, respectively, with a mean (median) of 7.1 (7.0) injections. The median time to retreatment was 42 days with 12 of 69 injection-free episodes (17%) lasting more than 3 months.

Conclusion

- Bevacizumab 1.25 mg intravitreous injections given as part of a 6 weekly variable retreatment regimen is superior to standard care (pegaptanib sodium, verteporfin, sham), with low rates of serious ocular adverse events. Treatment improved visual acuity on average at 54 weeks.
- Consistent with the visual acuity outcomes, bevacizumab improved the chances of a clinically relevant gain in contrast sensitivity in the study population. Given the association between contrast sensitivity and visual disability, the beneficial effects of bevacizumab therapy on contrast sensitivity outcomes are expected to have a favorable impact on patients' daily activities.
- Sustained improvements in structure and function were achieved using this 6 weekly variable-dosing regimen with intravitreal bevacizumab. Most retreatment decisions were based on qualitative interpretation of OCT scans.

RANIBIZUMAB VERSUS BEVACIZUMAB

Comparison of Age-related Macular Degeneration Treatments Trials (CATT)[28-30]

Purpose

To describe effects of Ranibizumab (RBZ) and bevacizumab when administered monthly or as needed for 2 years and to describe the impact of switching to as-needed treatment after 1 year of monthly treatment.

Background

Clinical trials have established the efficacy of RBZ for the treatment of neovascular AMD. In addition, bevacizumab is used off-label to treat AMD, despite the absence of similar supporting data. Bevacizumab and RBZ are derived from the same monoclonal antibody. Given its molecular similarity to RBZ, its low cost, and its availability, the interest in Bevacizumab has been considerable. Bevacizumab has not been evaluated relative to RBZ. In addition, previous studies do not answer the question of whether a reduced dosing schedule is as effective as a fixed schedule of monthly injections. Treatment dependent on clinical response has the potential to reduce the treatment burden to patients as well as to reduce the overall cost of therapy.

In a noninferiority trial, the aim is to determine whether one intervention (the new treatment) is at least almost as good as another intervention (the existing treatment). Noninferiority trials typically are conducted when the reference treatment is highly efficacious and, in particular, when the new treatment has some other desirable attribute (e.g., less toxic, less burdensome on the patient, greater availability, or less expensive).

Description

It was a prospective, multicenter, single blind, noninferiority randomized clinical trial. 1,208 patients with neovascular AMD were enrolled from February, 2008 and randomly assigned to receive intravitreal injections of RBZ (0.5 mg/0.05 mL) or bevacizumab (1.25 mg/0.05 mL) on either a monthly schedule or as needed with monthly evaluation. At enrollment, patients were assigned to 4 treatment groups defined by drug (RBZ or bevacizumab) and dosing regimen (monthly or as needed). Only a single eye in each patient was analyzed.

At 1 year, patients initially assigned to monthly treatment were reassigned randomly to monthly or as-needed treatment, without changing the drug assignment. 1,107 out of 1,185 patients were followed up during year 2.

Inclusion Criteria

Patients aged ≥50 years with active, subfoveal CNV, fibrosis <50% of total lesion area, VA 20/25-20/320 and at least 1 drusen (>63 µm) in either eye or late AMD in fellow eye were eligible.

Study Measures

The primary outcome was the mean change in visual acuity at 1 year, with a noninferiority limit of 5 letters on the eye chart.

Results

At 1 year:
- Bevacizumab administered monthly was equivalent to RBZ administered monthly, with 8.0 and 8.5 letters gained, respectively. Bevacizumab

administered as needed was equivalent to RBZ as needed, with 5.9 and 6.8 letters gained, respectively. RBZ as needed was equivalent to monthly RBZ, although the comparison between bevacizumab as needed and monthly bevacizumab was inconclusive.
- The mean decrease in central retinal thickness was greater in the RBZ-monthly group (196 µm) than in the other groups (152–168 µm, $p = 0.03$ by analysis of variance).
- For all treatment groups, older age, better baseline VA, larger CNV area, predominantly or minimally classic lesion, absence of RAP lesion, presence of geographic atrophy, greater total fovea thickness, and RPE elevation on OCT were independently associated with less improvement in VA at 1 year.
- Rates of death, myocardial infarction, and stroke were similar for patients receiving either bevacizumab or RBZ ($p > 0.20$). The proportion of patients with serious systemic adverse events (primarily hospitalizations) was higher with bevacizumab than with RBZ (24.1% vs. 19.0%; risk ratio, 1.29; 95% CI, 1.01 to 1.66), with excess events broadly distributed in disease categories not identified in previous studies as areas of concern.

At 2 years:
- Mean gain in visual acuity was similar for both drugs (bevacizumab-RBZ difference, -1.4 letters; 95% CI, -3.7 to 0.8; $p = 0.21$). Mean gain was greater for monthly than for as-needed treatment (difference, -2.4 letters; 95% CI, -4.8 to -0.1; $p = 0.046$).
- The proportion without fluid ranged from 13.9% in the bevacizumab-as-needed group to 45.5% in the RBZ monthly group (drug, $p = 0.0003$; regimen, $p < 0.0001$).
- Switching from monthly to as-needed treatment resulted in greater mean decrease in vision during year 2 (-2.2 letters; $p = 0.03$) and a lower proportion without fluid (-19%; $p < 0.0001$).
- Rates of death and arteriothrombotic events were similar for both drugs ($p > 0.60$). The proportion of patients with 1 or more systemic serious adverse events was higher with bevacizumab than RBZ (39.9% vs. 31.7%; adjusted risk ratio, 1.30; 95% CI, 1.07–1.57; $p = 0.009$). Most of the excess events have not been associated previously with systemic therapy targeting VEGF.

Conclusion

- At 1 year, bevacizumab and RBZ had equivalent effects on visual acuity when administered according to the same schedule. RBZ given as needed with monthly evaluation had effects on vision that were equivalent to those of RBZ administered monthly. Differences in rates of serious adverse events require further study.
- RBZ and bevacizumab had similar effects on visual acuity over a 2-year period. Treatment as needed resulted in less gain in visual acuity, whether instituted at enrollment or after 1 year of monthly treatment. There were

no differences between drugs in rates of death or arteriothrombotic events. The interpretation of the persistence of higher rates of serious adverse events with bevacizumab is uncertain because of the lack of specificity to conditions associated with inhibition of VEGF.

Inhibit VEGF in Age-related Choroidal Neovascularization (IVAN)[31]

Purpose
To compare the efficacy and safety of RBZ and bevacizumab intravitreal injections to treat neovascular AMD.

Description
It was a multicenter, noninferiority factorial trial with equal allocation to groups undertaken by the UK National Health Service (NHS). The noninferiority limit was 3.5 letters. The participants were from 23 teaching and general hospitals in the NHS.

Participants were randomized to four groups: RBZ or bevacizumab, given either every month (continuous) or as needed (discontinuous), with monthly review. Only one eye was studied per patient. As in CATT, the drug doses were 0.5 mg RBZ and 1.25 mg bevacizumab. All of the participants were treated at visits 0, 1 and 2. Participants randomized to the continuous regimen were treated monthly thereafter, while participants randomized to the discontinuous regimen were not retreated after visit 2, unless prespecified clinical and OCT criteria for active disease were met. If retreatment was needed, a further cycle of three doses delivered monthly was required. The retreatment criteria were
1. Any subretinal fluid, increasing intraretinal fluid, or fresh blood.
2. Visual acuity drop by ≥10 letters
3. Fluorescein leakage >25% of the lesion circumference or expansion of CNV

Between March 27, 2008 and October 15, 2010, 610 participants were randomized and treated. The primary outcome is at 2 years; an interim analysis was reported at 1 year. All outcomes, except for EQ-5D and serum VEGF, were measured at baseline and at visits 3, 6, and 12. EQ-5D was measured at baseline and at visits 3 and 12, and serum VEGF was measured at baseline and at visits 1, 11 and 12.

Inclusion Criteria
People >50 years of age with untreated neovascular AMD in the study eye who read ≥25 letters on the ETDRS chart were eligible. Participants without a subfoveal (within 200 μm) neovascular component were eligible if subretinal fluid or serous pigment epithelial detachment was subfoveal. To avoid including inactive or advanced disease, lesions comprising >50% fibrosis or blood were excluded.

Study Measures

The primary efficacy and safety outcome measures are distance visual acuity and arteriothrombotic events or heart failure. The secondary outcome measurements include: (1) adverse effects; (2) EQ-5D (generic health-related quality of life); (3) cumulative resource use and costs; (4) contrast sensitivity, near visual acuity, and reading index; (5) lesion morphology and metrics from angiograms and OCTs; and (6) serum VEGF levels.

Results

- 1 year after randomization, the comparison between bevacizumab and RBZ was inconclusive (bevacizumab minus RBZ -1.99 letters, 95% confidence interval [CI], -4.04 to 0.06).
- Discontinuous treatment was equivalent to continuous treatment (discontinuous minus continuous -0.35 letters; 95% CI, -2.40 to 1.70).
- Foveal total thickness did not differ by drug, but was 9% less with continuous treatment [geometric mean ratio (GMR), 0.91; 95% CI, 0.86–0.97; $p = 0.005$].
- Fewer participants receiving bevacizumab had an arteriothrombotic event or heart failure [odds ratio (OR), 0.23; 95% CI, 0.05–1.07; $p = 0.03$]. There was no difference between drugs in the proportion experiencing a serious systemic adverse event (OR, 1.35; 95% CI, 0.80–2.27; $p = 0.25$).
- Serum VEGF was lower with bevacizumab (GMR, 0.47; 95% CI, 0.41–0.54; $p < 0.0001$) and higher with discontinuous treatment (GMR, 1.23; 95% CI, 1.07–1.42; $p = 0.004$).
- Continuous and discontinuous treatment costs were £9656 and £6398 per patient per year for RBZ and £1654 and £1509 for bevacizumab; bevacizumab was less costly for both treatment regimens ($p < 0.0001$).

Conclusion

The comparison of visual acuity at 1 year between bevacizumab and RBZ was inconclusive. Visual acuities with continuous and discontinuous treatment were equivalent. Other outcomes are consistent with the drugs and treatment regimens having similar efficacy and safety.

Lucentis Compared to Avastin Study (LUCAS)[32]

Purpose

To compare the effects of intravitreal Bevacizumab (BVZ) with RBZ in patients of Wet AMD in Norway (treat and extend protocol).

Description

First randomized double blind prospective multicenter trial using a treat-and-extend protocol comparing the efficacy and safety of RBZ and BVZ for the treatment of neovascular AMD. 441 patients with age ≥50 years, previously untreated active neovascular AMD in 1 eye, and BCVA between 20/25 and 20/320 were recruited. Diagnosis was confirmed by choroidal neovascular leakage on fluorescein angiography (FA) and intraretinal or subretinal fluid as determined by OCT. Patients were examined and injected every 4 weeks until no signs of active AMD were found, as determined by OCT and biomicroscopic fundus examinations. If there were no signs of active neovascular disease, a new injection was given and the period to the next treatment was extended by 2 weeks at a time, up to a maximum interval of 12 weeks. Recurrent disease was defined as any fluid on OCT, new or persistent hemorrhage, or dye leakage, or increased lesion size on FA. In the event of recurrence, the interval was shortened by 2 weeks at a time, until the disease was inactive. Interval extension was then restarted, with the maximum final interval being 2 weeks less than the period when the previous recurrence was observed, to prevent multiple recurrences. Patients who developed wet AMD in the nonstudy eye received the same drug in both eyes.

Study Measures

Primary outcome measure was mean change in ETDRS BCVA at 1 year.

Secondary outcomes included the number of injections, change in CRT as measured with OCT, and change of lesion size as measured on FA. The safety outcome was the occurrence of arteriothrombotic events.

Results

- 431 patients were included for analysis, the mean increase in BCVA gained was 7.8 (BVZ) and 8.0 (RBZ) letters gained (95% CI of mean difference, −2.4 to 2.9; $p = 0.845$). The proportion of patients gaining ≥15 letters was similar between the treatment groups: 25.5% (BVZ) and 26.7% (RBZ). Thus at 1 year, bevacizumab was equivalent to ranibizumab when using a treat-and-extend protocol.
- There was a statistically significant difference between the drugs regarding mean number of treatments given, with 8.9±2.6 injections and visits for BVZ and 8.0±2.3 injections and visits for RBZ (95% CI of the mean difference, −1.3 to 0.3, $p = 0.001$).
- There were more patients receiving injections every 4 weeks in the BVZ group and more patients receiving injections with a 12-week interval in the RBZ group ($p = 0.020$).
- The mean CRT was similar and significantly reduced in both groups.
- Arteriothrombotic events causing death in the BVZ group ($n = 4$) was lower than in the RBZ ($n = 7$) group. Other serious adverse events, such as venous thrombotic events or gastrointestinal disorders, were infrequent and similar with both medications. 1 case had pseudo-endophthalmitis in the BVZ group.

Conclusion

BVZ and RBZ had equivalent effects on visual acuity at 1 year when administered according to a treat-and-extend protocol. The visual acuity results at 1 year were comparable to those of other clinical trials with monthly treatment with fewer treatments. The numbers of serious adverse events were small.

GEFAL[33]

Purpose

To evaluate the relative efficacy and safety profile of bevacizumab versus ranibizumab intravitreal injections for the treatment of neovascular age-related macular degeneration.

Description

A noninferiority, double-masked, randomized trial was designed to assess the relative efficacy and safety profile of ranibizumab and bevacizumab in neovascular AMD administered with an as-needed regimen over a 1-year period. The noninferiority limit was 5 letters. Patients aged ≥50 years were eligible if they presented with subfoveal neovascular AMD, with best-corrected visual acuity in the study eye of between 20/32 and 20/320 measured on the Early Treatment of Diabetic Retinopathy Study chart and a lesion area of less than 12 optic disc areas (DA).

Patients were randomly assigned to intravitreal administration of bevacizumab (1.25 mg) or ranibizumab (0.50 mg). Hospital pharmacies were responsible for preparing, blinding, and dispensing treatments. Patients were followed for 1 year, with a loading dose of 3 monthly intravitreal injections, followed by an as-needed regimen (1 injection in case of active disease) for the remaining 9 months with monthly follow-up.

Study Measure

Mean change in visual acuity at 1 year.

Results

Between June 2009 and November 2011, 501 patients were randomized. Bevacizumab was noninferior to ranibizumab (bevacizumab minus ranibizumab +1.89 letters; 95% CI, -1.16 to +4.93, p <0.0001) in per protocol analysis. The intention-to-treat analysis was concordant. The mean number of injections was 6.8 in the bevacizumab group and 6.5 in the ranibizumab group (p = 0.39). Both drugs reduced the central subfield macular thickness, with a mean decrease of 95 μm for bevacizumab and 107 μm for ranibizumab (p = 0.27). There were no significant differences in the presence of subretinal or intraretinal fluid at final evaluation, dye leakage on angiogram, or change in choroidal neovascular area. The proportion of patients with serious adverse events was 12.6% in the bevacizumab group and 12.1% in the ranibizumab group ($p = 0.88$). The proportion of patients with serious systemic or ocular adverse events was similar in both groups.

Conclusion
Bevacizumab was noninferior to ranibizumab for visual acuity at 1 year with similar safety profiles. Ranibizumab tended to have a better anatomic outcome. The results are similar to those of previous head-to-head studies.

The Treat-and-Extend Protocol in Patients with Wet Age-related Macular Degeneration (TREX-AMD)[34-36]

Purpose
To assess treat-and-extend (TREX) and compare it with monthly dosing of intravitreal ranibizumab in treatment-naïve neovascular age-related macular degeneration (AMD).

Background
Though PRN dosing reduces the treatment burden, many trials have shown superior results with fixed monthly dosing which is practically not that feasible. While PRN dosing allows disease recurrences, treat and extend (TREX) aims to keep the macula free of exudation. So, this study was done to directly compare the monthly and TREX protocols for AMD.

Description
It was a Phase IIIb, multicenter, randomized, controlled clinical trial between February 2013 and January 2014. Patients with treatment-naïve choroidal neovascularization secondary to exudative AMD with ETDRS BCVA between 78 and 18 and total area of subretinal hemorrhage and fibrosis comprising less than 50% of the total lesion were included. Sixty patients with treatment-naïve neovascular AMD were randomized 1:2 to monthly or TREX management.

All eyes received monthly intravitreal ranibizumab (0.5 mg) for three treatments. Patients in the monthly group (20) continued to receive monthly treatments. For eyes randomized to TREX (40), the subsequent treatments were tailored based on disease activity: eyes were treated at each visit, with extension of injection period by 2 weeks if the macula was dry. If the fluid was detected injection period was shortened by 2 weeks and subsequent extension by one week after the dry macula was achieved. In the third year, subjects randomized to monthly were managed PRN while subjects randomized to TREX were continued on TREX dosing or transitioned to PRN after achieving an interval of 12 weeks between visits.

Study Measures

The primary outcome measure was to assess mean BCVA change from baseline. Secondary outcome measures included mean change in CMT, total number of intravitreal injections, and percentage of patients with persistent exudative disease activity, percentage of patients gaining or losing 10 or 15 letters at 12 months and ocular and systemic adverse events.

Results

- At 12 months, mean BCVA improved by 9.2 and 10.5 letters in the monthly and TREX groups, respectively ($p = 0.60$). The mean number of injections administered by 12 months as was 13.0 and 10.1 in the monthly and TREX groups, respectively ($p < 0.0001$). The mean maximum extension interval between injections after the first 3 monthly doses was 8.4 weeks in TREX group.
- At 24 months, 50 patients completed follow-up. ETDRS BCVA letter gains were similar in two groups at 24 months: (10.5 and 8.7 for the monthly and TREX, respectively). The mean number of injections was 25.5 and 18.6 for the monthly and TREX groups.
- At 36 months, 46 patients completed follow-up. Transition from monthly to PRN was associated with a decline in BCVA. A mean of 6.1 injections during year 3 were administered in this group. TREX group required a small number (4%) of injections (those transitioned to PRN) and displayed an inferior BCVA trajectory compared with the other subjects.

Conclusion

Visual and anatomic results were comparable between monthly and TREX groups till 24 months. Upon transition to PRN, patients in monthly dosing experienced a decline in BCVA. Patients in TREX groups who transitioned to PRN after achieving a 12-week interval between visits, the overall need for additional treatment was low.

■ VEGF TRAP-EYE (AFLIBERCEPT, EYLEA)

CLEAR-IT-2 Trial[37]

Purpose

To evaluate anatomic outcomes and vision, injection frequency, and safety during the as-needed (PRN) treatment phase of a study evaluating a 12-week fixed dosing period followed by PRN dosing to week 52 with VEGF Trap-Eye for neovascular AMD.

Background

VEGF Trap-Eye (Regeneron Pharmaceuticals and Bayer Healthcare AG) is a 110 kDa fusion protein of portions of the extracellular binding domains of VEGF receptors 1 and 2 (VEGFR-1 and VEGFR-2) and the Fc region of human IgG1. Previous studies have found that one of the most potent ways to block VEGF signaling is to prevent VEGF from binding to its receptor by administering decoy VEGF receptors. VEGF Trap-Eye was engineered to have much higher affinity for VEGF-A (~1 pM), compared to bevacizumab (500–2,200 pM) and ranibizumab (140 pM). This may allow VEGF Trap-Eye to be more potent than either drug currently in use.

It is mathematically estimated that VEGF Trap-Eye will maintain significant intravitreal VEGF-binding activity for 10–12 weeks after a single intravitreal injection. Another possible advantage that VEGF Trap-Eye has over ranibizumab is that it blocks all isoforms of VEGF-A as well as placental growth factor (PlGF)-1 and 2. PlGF is a part of an independent angiogenesis cascade.

In November 2011, the US FDA approved EYLEA (aflibercept) injection, known in the scientific literature as VEGF Trap-Eye, for the treatment of patients with neovascular AMD. EYLEA is the only FDA-approved treatment for wet AMD labeled for less than monthly dosing that demonstrated clinical equivalence to the monthly standard of care.

Description

It was a phase II, multicenter, prospective, randomized, double-masked trial that included 159 patients with subfoveal CNV secondary to wet AMD. Patients were randomly assigned to 1 of 5 intravitreal VEGF Trap-Eye treatment groups: 0.5 mg or 2 mg every 4 weeks or 0.5 mg, 2 mg, 4 mg every 12 weeks during the fixed-dosing period (weeks 1–12). From weeks 16–52, patients were evaluated monthly and were retreated PRN with their assigned dose (0.5, 2, or 4 mg).

Study Measures

Change in central retinal/lesion thickness (CR/LT), change in total lesion and CNV size, mean change in best-corrected visual acuity (BCVA), proportion of patients with 15-letter loss or gain, time to first PRN injection, reinjection frequency, and safety at week 52 were the main outcome measures.

Results

The decrease in CR/LT at week 12 versus baseline remained significant at weeks 12–52 (-130 μm from baseline at week 52) and CNV size regressed from baseline by 2.21 mm^2 at 48 weeks. After achieving a significant improvement in BCVA during the 12-week, fixed-dosing phase for all groups combined,

PRN dosing for 40 weeks maintained improvements in BCVA to 52 weeks (5.3-letter gain; p <0.0001). The most robust improvements and consistent maintenance of visual acuity generally occurred in patients initially dosed with 2 mg every 4 weeks for 12 weeks, demonstrating a gain of 9 letters at 52 weeks. Overall, a mean of 2 injections was administered after the 12-week fixed-dosing phase, and the mean time to first reinjection was 129 days; 19% of patients received no injections and 45% received 1 or 2 injections. Treatment with VEGF Trap-Eye was generally safe and well tolerated, with few ocular or systemic adverse events.

Conclusion
PRN dosing with VEGF Trap-Eye at weeks 16–52 maintained the significant anatomic and vision improvements established during the 12-week fixed-dosing phase with a low frequency of reinjections. Repeated dosing with VEGF Trap-Eye was well-tolerated over 52 weeks of treatment.

VEGF Trap-Eye: Investigation of Efficacy and Safety in Wet AMD (VIEW 1 and 2)[38]

Purpose
To compare monthly and every-2-month dosing of intravitreal VEGF Trap-Eye with monthly RBZ.

Description
VIEW 1 and 2 were two similarly designed, phase III, double-masked, multicenter, parallel-group, active-controlled, randomized trials. VIEW 1 (n = 1,217) was performed at 188 sites in the United States and Canada, and VIEW 2 (n = 1,240) was performed at 190 sites in Europe, Asia, Japan, Australia and South America. Patients with active, subfoveal CNV lesions (or juxtafoveal lesions with leakage affecting the fovea) secondary to AMD were randomized to intravitreal VEGF Trap-Eye 0.5 mg monthly (0.5q4), 2 mg monthly (2q4), 2 mg every 2 months after 3 initial monthly doses (2q8), or RBZ 0.5 mg monthly (Rq4).

Study Measures
The primary end point was noninferiority (margin of 10%) of the VEGF Trap-Eye regimens to RBZ in the proportion of patients maintaining vision at week 52 (losing <15 letters on ETDRS chart). Other key end points included change in BCVA and anatomic measures.

Results
- All VEGF Trap-Eye groups were noninferior and clinically equivalent to monthly RBZ for at 1 year (the 2q4, 0.5q4, and 2q8 regimens were 95.1%,

95.9%, and 95.1%, respectively, for VIEW 1, and 95.6%, 96.3%, and 95.6%, respectively, for VIEW 2, whereas monthly RBZ was 94.4% in both studies).
- In a prespecified integrated analysis of the 2 studies, all VEGF Trap-Eye regimens were within 0.5 letters of the reference RBZ for mean change in BCVA; all VEGF Trap-Eye regimens also produced similar improvements in anatomic measures.
- Ocular and systemic adverse events were similar across treatment groups.

Conclusion

Intravitreal VEGF Trap-Eye dosed monthly or every 2 months after 3 initial monthly doses produced similar efficacy and safety outcomes as monthly RBZ. These studies demonstrate that VEGF Trap-Eye is an effective treatment for AMD, with the every-2-month regimen offering the potential to reduce the risk from monthly intravitreal injections and the burden of monthly monitoring.

VIEW 1 and 2 Extension Studies (VEGF Trap-Eye: Investigation of Efficacy and Safety in Wet AMD)[39]

Purpose

To determine the efficacy and safety of intravitreal aflibercept in neovascular AMD during a second year of variable dosing after a first-year fixed-dosing period.

Description

This was an extension study of two randomized, double-masked, active-controlled, phase 3 trials (View 1 and View 2). 2,457 patients with neovascular AMD received their original dosing assignment using an as-needed regimen with defined retreatment criteria and mandatory dosing at least every 12 weeks during weeks 52 through 96.

Outcome Measures

Proportion of eyes at week 96 that maintained best-corrected visual acuity (BCVA; lost <15 letters from baseline); change from baseline in BCVA.

Results

- 94.4% to 96.1% of eyes at week 52 and 91.5% to 92.4% of eyes at week 96 maintained BCVA. Mean BCVA gains were 8.3 to 9.3 letters at week 52 and 6.6 to 7.9 letters at week 96.
- Proportions of eyes without retinal fluid decreased from week 52 (60.3–72.4%) to week 96 (44.6–54.4%), and more 2q4 eyes were without fluid at weeks 52 and 96 than Rq4 eyes.

- Patients received on average 4.7, 4.1, 4.6, and 4.2 injections during weeks 52 through 96 in the Rq4, 2q4, 0.5q4, and 2q8 groups, respectively.
- Arterial thromboembolic events were similar across groups (2.4–3.8%) from baseline to week 96.

Conclusion

All aflibercept and ranibizumab groups were equally effective in improving BCVA and preventing BCVA loss at 96 weeks. The 2q8 aflibercept group was similar to ranibizumab in visual acuity outcomes during 96 weeks, but with an average of 5 fewer injections. Small losses at 96 weeks in the visual and anatomic gains seen at 52 weeks in all arms were in the range of losses commonly observed with variable dosing.

Conbercept for Treatment of Neovascular Age-related Macular Degeneration: Results of the Randomized Phase 3 PHOENIX Study[40]

Purpose

To evaluate the efficacy and safety of intravitreal injections of 0.5 mg conbercept, for the treatment of AMD.

Background

Conbercept (Lumitin, Chengdu Kanghong Biotech Co., Ltd, P. R. China), an anti-VEGF agent (VEGF trap) developed in China is a 141 k-Da engineered fusion protein produced by the gene recombination of VEGF receptor domains with the Fc fragment of human immunoglobulin. Compared to aflibercept, it has 4th binding domain of VEGF receptor 2 stabilize the receptor-ligand complex and enhance dimerization extending its half-life to allow quarterly (q3M) dosing.

Description

A 12-month prospective, double-masked, multicenter, sham-controlled, phase III randomized trial. Patients with neovascular AMD with BCVA 20/40–20/400 were enrolled and randomized 2:1 to the conbercept group or the sham control group.

The conbercept group received intravitreal injections of conbercept 0.5 mg once monthly for the first 3 months, then quarterly until month 12 (3 + q3M). The sham group received first 3 monthly sham injections and then 3 monthly injections of conbercept (0.5 mg) followed by quarterly administrations until month 12.

Main Outcome Measures

The primary endpoint was mean change from baseline in best-corrected visual acuity at month 3.

Results

- A total of 114 patients (91.9%) from 9 sites in China completed the 12-month study.
- At the 3-month primary endpoint, the mean changes in BCVA from baseline were +9.20 letters in the conbercept group and +2.02 letters in the sham group, respectively ($p < 0.001$).
- At 12 months, the mean changes from baseline in BCVA letter score were +9.98 letters in the conbercept group and +8.81 letters in the sham group ($p = 0.64$).
- The most common ocular adverse events were associated with intravitreal injections, such as conjunctival hemorrhage, and increased intraocular pressure.

Conclusion

A conbercept dosing regimen of 3 initial monthly administrations followed by quarterly treatments is effective for treatment of AMD. In previous reports, other anti-VEGF agents were unable to maintain similar clinical benefits with the same regimen.

Comment

Due to stock of ICG running out in China, some PCV patients might have been included in study. Studies with longer follow-up and direct comparison with other anti-VEGF are needed to make any treatment recommendation.

BROLUCIZUMAB

HAWK and HARRIER: Phase 3, Multicenter, Randomized, Double-masked Trials of Brolucizumab for Neovascular Age-related Macular Degeneration[41]

Purpose

To compare brolucizumab with aflibercept to treat nAMD.

Background

Though monthly anti-VEGF injections have provided 1–2 lines of improvement in vision in nAMD patients in clinical trials the same has not translated in the real-world scenario. A major problem may be the frequent requirement of patient visits and injections.

Brolucizumab (formerly ESBA1008 and RTH258) is a single chain antibody fragment. Single-chain antibody fragments (scFv) are the smallest functional unit of an antibody. This allows a greater molar dose to be delivered in a single shot, which can increase the duration of action. A smaller molecule also allows better tissue penetration.

Description

HAWK and HARRIER were double-masked, multicenter, active-controlled, randomized, 24-month trials conducted over 408 sites all over the world.

These included 1,817 eyes with treatment naive active choroidal neovascularization due to nAMD affecting central 1 mm of fovea. The included eyes had BCVA between 20/32 and 20/400 and no fibrosis or geographic atrophy affecting the central 1 mm.

Patients were randomized to intravitreal brolucizumab 3 mg (in HAWK trial only) or 6 mg or aflibercept 2 mg. After 3 monthly loading injections, brolucizumab-treated eyes received an injection every 12 weeks. The interval was adjusted to every 8 weeks if disease activity was present; aflibercept-treated eyes received injection every 8 weeks.

Study Measures

The primary outcome was to show noninferiority in mean BCVA change from baseline to week 48. Other main end points included the percentage of patients who maintained quarterly dosing till week 48 and anatomic outcomes.

Results

- At 48 weeks, each brolucizumab arm demonstrated noninferiority to aflibercept in BCVA change from baseline.
- Greater than 50% of brolucizumab 6 mg treated eyes were maintained on quarterly dosing at 48 weeks (56% and 51% in HAWK and HARRIER, respectively).
- At week 16, after loading treatment, fewer brolucizumab 6 mg treated eyes had disease activity versus aflibercept in HAWK (24.0% vs. 34.5%) and HARRIER (22.7% vs. 32.2%).
- Greater central subfield thickness reductions were observed with brolucizumab 6 mg versus aflibercept in HAWK and HARRIER.
- Adverse event rates were generally similar in two groups.

Conclusion

Brolucizumab was noninferior to aflibercept in terms of improvement in BCVA at 48 weeks and more than 50% of the eyes treated with 6 mg brolucizumab were maintained on quarterly dosing interval. Anatomic outcomes were better with brolucizumab than aflibercept.

Table 1: Summary of clinical trials in age-related macular degeneration–II.

Title	Purpose	No. of Patients	Inclusion criteria	Outcome measure	Result/conclusion
VISION	Pegaptanib Sodium in early subfoveal CNV secondary to AMD	1,186	All angiographic CNV lesion compositions of AMD	Proportion of patients avoiding three lines of vision loss at one year	• Continuing visual benefit was observed in patients who were randomized to receive therapy with pegaptanib in year 2 compared to 2 years' usual care or cessation of therapy at year 1 • 3 year safety profile was favorable
ANCHOR	RBZ vs. PDT in predominantly classic neovascular AMD	423	• Predominantly classic, subfoveal CNV not previously treated with PDT or anti-angiogenic drugs, total size <5,400 µm, BCVA of 20/40 to 20/320	Percentage losing <15 letters and percentage gaining ≥15 letters from baseline	RBZ over a 24-month period was effective and superior to PDT treatment in maintaining or improving VA and lesion characteristics
MARINA	RBZ in minimally classic/ occult neovascular ARMD	716	• BCVA 20/40 to 20/320; primary or recurrent subfoveal CNV due to AMD, minimally classic or occult with no classic CNV; maximum lesion size of 12 DA, and presumed recent progression	Percentage losing <15 letters, percentage gaining ≥15 letters from baseline. Primary efficacy analysis was at 12 months, with continued measurements to month 24	• RBZ for nonclassic neovascular AMD had substantially better VA outcomes compared to sham injections • RBZ treatment showed stabilization of lesion size

Contd...

Contd...

Title	Purpose	No. of Patients	Inclusion criteria	Outcome measure	Result/conclusion
PIER	RBZ given monthly for 3 months and then quarterly in patients with subfoveal CNV due to AMD	184	All lesion types due to ARMD if the active CNV accounted for at least 50% of the total lesion	Mean change from baseline visual acuity at month 12 and at month 24	• RBZ provided significant VA benefit • With quarterly dosing, there was a steady decline in VA during months 4 through 24 in PIER compared to the VA stabilization achieved in ANCHOR and MARINA with monthly injections
EXCITE	Quarterly versus monthly regimen of RBZ in subfoveal CNV secondary to AMD (PIER vs. MARINA/ANCHOR) regimen	353	Classic and nonclassic subfoveal neovascular AMD	Mean change in BCVA central retinal thickness (CRT) from baseline to month 12	At month 12, BCVA gain in the monthly regimen was higher than that of the quarterly regimens
PrONTO	OCT-guided, variable-dosing regimen RBZ for patients with neovascular AMD	37	AMD patients with subfoveal CNV and a CRT of at least 300 microns	Change in VA scores and OCT measurements from baseline at 24 months	OCT-guided variable-dosing regimen with RBZ resulted in VA outcomes similar to results from the Phase III MARINA and ANCHOR studies
SUSTAIN	Individualized RBZ (PRN regime) in patients with neovascular AMD	513	AMD patients with subfoveal CNV naive to RBZ treatment	Frequency of adverse events, monthly change of BCVA and CRT from baseline	Like PrONTO, results from the SUSTAIN trial showed a rapid increase in VA in the first 3 months, which deteriorated, but not nearly as much as in PIER, over the nine months of PRN dosing

Contd...

Contd...

Title	Purpose	No. of Patients	Inclusion criteria	Outcome measure	Result/conclusion
HARBOR	RBZ 0.5 mg and 2.0 mg monthly vs on PRN basis in treatment-naïve subfoveal neovascular AMD	1,098	Subfoveal CNV due to ARMD, lesions <12 disc areas and BCVA 20/40–20/320	Mean change from baseline in BCVA at month 12	RBZ 0.5 mg dosed monthly provides optimum results in patients with wet AMD. There is no additional benefit from the high dose in treatment-naïve wet AMD
SAILOR	RBZ in a large population of subjects with neovascular AMD	4,300	Angiographically determined subfoveal CNV secondary to AMD	Safety outcomes included the incidence of ocular and nonocular adverse events. Efficacy outcomes included changes in BCVA	• Intravitreal RBZ was safe and well-tolerated in a large population with neovascular AMD • Although the risks of arterial thrombolic events related to RBZ are low, they were similar to that observed in previous RBZ studies and ophthalmologists should be aware of these risks
HORIZON	Long-term safety and efficacy of RBZ injections in patients with CNV secondary to AMD	853	Patients who completed the controlled treatment phase of 1 of 3, 2-year clinical trials (ANCHOR, MARINA or FOCUS)	Incidence and severity of ocular and nonocular adverse events	The incidence of serious ocular and nonocular adverse effects during the 2-year study period of HORIZON trial were low and consistent with those observed during the 24 months of treatment in the prior Phase III trials
SANA	Systemic bevacizumab (BVZ) for the treatment of subfoveal CNV in neovascular AMD	18	AMD with subfoveal CNV, BCVA letter scores of 70 to 20 and a central retinal thickness of 300 microns	Safety assessments, changes from baseline in VA scores, OCT measurements and angiographic lesion characteristics	Systemic BVZ for neovascular AMD was well-tolerated and effective for all 18 patients through 24 weeks, with an improvement in VA, OCT, and angiographic outcomes

Contd...

Title	Purpose	No. of Patients	Inclusion criteria	Outcome measure	Result/conclusion
ABC	Intravitreal BVZ vs PDT (for classic) or pagaptanib (for occult/minimally classic) for the treatment of neovascular AMD	131	Predominantly classic or occult or minimally classic type neovascular AMD	Proportion of patients gaining ≥15 letters of visual acuity at 1 year	• BVZ retreatment regimen is superior to standard care (pegaptanib sodium, verteporfin, sham), with low rates of serious ocular adverse events • Treatment improved visual acuity on average at 54 weeks
CATT	RBZ versus BVZ administered monthly or as needed for 2 years in neovascular ARMD	1,208	Active, subfoveal CNV, fibrosis <50% of total lesion area, VA 20/25–20/320 and at least 1 drusen in either eye or late AMD in fellow eye	Mean change in visual acuity at 1 year	• RBZ and BVZ had similar effects on visual acuity over a 2-year period. • Treatment as needed resulted in less gain in visual acuity. • No differences between drugs in rates of death or arteriothrombotic events
IVAN	RBZ versus BVZ intravitreal injections to treat neovascular AMD	610	Untreated subfoveal neovascular AMD in the study eye with VA ≥25 letters	Distance visual acuity (efficacy) and arteriothrombotic events or heart failure (safety)	• The comparison of visual acuity at 1 year between BVZ and RBZ was inconclusive. • Visual acuities with continuous and discontinuous treatment were equivalent
CLEAR-IT 2	VEGF Trap-Eye for neovascular AMD	159	Subfoveal CNV secondary to wet AMD	Change in central retinal/lesion thickness (CR/LT), change in total lesion and CNV size, mean change in BCVA, proportion of patients with 15-letter loss or gain, time to first PRN injection, reinjection frequency, and safety at week 52	PRN dosing with VEGF Trap-Eye at weeks 16–52 maintained the significant anatomic and vision improvements established during the 12-week fixed-dosing phase with a low frequency of reinjections

Contd...

Title	Purpose	No. of Patients	Inclusion criteria	Outcome measure	Result/conclusion
VIEW 1 and 2	Monthly and every-2-month dosing of intravitreal VEGF Trap-Eye versus monthly RBZ in subfoveal CNV secondary to ARMD	2,419	Subfoveal CNV secondary to ARMD	Noninferiority (margin of 10%) of the VEGF Trap-Eye regimens to RBZ in the proportion of patients maintaining vision at week 52	VEGF Trap-Eye dosed monthly or every 2 months after 3 initial monthly doses produced similar efficacy and safety outcomes as monthly RBZ
HAWK and HARRIER	To compare brolucizumab with aflibercept in nAMD	1,817	Treatment naive active CNV due to nAMD affecting central 1 mm of fovea	Noninferiority in mean BCVA change from baseline to week 48 and percentage of patients who maintained quarterly dosing till week 48 and anatomic outcomes	• Intravitreal brolucizumab 3 mg (in HAWK trial only) and 6 mg noninferior to aflibercept 2 mg. • Greater than 50% of brolucizumab 6 mg treated eyes were maintained on quarterly dosing at 48 weeks. • Greater CMT reduction than aflibercept
GEFAL	To compare bevacizumab versus ranibizumab for neovascular age-related macular degeneration	501	Subfoveal neovascular AMD, with BVCA in the study eye of between 20/32 and 20/320	Bevacizumab was noninferior to ranibizumab in terms of BCVA improvement and reduction in macular thickness	Bevacizumab was noninferior to ranibizumab for visual acuity at 1 year with similar safety profiles

DA: disc area
AMD: age-related macular degeneration
VEGF: vascular endothelial growth factor
CNV: choroidal neovascularization

REFERENCES

1. VISION Clinical Trial Group. Pegaptanib for neovascular age-related macular degeneration. N Engl J Med. 2004;351:2805-16.
2. VISION Clinical Trial Group. Year 2 efficacy results of 2 randomized controlled clinical trials of pegaptanib for neovascular age-related macular degeneration. Ophthalmology. 2006;113:1508.e1-25.
3. Singerman LJ, Masonson H, Patel M, Adamis AP, Buggage R, Cunningham E, et al. Pegaptanib sodium for neovascular age-related macular degeneration: third-year safety results of the VEGF Inhibition Study in Ocular Neovascularisation (VISION) trial. Br J Ophthalmol. 2008;92:1606-11.
4. ANCHOR Study Group. Ranibizumab versus verteporfin for neovascular age-related macular degeneration. N Engl J Med. 2006;355:1432-44.
5. ANCHOR Study Group. Ranibizumab versus verteporfin photodynamic therapy for neovascular age-related macular degeneration: Two-year results of the ANCHOR study. Ophthalmology. 2009;116:57-65.e5.
6. Sadda SR, Stoller G, Boyer DS, Heier JS, Sy JP, Ianchulev T, et al. Anatomical benefit from ranibizumab treatment of predominantly classic neovascular age-related macular degeneration in the 2-year ANCHOR study. Retina. 2010;30:1390-9.
7. MARINA Study Group. Ranibizumab for neovascular age-related macular degeneration. N Engl J Med. 2006;355:1419-31.
8. MARINA Study Group. Angiographic and optical coherence tomographic results of the MARINA study of ranibizumab in neovascular age-related macular degeneration. Ophthalmology. 2007;114:1868-75.
9. MARINA Study Group. Subgroup analysis of the MARINA study of ranibizumab in neovascular age-related macular degeneration. Ophthalmology. 2007;114:246-52.
10. Regillio CD, Brown DM, Abraham P, Yue H, Ianchulev T, Schneider S, et al. Randomized double-masked, sham-controlled trial of ranibizumab for neovascular age-related macular degeneration: PIER Study year 1. Am J Ophthalmol. 2008;145:239-48.
11. Abraham P, Yue H, Wilson L. Randomized, double-masked, sham-controlled trial of ranibizumab for neovascular age related macular degeneration: PIER study year 2. Am J Ophthalmol. 2010;150:315-24.
12. EXCITE Study Group. Efficacy and safety of monthly versus quarterly ranibizumab treatment in neovascular age-related macular degeneration: the EXCITE study. Ophthalmology. 2011;118:831-9.
13. Fung AE, Lalwani GA, Rosenfeld PJ, Dubovy SR, Michels S, Feuer WJ, et al. An optical coherence tomography-guided, variable dosing regimen with intravitreal ranibizumab (Lucentis) for neovascular age-related macular degeneration. Am J Ophthalmol. 2007;143:566-83.
14. Lalwani GA, Rosenfeld PJ, Fung AE, Dubovy SR, Michels S, Feuer W, et al. A variable-dosing regimen with intravitreal ranibizumab for neovascular age related macular degeneration: year 2 of the PrONTO Study. Am J Ophthalmol. 2009;148:43-58.
15. SUSTAIN Study Group. Safety and efficacy of a flexible dosing regimen of ranibizumab in neovascular age-related macular degeneration: the SUSTAIN study. Ophthalmology. 2011;118:663-71.
16. HARBOR Study Group. Twelve-month efficacy and safety of 0.5 mg or 2.0 mg Ranibizumab in patients with subfoveal neovascular age-related macular degeneration. Ophthalmology. 2013;pii: S0161-6420(12)00986-4.
17. Boyer DS, Heier JS, Brown DM, Francom SF, Ianchulev T, Rubio RG. A Phase IIIb study to evaluate the safety of ranibizumab in subjects with neovascular age-related macular degeneration. Ophthalmology. 2009;116:1731-9.

18. Mitchell P, Korobelnik JF, Lanzetta P, Holz FG, Prünte C, Schmidt-Erfurth U, et al. Ranibizumab (Lucentis) in neovascular age-related macular degeneration: Evidence from clinical trials. Br J Ophthalmol. 2010;94:2-13.
19. Singer MA, Awh CC, Sadda S, Freeman WR, Antoszyk AN, Wong P, et al. HORIZON: an open-label extension trial of ranibizumab for choroidal neovascularization secondary to age-related macular degeneration. Ophthalmology. 2012;119:1175-83.
20. Rofagha S, Bhisitkul RB, Boyer DS, Sadda SR, Zhang K, Seven-Up Study Group. Seven-year outcomes in ranibizumab-treated patients in ANCHOR, MARINA, and HORIZON: a multicenter cohort study (SEVEN-UP). Ophthalmology. 2013;120:2292-9.
21. Bhisitkul RB, Mendes TS, Rofagha S, Enanoria W, Boyer DS, Sadda SR, et al. Macular atrophy progression and 7-year vision outcomes in subjects from the ANCHOR, MARINA, and HORIZON studies: the SEVEN-UP study. Am J Ophthalmol. 2015;159:915-24.
22. Campochiaro PA, Marcus DM, Awh CC, Regillo C, Adamis AP, Bantseev V, et al. The port delivery system with ranibizumab for neovascular age-related macular degeneration: results from the randomized phase 2 Ladder Clinical Trial. Ophthalmology. 2019;126:1141-54.
23. Michels S, Rosenfeld PJ, Puliafito CA, Marcus EN, Venkatraman AS. Systemic bevacizumab (Avastin) therapy for neovascular age-related macular degeneration twelve-week results of an uncontrolled open-label clinical study. Ophthalmology. 2005;112:1035-47.
24. Moshfeghi AA, Rosenfeld PJ, Puliafito CA, Michels S, Marcus EN, Lenchus JD, et al. Systemic bevacizumab (Avastin) therapy for neovascular age-related macular degeneration: twenty-four-week results of an uncontrolled open-label clinical study. Ophthalmology. 2006;113: 2002.e1-12.
25. ABC Trial Investigators. Bevacizumab for neovascular age-related macular degeneration (ABC Trial): multicentre randomised double masked study. BMJ. 2010;340:c2459.
26. ABC Trial Study Group. Contrast sensitivity outcomes in the ABC Trial: a randomized trial of bevacizumab for neovascular age-related macular degeneration. Invest Ophthalmol Vis Sci. 2011;52:3089-93.
27. Patel PJ, Tufail A, ABC Trial Investigators. Optimizing individualized therapy with bevacizumab for neovascular age-related macular degeneration. Retina. 2012.
28. CATT Research Group. Ranibizumab and bevacizumab for neovascular age-related macular degeneration. N Engl J Med. 2011;364:1897-908.
29. CATT Research Group. Ranibizumab and bevacizumab for treatment of neovascular age-related macular degeneration: two-year results. Ophthalmology. 2012;119:1388-98.
30. CATT Research Group. Baseline predictors for one-year visual outcomes with ranibizumab or bevacizumab for neovascular age-related macular degeneration. Ophthalmology. 2013;120:122-9.
31. IVAN Study Investigators. Ranibizumab versus bevacizumab to treat neovascular age-related macular degeneration: one-year findings from the IVAN randomized trial. Ophthalmology. 2012;119:1399-411.
32. Berg K, Pedersen TR, Sandvik L, Bragadóttir R. Comparison of ranibizumab and bevacizumab for neovascular age-related macular degeneration according to LUCAS treat-and-extend protocol. Ophthalmology. 2015;122(1):146-52.
33. Kodjikian L, Souied EH, Mimoun G, Mauget-Faÿsse M, Behar-Cohen F, Decullier E, et al. Ranibizumab versus bevacizumab for neovascular age-related macular degeneration: results from the GEFAL noninferiority randomized trial. Ophthalmology. 2013;120:2300-9.
34. Wykoff CC, Croft DE, Brown DM, Wang R, Payne JF, Clark L, et al. Prospective trial of treat-and-extend versus monthly dosing for neovascular age-related macular degeneration: TREX-AMD 1-year results. Ophthalmology. 2015; 22:2514-22.

35. Wykoff CC, Ou WC, Brown DM, Croft DE, Wang R, Payne JF, et al. Randomized trial of treat-and-extend versus monthly dosing for neovascular age-related macular degeneration: 2-year results of the TREX-AMD study. Ophthalmol Retina. 2017;1:314-21.
36. Wykoff CC, Ou WC, Croft DE, Payne JF, Brown DM, Clark WL, et al. Neovascular age-related macular degeneration management in the third year: final results from the TREX-AMD randomised trial. Br J Ophthalmol. 2018;102:460-4.
37. CLEAR-IT 2 Investigators. The 1-year results of CLEAR-IT 2, a phase 2 study of vascular endothelial growth factor trap-eye dosed as-needed after 12-week fixed dosing. Ophthalmology. 2011;118:1098-106.
38. VIEW 1 and VIEW 2 Study Groups. Intravitreal aflibercept (VEGF trap-eye) in wet age-related macular degeneration. Ophthalmology. 2012;119: 2537-48.
39. Schmidt-Erfurth U, Kaiser PK, Korobelnik JF, Brown DM, Chong V, Nguyen QD, et al. Intravitreal aflibercept injection for neovascular age-related macular degeneration: ninety-six-week results of the VIEW studies. Ophthalmology. 2014;121:193-201.
40. Liu K, Song Y, Xu G, Ye J, Wu Z, Liu X, et al. Conbercept for Treatment of Neovascular Age-related Macular Degeneration: Results of the Randomized Phase 3 PHOENIX Study. Am J Ophthalmol. 2019;197:156-67.
41. Dugel PU, Koh A, Ogura Y, Jaffe GJ, Schmidt-Erfurth U, Brown DM, et al. HAWK and HARRIER: phase 3, multicenter, randomized, double-masked trials of brolucizumab for neovascular age-related macular degeneration. Ophthalmology. 2020;127:72-84.

Clinical Trials in Age-related Macular Degeneration–III

Pooja Shah, Vinod Kumar

■ INTRODUCTION

The combination of therapeutic modalities targeting different molecular pathways or different aspects of a pathological process is believed to enhance treatment efficacy through additive or synergistic effects. This principle is applied in the management of numerous pathological states, including systemic hypertension, diabetes mellitus, pain, infection and cancer. In the management of exudative age-related macular degeneration (AMD), combination approaches are currently being investigated as a means of improving treatment efficacy as well as reducing treatment frequency. The concept of combination therapy for AMD has become possible only within the past decade as a result of the introduction of important treatment modalities such as verteporfin (Visudyne) photodynamic therapy (PDT) and inhibitors of vascular endothelial growth factor (VEGF) such as pegaptanib (Macugen), ranibizumab (RBZ) (Lucentis), aflibercept (Eylea), brolucizumab (Pagenex) and bevacizumab (Avastin). Prior to the use of VEGF inhibitors for AMD, studies reported successful treatment using combinations of PDT and corticosteroids using various doses and delivery modalities.

There is a sound biological rationale for combining verteporfin PDT (vPDT) with anti-VEGF agents. Their actions complement each other and may be synergistic. PDT causes photothrombosis and occlusion of new vessels, while anti-VEGF agents inhibit vasopermeability and angiogenesis. One of the reasons why PDT does not result in significant improvement in vision despite closure of choroidal neovascularization (CNV) is the upregulation of VEGF that occurs within hours following its administration because of temporary hypoxia within the treatment zone. This upregulation of VEGF is an undesirable negative effect, which may be countered by same-day administration of an anti-VEGF agent.

■ RhuFab V2 OCULAR TREATMENT COMBINING THE USE OF VISUDYNE TO EVALUATE SAFETY (FOCUS)[1,2]

Purpose

To investigate the safety and efficacy of intravitreal RBZ treatment combined with vPDT in patients with predominantly classic CNV secondary to AMD.

Description

In this 2-year, phase I/II, multicenter, randomized, single-masked, controlled study, patients received monthly RBZ (0.5 mg) ($n = 106$) or sham ($n = 56$) injections. The PDT was performed 7 days before initial RBZ or sham treatment and then quarterly as needed.

Study Measures

Efficacy assessment included changes in visual acuity (VA) and lesion characteristics and PDT frequency. Proportion of patients losing fewer than 15 letters from baseline VA at 12 months was the primary efficacy outcome. Adverse events were summarized by incidence and severity.

Results

At 12 months
- 90.5% of the RBZ-treated patients and 67.9% of the control patients had lost fewer than 15 letters ($p < 0.001$).
- The most frequent RBZ-associated serious ocular adverse events were intraocular inflammation (11.4%) and endophthalmitis (1.9%; 4.8% if including presumed cases). On average, patients with serious inflammation had better VA outcomes at 12 months than did controls. Key serious nonocular adverse events included myocardial infarctions in the PDT-alone group (3.6%) and cerebrovascular accidents in the RBZ-treated group (3.8%).

At month 24
- 88% of RBZ + PDT patients had lost <15 letters from baseline VA (vs. 75% for PDT alone), 25% had gained ≥15 letters (vs. 7% for PDT alone), and the two treatment arms differed by 12.4 letters in mean VA change ($p < 0.05$ for all between-group differences).
- On average, RBZ + PDT patients exhibited less lesion growth and greater reduction of CNV leakage and subretinal fluid (SRF) accumulation, and required fewer PDT retreatments, than PDT-alone patients (mean = 0.4 vs. 3.0 PDT retreatments).
- Endophthalmitis and serious intraocular inflammation occurred, respectively, in 2.9% and 12.4% of RBZ + PDT patients and 0% of PDT-alone patients. Incidences of serious nonocular adverse events were similar in the two treatment groups.

Conclusion

Ranibizumab + PDT was more efficacious than PDT alone for treating neovascular AMD. Although RBZ treatment increased the risk of serious intraocular inflammation, affected patients on an average still experienced VA benefit.

PROTECT STUDY[3]

Purpose
To evaluate safety of same-day administration of verteporfin and RBZ.

Description
It was a prospective, open-label, multicenter study. Patients with predominantly classic ($n = 13$) or occult ($n = 19$) CNV secondary to AMD received standard-fluence verteporfin at baseline and months 3, 6, and 9, based on fluorescein angiography (FA). RBZ 0.5 mg was administered at baseline and months 1, 2, and 3.

Study Measures
The incidence of severe vision loss [best corrected visual acuity (BCVA loss ≥30 letters; primary safety assessment)] was the main outcome measure.

Results
No severe vision loss due to ocular inflammation or uveitis occurred. One patient had moderate vision loss (BCVA loss ≥15 letters). Three patients had mild/moderate uveitis. Two serious ocular adverse events occurred (retinal pigment epithelial tear and moderate BCVA decrease). No systemic adverse events occurred. At 9 months, all lesions were inactive with no recurrent leakage on FA and optical coherence tomography (OCT); macular edema and SRF resolved. The mean BCVA measured at 2 m improved by 6.9 letters at 4 months and 2.4 letters at 9 months.

Conclusion
Same-day verteporfin and RBZ was safe and not associated with severe vision loss or severe ocular inflammation. Lesions stabilized, with minimal treatment required after 3 months.

TORPEDO TRIAL[4]

Purpose
To demonstrate long-term prevention of vision loss and improvement in BCVA after treatment with one-time reduced-fluence-rate PDT followed by administration of RBZ on a variable dosing regimen over 24 months in patients with neovascular AMD.

Description
This prospective, nonrandomized, open-label, single-center study enrolled 27 consecutive patients (27 eyes) presenting at the Leuven University Eye Hospital, Belgium with previously untreated, active neovascular AMD

between September 2006 and January 2007. All patients were treated with one-time, reduced-fluence-rate vPDT, followed by intravitreal RBZ 0.5 mg on the same day. A second and third RBZ injection were given at weeks 4 and 8, respectively, after which patients were followed up monthly for 24 months. Additional treatment with RBZ was administered to eyes with active neovascularization as indicated clinically and on imaging studies. Retreatment was based on the following criteria:

- Presence of SRF, intraretinal edema or subretinal pigment epithelial fluid, as seen on OCT
- Increase of central macular thickness (CMT) by >100 μm on OCT
- Signs of active CNV leakage on FA
- New sub- or intraretinal hemorrhage
- Decrease in best corrected visual acuity of ≥5 letters on the Early Treatment Diabetic Retinopathy Study (ETDRS) chart.

If any single criterion for reinjection was fulfilled, retreatment with RBZ was administered.

Study Measures

Improvement in BCVA was the primary outcome measure. Secondary outcome measures included the change in CMT, reinjection frequency, and safety.

Results

Twenty-five patients completed the 2-year study. Occult CNV was present in 64% and retinal angiomatous proliferative (RAP) lesions were present in 24% of the study eyes. The remaining three eyes had lesions classified as classic (one eye) or predominantly classic (two eyes) CNV.

- Mean baseline VA was 58.6 letters (range: 35–70; SD = 8.4); 24-month VA was 66.2 letters (35–82; 12.7), not including one warfarin-treated patient who suffered vitreous hemorrhage. The mean VA improved by 7.2 letters ($p <0.05$) and the mean CMT decreased by 146 μm. VA improved >3 lines (15 letters) in 16%; improved 1–3 lines in 20%; remained within one line of baseline in 32%, decreased 1–3 lines in 16%, and decreased >3 lines in 16%. Losses of >3 lines were due to vitreous hemorrhage, geographic atrophy, fibrosis, and growth of an initially small CNV lesion.
- An average of 5.1 injections (range: 3–9) were administered during the first 12 months, and 7.1 injections (3–13) over 24 months. A total of 178 injections were performed; no systemic side-effects, uveitis, or choroidal collateral vascular damage were observed.

Conclusion

Combined PDT and RBZ injection the same day was well tolerated in all patients. Eighty-four percent of patients had stable or improved vision at month 24.

SUMMIT TRIALS

The SUMMIT trial program was designed to explore the efficacy and safety of combination therapy of vPDT and RBZ compared with RBZ monotherapy in patients with subfoveal CNV due to AMD, as well as the impact of the combination on treatment burden and health economics outcomes. The SUMMIT program consisted of three randomized clinical trials—(1) DENALI, (2) EVEREST, and (3) MONT BLANC. The DENALI study was a 2-year, randomized, double-masked multicenter study conducted at 45 centers in the United States and five centers in Canada, enrolling subjects with subfoveal CNV of all angiographic subtypes who were randomized to receive either RBZ monotherapy, a combination of RBZ and standard fluence (SF) PDT or a combination of RBZ and reduced-fluence (RF) PDT. MONT BLANC was a similar study conducted at 50 centers throughout Europe, enrolling subjects with subfoveal CNV of all angiographic subtypes who were randomized to receive either RBZ monotherapy or RBZ in combination with SF PDT. EVEREST was performed in Asia and was designed to evaluate combination therapy versus PDT or RBZ monotherapy in patients with polypoidal choroidal vasculopathy (PCV).

Verteporfin Plus Ranibizumab for Choroidal Neovascularization in Age-related Macular Degeneration: DENALI Study[5]

Purpose

To demonstrate noninferiority of RBZ in combination with vPDT versus RBZ monotherapy in patients with subfoveal CNV secondary to AMD.

Description

It was a prospective, multicenter, double-masked, randomized, phase IIIb clinical trial. 321 patients were randomized to receive either RBZ 0.5 mg monotherapy ($n = 112$), SF, (light dose 50 J/cm^2) vPDT combination therapy ($n = 104$), or (RF, light dose 25 J/cm^2) vPDT combination therapy ($n = 105$). RBZ was administered monthly in the monotherapy group. In both combination therapy groups, RBZ was initiated with 3 consecutive monthly injections, followed from month 3 by RBZ as needed [pro re nata (PRN)] and verteporfin standard or RF as needed, with monthly monitoring. All patients were evaluated monthly for 12 months.

Inclusion Criteria

Enrollment criteria were 50 years of age, with any type of subfoveal CNV secondary to AMD, lesion size <9 DA, naïve to AMD treatment, and a BCVA letter score of 73–24 (Snellen equivalent 20/40–20/320).

Study Measures

Study outcomes included efficacy and safety (mean change in BCVA from baseline at month 12, FA, and OCT measurements), treatment burden of combination therapy (number of retreatments, time to first retreatment, RBZ treatment-free interval of 3 months or longer), and health economics outcomes.

Results

Two hundred eighty-six patients (89.1%) completed the 12-month study.
- Mean BCVA change at month 12 was + 5.3 and + 4.4 letters with verteporfin SF (n = 103) or verteporfin RF (n = 105) plus RBZ, respectively, compared with + 8.1 letters with RBZ monotherapy [n = 110; adjusted 97.5% confidence interval (CI), (-7.90 to infinity)]; p = 0.0666; and 97.5% CI, (-8.51 to infinity); p = 0.1178; for combination regimens versus monotherapy, respectively). Noninferiority of either combination regimen to monthly RBZ monotherapy was not demonstrated (primary end point).
- A RBZ treatment-free interval of 3 months or longer was achieved in 92.6% and 83.5% of the patients randomized to verteporfin SF or verteporfin RF groups, respectively, with a mean of 5.1 and 5.7 RBZ injections, respectively, and patients in the RBZ monotherapy arm received 10.5 injections.
- At month 12, mean central retinal thickness decreased by 151.7 µm and 140.9 µm for the verteporfin SF and RF groups, respectively, and by 172.2 µm with RBZ monotherapy.
- Safety and tolerability of all 3 regimens were similar to and consistent with previous studies in neovascular AMD. The number of ocular serious adverse events was low and occurred largely as single cases.

Conclusion

Ranibizumab monotherapy or combined with vPDT improved BCVA at month 12; however, noninferiority (7-letter margin) of combination regimens to RBZ monotherapy was not demonstrated. Verteporfin RF did not confer clinical benefits over verteporfin SF. All treatments were well tolerated.

Verteporfin Plus Ranibizumab for Choroidal Neovascularization in Age-related Macular Degeneration: MONT BLANC Study[6]

Purpose

To compare the efficacy and safety of same-day vPDT and intravitreal RBZ combination treatment versus RBZ monotherapy in neovascular AMD.

Description
It was a prospective, multicenter, double-masked, randomized, active-controlled trial. 255 patients with all types of active subfoveal CNV were included. Patients were randomized 1:1 to as-needed (PRN) combination (SF verteporfin 6 mg/m^2 PDT and RBZ 0.5 mg) or PRN RBZ monotherapy [sham infusion (5% dextrose) PDT and RBZ 0.5 mg]. Patients received 3 consecutive monthly injections followed by PRN retreatments based on protocol-specific retreatment criteria.

Inclusion Criteria
Enrollment criteria were 50 years of age, with any type of subfoveal CNV secondary to AMD, lesion size <9 DA, naïve to AMD treatment, and a BCVA letter score of 73–24 (Snellen equivalent 20/40–20/320).

Study Measures
Study outcomes include efficacy and safety (mean change in BCVA from baseline to month 12, FA, and OCT measurements), treatment burden of combination therapy (number of retreatments, time to first retreatment, and the proportion of patients with treatment-free interval ≥3 months at any time point after month 2), and health economics outcomes.

Results
- The mean change in BCVA at month 12 was + 2.5 and + 4.4 letters in the combination and monotherapy groups, respectively ($p = 0.0048$; difference: –1.9 letters (95% confidence interval, –5.76 to 1.86), for having achieved noninferiority with a margin of 7 letters).
- The proportion of patients with a treatment-free interval of ≥3 months at any time point after month 2 was high, but did not show a clinically relevant difference between the treatment groups.
- Secondary efficacy endpoints included the mean number of RBZ retreatments after month 2 [1.9 and 2.2 with combination and monotherapy, respectively ($p = 0.1373$)]. The time to first RBZ retreatment after month 2 was delayed by 34 days (about 1 monthly visit) with combination (month 6) versus monotherapy (month 5).
- At month 12, mean ± standard error central retinal thickness decreased by 115.3 ± 9.04 µm in the combination group and 107.7 ± 11.02 µm in the monotherapy group.
- The mean number of verteporfin/sham PDT treatments was comparable in the 2 groups (combination, 1.7; monotherapy, 1.9).
- The safety profiles of the 2 groups were comparable, with a low incidence of ocular serious adverse events.

Conclusion

The combination PRN treatment regimen with vPDT and RBZ was effective in achieving BCVA gain comparable with RBZ monotherapy; however, the study did not show benefits with respect to reducing the number of RBZ retreatment over 12 months. The combination therapy was well tolerated.

Efficacy and Safety of Verteporfin Photodynamic Therapy in Combination with Ranibizumab or Alone Versus Ranibizumab Monotherapy in Patients with Symptomatic Macular Polypoidal Choroidal Vasculopathy: EVEREST Study[7]

Purpose

To assess the effects of vPDT combined with RBZ or alone versus RBZ monotherapy in patients with symptomatic macular PCV.

Background

In Asia, especially among patients of East Asian descent, PCV has been reported to account for at least 30% of all cases of serosanguineous maculopathy. In contrast, the prevalence of PCV is only about 10% in nonAsian populations. Thus, the diagnosis of PCV might not be made in a significant proportion of Asian patients of Western retina practices if indocyanine green angiography (ICGA) is not performed due to lack of availability, accessibility, or awareness on the part of the physician.

The response of PCV to anti-VEGF monotherapy is unsatisfactory; one-third of patients do not respond, and polypoidal lesions persist in 9 of 10 cases. VPDT has been shown to be effective in achieving polyp closure when used alone or in combination with RBZ. The EVEREST trial was a part of the SUMMIT clinical trial series that specifically evaluated the efficacy of PDT in angiographic closure of PCV.

Description

In this multicenter, double-masked, primarily ICGA-guided trial, 61 Asian patients were randomized to vPDT (SF), RBZ 0.5 mg, or the combination. Patients were administered with vPDT/placebo and initiated with three consecutive monthly RBZ/sham injections starting Day 1, and retreated (months 3–5) as per predefined criteria.

Study Measures

The primary endpoint was the proportion of patients with ICGA-assessed complete regression of polyps at month 6. Secondary endpoints included mean change in BCVA at month 6 and safety.

Results

At month 6, verteporfin combined with RBZ or alone was superior to RBZ monotherapy in achieving complete polyp regression (77.8% and 71.4% vs. 28.6%; $p <0.01$); mean change ± standard deviation in BCVA (letters) was 10.9 ± 10.9 (vPDT + RBZ), 7.5 ± 10.6 (vPDT), and 9.2 ± 12.4 (RBZ). There were no new safety findings with either drug used alone or in combination.

Conclusion

Verteporfin PDT combined with RBZ 0.5 mg or alone was superior to RBZ monotherapy in achieving complete regression of polyps in this 6-month study in patients with symptomatic macular PCV. All treatments were well tolerated over 6 months.

Efficacy and Safety of Ranibizumab with or without Verteporfin Photodynamic Therapy for Polypoidal Choroidal Vasculopathy: A Randomized Clinical Trial: EVEREST 2 Study[8]

Purpose

To compare the efficacy and safety of combination therapy of RBZ and vPDT with RBZ monotherapy in PCV.

Background

The EVEREST study showed that combination therapy was significantly better than RBZ alone for complete polyp regression over the study period (6 months). Although BCVA improved in patients in both the groups, the study was not powered to compare these treatment modalities in terms of BCVA gains and the study period was limited to 6 months. Therefore, EVEREST II trial was conducted to compare the long-term effect of combination therapy versus RBZ monotherapy in symptomatic macular PCV over 24 months (2017).

Description

This was a 24-month multicenter, randomized, double-masked study conducted over several centers in Asia and included 322 patients with symptomatic macular PCV. The patients were recruited according to predefined criteria at a central reading center. Participants were randomized to combination therapy (RBZ, 0.5 mg and vPDT, $n = 168$) or RBZ, 0.5 mg, and sham PDT ($n = 154$). All participants received 3 consecutive monthly RBZ injections, followed by a PRN regimen. vPDT/sham PDT was done on day 1. The repeat vPDT/sham PDT was done on PRN regimen based on the presence of active polypoidal lesions but not before 3 months.

Study Measures

The primary objective was to demonstrate that:
- Combination therapy was noninferior to RBZ monotherapy in terms of change in BCVA from baseline to month 12
- Combination therapy was superior with respect to complete polyp regression (on ICGA) at month 12.

The secondary objectives included additional functional and anatomical outcomes, treatment exposure, and safety and tolerability for both treatments.

Results

- At 12 months, mean improvement from baseline was more ($p = 0.01$) with combination therapy (8.3 letters) than with monotherapy (5.1 letters) ($p = 0.01$).
- Combination therapy was also superior to monotherapy in achieving complete polyp regression (69.3% vs. 34.7%; $p < 0.001$)
- Combination therapy group received a median of 4 RBZ injections compared with 7 in the monotherapy group.
- Vitreous hemorrhage was more common in monotherapy group (2% vs. 0.6% in combination therapy group).

Conclusion

Combination therapy should be considered for treatment of PCV as it is superior to monotherapy in terms of BCVA and complete polyp regression while requiring fewer injections.

■ RADICAL (REDUCED FLUENCE VISUDYNE-ANTI-VEGF-DEXAMETHASONE IN COMBINATION FOR AMD LESIONS)[9]

Purpose

To determine if combination therapy [RF vPDT followed by RBZ (within 2 hours) or either of two regimens of RF vPDT followed by RBZ-dexamethasone triple therapy (within 2 hours)] reduces retreatment rates compared with RBZ monotherapy while maintaining similar vision outcomes and an acceptable safety profile.

Description

It was a Phase II, randomized, multicenter, single masked study conducted from 2007 to 2010, sponsored by QLT Inc. (Vancouver, Canada). 162 patients with CNV due to AMD were randomized into one of four treatment groups:

1. Quarter-fluence PDT (180 mW/cm^2 for 83 seconds to deliver 15 J/cm^2) followed within 2 hours by RBZ (0.5 mg) and dexamethasone (0.5 mg)

2. Half-fluence PDT (300 mW/cm^2 for 83 seconds to deliver 25 J/cm^2) followed within 2 hours by RBZ (0.5 mg) and dexamethasone (0.5 mg)
3. Half-fluence PDT (300 mW/cm^2 for 83 seconds to deliver 25 J/cm^2) followed within 2 hours by RBZ (0.5 mg)
4. RBZ monotherapy (0.5 mg) administered for the first 2 months followed by injections on an as-needed basis.

Initial treatment in the combination therapy groups was mandatory. The RBZ monotherapy group received mandatory injections for initial treatment and the first 2 months. After mandatory treatment, all groups received subsequent treatment on an as-needed basis. Patients were assessed to determine if retreatment was needed at each follow-up visit from month 1 (combination therapy groups) or month 3 (RBZ monotherapy group), except for the final visit. The study duration was 24 months with a planned primary analysis when all subjects completed 12 months of follow-up.

The treatments received in all groups were experimental: RF vPDT and as-needed RBZ are not standard regimens, while dexamethasone and combination therapies for AMD are not approved for marketing by regulatory agencies.

Inclusion Criteria

Patients aged 50 years or older with subfoveal CNV due to AMD and fulfilling the following criteria were eligible:
- Treatment naive except for laser treatment outside the subfoveal area
- Choroidal neovascularization ≥50% of the entire lesion
- All lesion composition types with a lesion greatest linear dimension (GLD) <5400 microns [approximately ≤9 disc areas (DA)]
- Best-corrected ETDRS VA score of 25–73 letters (approximate Snellen equivalent of 20/40 –20/320).

Study Measures

The primary outcome measures were the mean number of retreatments and the mean change in BCVA (ETDRS chart) from baseline in the study eye. Secondary outcome measures included percentage of subjects with ≥15 letters of VA gained from baseline, percentage of subjects with ≥0 letter gain of VA from baseline, percentage of subjects with ≥15 letters of VA lost from baseline, mean change from baseline in central retinal thickness and mean change from baseline in lesion size.

Results
- 12-month results showed that statistically significantly fewer retreatments were required with the combination therapies than with RBZ monotherapy. Of the four treatment groups, the triple therapy half-fluence group demonstrated superior results, with the fewest retreatment

visits (three) and mean VA improvement most comparable to PDT monotherapy.
- Through 24 months, patients in the triple therapy half-fluence group had a mean of 4.2 retreatment visits compared with 8.9 for patients who received RBZ monotherapy ($p < 0.001$). In the second year, the average number of retreatment visits in the triple therapy half-fluence group (1.2) was approximately one-third that of the RBZ monotherapy group (3.0). At the month 24 examination, mean VA in the triple therapy half-fluence group improved 1.8 letters fewer (95% confidence interval 11.1 letters fewer to 7.6 letters better) compared with the RBZ monotherapy group ($p = 0.71$).
- Ocular adverse events considered associated with treatment were reported for 30–38% of patients in the combination therapy groups, compared with 27% of patients in the RBZ monotherapy group. The higher incidence of these events with combination therapy is primarily due to vision disturbance events, which are transient and known to be associated with vPDT therapy.

Conclusion

The 24-month results showed that significantly fewer retreatment visits were required with combination therapies than with RBZ monotherapy. Mean VA change from baseline was not statistically different among the treatment groups, although the sample sizes were insufficient to draw definitive conclusions regarding VA outcomes. Overall adverse event incidence was similar across treatment groups, with no unexpected safety findings.

CABERNET (THE CHOROIDAL NEOVASCULARIZATION SECONDARY TO AMD TREATED WITH BETA RADIATION EPIRETINAL THERAPY)[10]

Purpose

To evaluate the safety and efficacy of epimacular brachytherapy (EMBT) for the treatment of CNV in neovascular AMD.

Background

Radiation therapy is being investigated for the treatment of neovascular AMD. The Epi-Rad90™ Ophthalmic System treats neovascularization of retinal tissue by means of a focal, directional delivery of radiation to the target tissues in the retina. Using standard vitreoretinal surgical techniques, the sealed radiation source is placed temporarily over the retinal lesion by means of a handheld medical device.

Description
It was a multicenter, randomized, active-controlled, phase III clinical trial of 494 participants with treatment-naïve neovascular AMD conducted from 2007 to 2012. Participants with classic, minimally classic, and occult lesions were randomized in a 2:1 ratio to EMBT or a RBZ monotherapy control arm. The EMBT arm received 2 mandated, monthly loading injections of 0.5 mg RBZ. The control arm received 3 mandated, monthly loading injections of RBZ then quarterly injections. Both arms also received monthly as needed (PRN) retreatment.

Inclusion Criteria
Patients aged 50 years or older with predominantly classic, minimally classic, or occult with no classic lesions, secondary to AMD, with a total lesion size (including blood, scarring, and neovascularization) of <12 total DA (21.24 mm^2), and a GLD ≤5.4 mm were included.

Study Measures
The proportion of participants losing fewer than 15 ETDRS letters from baseline VA and the proportion gaining more than 15 ETDRS letters from baseline VA were evaluated.

Results
At 24 months, 77% of the EMBT group and 90% of the control group lost fewer than 15 letters. This difference did not meet the prespecified 10% noninferiority margin. This end point was noninferior using a 20% margin and a 95% confidence interval for the group as a whole and for classic and minimally classic lesions, but not for occult lesions. The EMBT did not meet the superiority end point for the proportion of participants gaining more than 15 letters (16% for the EMBT group vs. 26% for the control group): this difference was statistically significant (favoring controls) for occult lesions, but not for predominantly classic and minimally classic lesions. Mean VA change was -2.5 letters in the EMBT arm and +4.4 letters in the control arm. Participants in the EMBT arm received a mean of 6.2 RBZ injections versus 10.4 in the control arm. At least 1 serious adverse event occurred in 54% of the EMBT arm, most commonly postvitrectomy cataract, versus 18% in the control arm. Mild, nonproliferative radiation retinopathy occurred in 3% of the EMBT participants, but no case was vision threatening.

Conclusion
The 2-year efficacy data do not support the routine use of EMBT for treatment-naïve wet AMD, despite an acceptable safety profile. Further safety review is required.

INITIAL VERSUS DELAYED PHOTODYNAMIC THERAPY IN COMBINATION WITH RANIBIZUMAB FOR TREATMENT OF POLYPOIDAL CHOROIDAL VASCULOPATHY: THE FUJISAN STUDY[11]

Purpose

To compare the results of initial or deferred vPDT combined with intravitreal ranibizumab (IVR) for PCV.

Background

Though vPDT is known to resolve the polyps well in the setting of PCV, anti-VEGF also work well in maintaining the vision in these patients. However, anti-VEGFs especially, RBZ have limited ability to regress the polyps. The both modalities can thus be combined to get good results. The exact timing of vPDT (at the beginning or after anti-VEGF therapy) is not known which this study (2015) has tried to address.

Description

This was a prospective, multicenter, randomized trial and was conducted at six Japanese centers from January 2011 to October 2012. 72 eyes with treatment naive PCV were randomized to initial or deferred PDT combined with IVR. In both groups, 2 additional monthly IVR followed. From month 3, PDT and IVR were administered according to the retreatment criteria.

Inclusion and exclusion criteria: PCV was diagnosed based on polypoidal lesions or polyps with or without a branching vascular network on ICGA, BCVA range from 0.1 to 0.7 using a Landolt C chart and greatest lesion size less than 12 macular photocoagulation study disc areas. Eyes with central serous chorioretinopathy, retinal vascular disease, any neovascular maculopathy, glaucoma, or a history of intraocular surgery other than phacoemulsification were excluded.

Study Measures

The primary outcome was to assess difference in BCVA at 12 months from baseline between the two groups. Secondary outcomes were to compare mean central retinal thickness, regression of polypoidal lesions and number of additional treatments.

Results

- Best corrected visual acuity improved by a mean of 8.1 and 8.8 ETDRS letters in the initial and later PDT group, and these were comparable ($p = 0.59$).
- The mean central retinal thickness decreased significantly in both groups though it was more with combination therapy within the first 4 months

(at each visit); the difference was not statistically significant at 12 months ($p = 0.30$).
- Regression of polypoidal lesions at 12 months was 62.1% in the initial PDT group and 54.8% in the later PDT group, this was not statistically significant ($p = 0.53$).
- The mean number of additional IVR was 1.5 in initial PDT and 3.8 in later PDT; additional PDTs were 0.14 and 0.45, respectively, and they were significantly different.

Conclusion

Both initial and deferred PDT combined with IVR show the similar visual and anatomical improvements at 12 months in PCV treatment. Initial PDT combination leads to significantly fewer additional treatments.

AFLIBERCEPT IN POLYPOIDAL CHOROIDAL VASCULOPATHY (PLANET) STUDY [12,13]

Efficacy and Safety of Intravitreal Aflibercept for Polypoidal Choroidal Vasculopathy in the PLANET Study: A Randomized Clinical Trial

Purpose

To evaluate intravitreal aflibercept (IVA) in patients with PCV and compare IVA monotherapy with IVA plus rescue vPDT.

Background

While vPDT has been the first widely used treatment for PCV, it is associated with several other complications including recurrent hemorrhages, exudation, atrophy and choroidal ischemia. Anti-VEGF monotherapy is currently the gold standard for other forms of neovascular AMD. Therefore, this study was conducted to assess IVA in PCV.

Description

This 96-week, double-masked, sham-controlled phase 3b/4 randomized clinical trial was conducted at multiple centers in Australia, Germany, Hong Kong, Hungary, Japan, Singapore, South Korea, and Taiwan from May 2014 to August 2016.

The study included adults ≥50 years with symptomatic macular PCV (GLD <5400 mm) and BCVA of 73–24 ETDRS letters (Snellen equivalent 20/40–20/320). Eyes with prior use of intravitreal or subtenon corticosteroids, intraocular anti-VEGF agents or macular laser in the study eye or systemic use of anti-VEGF products within 3 months prior to study were excluded.

All patients received three IVAs at 0, 4, and 8 weeks. At week 12, patients were randomized to IVA monotherapy or IVA combined with vPDT. In both the groups patient not meeting rescue criteria were given 8 weekly IVA. Eyes with suboptimal response (meeting rescue criteria) were to receive IVA 4 weekly plus sham vPDT (in IVA monotherapy group) or IVA 4 weekly plus rescue PDT (in combined group). When the rescue criteria were no longer met, injection intervals were gradually extended to 8 weeks.

Study Measures

Primary objective of the study was to evaluate efficacy and safety of IVA monotherapy and noninferiority of IVA monotherapy to IVA/vPDT for mean change in BCVA from baseline to 52 weeks. Secondary objectives were to estimate the proportion of patients who required active PDT and whether active PDT was beneficial in eyes with suboptimal response to IVA monotherapy.

Results

A total of 318 patients with mean age of 70.6 years were included of whom, 30.2% were women, and 47.8% were Japanese.

Intravitreal aflibercept (IVA) monotherapy was noninferior to IVA/vPDT for the primary end point with few participants requiring rescue therapy (12.1% vs. 14.3% respectively).

- Participants in both treatment groups had similar reductions in CMT from baseline to week 52.
- At week 52, 38.9% and 44.8% had no polypoidal lesions observed on ICGA in the IVA monotherapy and combined therapy groups, respectively. 81.7% and 88.9% respectively had no polypoidal lesions with leakage.

Conclusion

Visual and/or functional outcomes improved in more than 85% of patients receiving IVA monotherapy. More than 80% eyes showed no signs of leakage from polypoidal lesions. As <15% met the criteria of a suboptimal response to receive PDT, the potential benefit of adding PDT cannot be determined.
2-year result:
- Over 96 weeks, 17.0% met rescue criteria.
- Intravitreal aflibercept monotherapy was noninferior to IVA/vPDT in terms of BCVA.
- Proportions of patients with complete polyp regression (33.1% vs. 29.1%) or without active polyps (82.1% vs. 85.6%) were similar.
- In year 2, the mean number of injections was 4.6 in both arms.

The other Trials in PCV that readers may be interested in are LAPTOP, APOLLO, VAULT, ALTAIR and DRAGON.

Table 1: Clinical trials in ARMD III.

Title	Purpose	No. of Patients	Inclusion criteria	Outcome measure	Result/Conclusion
FOCUS	RBZ combined with verteporfin PDT in predominantly classic CNV in AMD	162	Predominantly classic CNV in AMD (PDT was performed 7 days before initial RBZ or sham treatment)	Proportion of patients losing fewer than 15 letters from baseline visual acuity at 12 months	RBZ + PDT were more efficacious than PDT alone for treating neovascular AMD, though RBZ treatment increased the risk of serious intraocular inflammation
PROTECT	Safety of same-day administration of verteporfin PDT (standard fluence) and RBZ	32	Predominantly classic or occult CNV secondary to AMD	Incidence of severe vision loss (BCVA loss ≥30 letters)	Same day verteporfin and RBZ was safe and not associated with severe vision loss or severe ocular inflammation
TORPEDO	One-time reduced-fluence-PDT followed by RBZ on a variable dosing regimen in neovascular AMD	27	Previously untreated, active neovascular AMD	Improvement in BCVA over 2 years	Combined PDT and RBZ injection the same day were well tolerated in all patients. 84% of patients had stable or improved vision at month 24
DENALI	RBZ in combination with verteporfin PDT versus RBZ monotherapy in subfoveal CNV in AMD	321	Subfoveal CNV in AMD, lesion size <9 DA, naïve to AMD treatment, and a BCVA letter score of 73–24	Mean change in BCVA from baseline at month 12	• RBZ monotherapy or combined with verteporfin PDT improved BCVA at month 12 • Verteporfin reduced fluence did not confer clinical benefits over verteporfin standard fluence
MONT BLANC	Same-day verteporfin PDT and intravitreal RBZ versus RBZ monotherapy in neovascular AMD	255	Subfoveal CNV secondary to AMD, lesion size <9 DA, naïve to AMD treatment, and a BCVA letter score of 73–24	Mean change in BCVA from baseline to month 12	• The combination was effective in achieving BCVA gain comparable with RBZ monotherapy • Study did not show benefits with respect to reducing the number of RBZ retreatment over 12 months

Contd...

Contd...

Title	Purpose	No. of Patients	Inclusion criteria	Outcome measure	Result/Conclusion
EVEREST	Verteporfin PDT combined with RBZ or alone versus RBZ monotherapy in symptomatic macular PCV	61	PCV with BCVA letter score between 73–24, greatest linear dimension of the total lesion area <5400 μm	Proportion of patients with ICGA-assessed complete regression of polyps at month 6	At month 6, verteporfin combined with RBZ or alone was superior to RBZ monotherapy in achieving complete polyp regression
EVEREST 2	vPDT at baseline combined with RBZ versus RBZ monotherapy in PCV	322 Asian patients	Symptomatic macular PCV confirmed by the central reading center using ICGA	Change in BCVA from baseline to month 12 Complete regression of polyp	Combination therapy of RBZ + vPDT was not only noninferior but also superior to RBZ monotherapy in BCVA and superior in complete polyp regression while requiring fewer injections
RADICAL	RF PDT+RBZ versus either of two regimens of RF PDT + RBZ + Dexamethasone versus RBZ monotherapy	162	Treatment naive subfoveal CNV due to AMD, GLD <9 DA, BCVA score of 25–73 letters	Mean number of retreatments and the mean change in BCVA from baseline at 24 months	• Significantly fewer retreatment visits were required with combination therapies than with RBZ monotherapy. • Mean VA change from baseline was not statistically different among the treatment groups
CABERNET	Safety and efficacy of epimacular brachytherapy (EMBT) for the treatment of CNV in neovascular AMD	494	Predominantly classic, minimally classic, or occult with no classic lesions, secondary to AMD, with a total lesion size of <12 DA, and a GLD ≤5.4 mm	Proportion of patients losing fewer than 15 letters from baseline and the proportion gaining more than 15 letters	The 2-year efficacy data do not support the routine use of EMBT for treatment-naïve wet AMD, despite an acceptable safety profile

Contd...

Contd...

Title	Purpose	No. of Patients	Inclusion criteria	Outcome measure	Result/Conclusion
Fujisan	Compare initial or deferred vPDT combined with IVR for PCV	72	Treatment naïve PCV BCVA range from 0.1 to 0.7 on Landolt C chart GLD <12 MPS disk area	Mean change in BCVA from baseline to month 12	• Both initial and deferred PDT combined with IVR show the similar visual and anatomical improvements at 12 months • Initial PDT combination leads to significantly fewer additional treatments
PLANET	Compare IVA monotherapy with IVA plus rescue vPDT in PCV	318	Symptomatic macular PCV ≥50 year and BCVA 20/40–20/320	Mean change in BCVA from baseline to week 52	Monotherapy with IVA was noninferior to IVA/PDT with few participants requiring rescue therapy (12.1% vs. 14.3%, respectively)

(IVA: intravitreal aflibercept; PCV: polypoidal choroidal vasculopathy; BCVA: best corrected visual acuity; PDT: photodynamic therapy; vPDT: verteporfin photodynamic therapy; GLD: greatest linear dimension; IVR: intravitreal ranibizumab; RBZ: ranibizumab; AMD: age-related macular degeneration; CNV: choroidal neovascularization; ICGA: indocyanine green angiography)

REFERENCES

1. Heier JS, Boyer DS, Ciulla TA, Ferrone PJ, Jumper JM, Gentile RC, et al. Ranibizumab combined with verteporfin photodynamic therapy in neovascular age-related macular degeneration: year 1 results of the FOCUS Study. Arch Ophthalmol. 2006;124(11):1532-42.
2. Antoszyk AN, Tuomi L, Chung CY, Singh A. Ranibizumab combined with verteporfin photodynamic therapy in neovascular age-related macular degeneration (FOCUS): year 2 results. Am J Ophthalmol. 2008;145(5):862-74.
3. Schmidt-Erfurth U, Wolf S. Same-day administration of verteporfin and ranibizumab 0.5 mg in patients with choroidal neovascularisation due to age-related macular degeneration. Br J Ophthalmol. 2008;92(12):1628-35.
4. Spielberg L, Leys A. Treatment of neovascular age-related macular degeneration with a variable ranibizumab dosing regimen and one-time reduced-fluence photodynamic therapy: the TORPEDO trial at 2 years. Graefes Arch Clin Exp Ophthalmol. 2010;248(7):943-56.
5. Kaiser PK, Boyer DS, Cruess AF, Slakter JS, Pilz S, Weisberger A. Verteporfin plus ranibizumab for choroidal neovascularization in age-related macular degeneration: twelve-month results of the DENALI study. Ophthalmology. 2012;119(5):1001-10.
6. Larsen M, Schmidt-Erfurth U, Lanzetta P, Wolf S, Simader C, Tokaji E, et al. Verteporfin plus ranibizumab for choroidal neovascularization in age-related macular degeneration: twelve-month MONT BLANC study results. Ophthalmology. 2012;119(5):992-1000.
7. Koh A, Lee WK, Chen LJ, Chen SJ, Hashad Y, Kim H, et al. EVEREST study: efficacy and safety of verteporfin photodynamic therapy in combination with ranibizumab or alone versus ranibizumab monotherapy in patients with symptomatic macular polypoidal choroidal vasculopathy. Retina. 2012;32(8):1453-64.
8. Koh A, Lai TY, Takahashi K, Wong TY, Chen LJ, Ruamviboonsuk P, et al. Efficacy and safety of ranibizumab with or without verteporfin photodynamic therapy for polypoidal choroidal vasculopathy: a randomized clinical trial. JAMA Ophthalmol. 2017;135(11):1206-13.
9. Drugs.com. QLT announces final results: Radical study evaluating verteporfin PDT visudyne combination therapy. [online] Available from http://www.drugs.com/clinical_trials/qlt-announces-final-results-radical-study-evaluating-verteporfin-pdt-visudyne-combination-therapy-9675.html. [Last accessed January, 2021]
10. Dugel PU, Bebchuk JD, Nau J, Reichel E, Singer M, Barak A, et al. Epimacular brachytherapy for neovascular age-related macular degeneration: a randomized, controlled trial (CABERNET). Ophthalmology. 2013;120(2):317-27.
11. Gomi F, Oshima Y, Mori R, Kano M, Saito M, Yamashita A, et al. Initial versus delayed photodynamic therapy in combination with ranibizumab for treatment of polypoidal choroidal vasculopathy: The Fujisan Study. Retina. 2015;35(8):1569-76.
12. Lee WK, Iida T, Ogura Y, Chen SJ, Wong TY, Mitchell P, et al. Efficacy and safety of intravitreal aflibercept for polypoidal choroidal vasculopathy in the PLANET study: a randomized clinical trial. JAMA Ophthalmol. 2018;136(7):786-93.
13. Wong TY, Ogura Y, Lee WK, Iida T, Chen SJ, Mitchell P, et al. Efficacy and safety of intravitreal Aflibercept for polypoidal choroidal vasculopathy: two-year results of the Aflibercept in polypoidal choroidal vasculopathy study. Am J Ophthalmol. 2019;204:80-9.

Clinical Trials in Age-related Macular Degeneration-IV

Pooja Shah, Arpit Sharma, Neha Goel

AGE-RELATED EYE DISEASE STUDY (AREDS)[1,2]

Purpose

1. To assess the clinical course, prognosis, and risk factors of age-related macular degeneration (AMD) and cataract.
2. To evaluate the effects of high doses of antioxidants and zinc on the progression of AMD and vision loss.
3. To evaluate the effects of high doses of antioxidants on the development and progression of cataract and vision loss.

Background

Age-related macular degeneration (AMD) and cataract are the leading causes of visual impairment and blindness.

Risk factors for AMD include older age, Caucasian race, family history of AMD, hypermetropia, cardiovascular disease, smoking, and hypertension. Treatments for advanced AMD are very limited, and there has been no treatment to slow the progression of intermediate AMD. As the average lifespan of population increases, the number of people who develop AMD will increase dramatically. Unless successful means of prevention or treatment are developed, blindness from AMD and its importance as a public health problem will increase.

Animal studies, observational epidemiologic studies, and a few small clinical trials had previously suggested that antioxidants and the trace elements zinc and selenium may be associated with the risk of AMD and cataract development. Also, a small, randomized clinical trial of zinc supplementation found a statistically significant reduction in vision loss in a group treated with zinc compared with a group treated with a placebo, a harmless substance that has no effect on eye disease. The conclusion of the pilot study was that a more definitive study was necessary.

Description

The AREDS included two long term, multicenter, prospective, double masked clinical trials—one for AMD and one for cataract—that generally shared one pool of participants. There were 4,757 participants, aged 55–80 years, enrolled in the study. The participants were enrolled in 11 clinics nationwide. Enrolment began in November 1992 and ended in January 1998. About 90% of all participants were followed for a minimum of 5 years.

Because 1,117 participants did not have at least early stages of AMD, the AMD trial included only the 3,640 participants who had at least early AMD. The cataract results are based on 4,629 enrollees; 128 of the 4,757 participants had cataract surgery on both eyes prior to enrolment and therefore were ineligible for the cataract clinical trial.

The participants' stages of disease ranged from no evidence of AMD in either eye, to advanced AMD with vision loss in one eye but good vision (at least 20/30) in the other eye. Depending on their stages of AMD, the AREDS participants were placed in one of four categories. The one constant was that at least one eye of each participant had to be free from any vision-threatening eye disease other than AMD or cataract, and that eye could not have had previous surgery, except for cataract surgery.

1. *In category one*, participants had *no AMD* and a few small or no drusen —tiny yellow deposits in the retina—in either eye.
2. In *category two*, participants had *early AMD*—either several small drusen or a few medium-sized drusen in one or both eyes.
3. *Category three* participants had intermediate AMD—either many medium-sized drusen or one or more large drusen in one or both eyes; these participants were at high risk for developing advanced AMD, which is generally defined as either a breakdown of light-sensitive cells and supporting tissue in the central retinal area (advanced dry form), or abnormal and fragile blood vessels under the retina (wet form).
4. *Category four* participants already had *advanced AMD* in one eye, and in the other eye had good vision with no sign of advanced AMD. Previous studies had shown that the eye without AMD was at high risk for developing advanced AMD.

The participants in each category were randomly selected to receive daily oral tablets for one of four treatments: (1) zinc alone; (2) antioxidants alone; (3) a combination of antioxidants and zinc; or (4) a placebo. The specific daily amounts of antioxidants and zinc used by the AREDS researchers were 500 mg of vitamin C; 400 IU of vitamin E; 15 mg of beta-carotene; 80 mg of zinc as zinc oxide; and 2 mg of copper as cupric oxide.

Baseline and annual (starting at year 2) lens photographs were graded at a reading center for the severity of lens opacities using the AREDS cataract grading scale.

Inclusion Criteria

The study enrolled participants in an AMD trial if they had extensive small drusen, intermediate drusen, large drusen, noncentral geographic atrophy, or pigment abnormalities in one or both eyes, or advanced AMD or vision loss due to AMD in one eye. At least one eye had best-corrected visual acuity of 20/32 or better.

Study Measures

Primary outcomes were—(1) an increase from baseline in nuclear, cortical, or posterior subcapsular opacity grades or cataract surgery, and (2) at least moderate visual acuity loss from baseline (≥15 letters). Primary analyses used repeated-measures logistic regression with a statistical significance level of $p = 0.01$. Serum level measurements, medical histories, and mortality rates were used for safety monitoring.

Results

Age-related macular degeneration (AMD): Average follow-up of the 3,640 enrolled study participants, aged 55–80 years, was 6.3 years, with 2.4% lost to follow-up.

- AREDS scientists found that people at high risk for developing advanced ARMD—those with intermediate AMD, and those with advanced ARMD in one eye only *(Category 3 and 4)*—reduced their risk of developing advanced stages of ARMD by about 25% when treated with the combination of "antioxidants plus zinc". The combination of "antioxidants plus zinc" also reduced the risk of central vision loss by 19% in the same group. Participants at high risk for developing advanced AMD who were treated with "zinc alone" reduced their risk of developing advanced AMD by about 21% and their risk of vision loss by about 11%. Participants who were treated with "antioxidants alone" reduced their risk of developing advanced stages of AMD by about 17% and their risk of vision loss by about 10%.
- The study was not designed to evaluate the effect of the antioxidants and zinc in study participants who initially had no AMD (*Category One*). This is because previous studies had indicated that people aged 60 and over with no AMD have a very low risk for developing a clear progression of AMD within a 7-year period (the life of the AREDS clinical trial). The AREDS confirmed this low risk—participants with no AMD had less than a 1% chance of losing vision from AMD during the study.
- For those study participants who initially had early AMD (*Category Two*), the antioxidants and zinc used by the AREDS researchers did not slow the disease's progression to intermediate AMD. Consequently, there is no apparent need for those diagnosed with early AMD to take the combination studied in the AREDS. However, those with early AMD should get dilated eye examinations every year to determine if the disease is progressing.

Cataract: Of 4,757 participants enrolled, 4,629 who were aged from 55 to 80 years had at least 1 natural lens present and were followed up for an average of 6.3 years. No statistically significant effect of the antioxidant formulation was seen on the development or progression of age-related lens opacities (odds ratio = 0.97, p = 0.55). There was also no statistically significant effect of treatment in reducing the risk of progression for any of the 3 lens opacity types or for cataract surgery. No statistically significant serious adverse effect was associated with treatment.

Conclusion

- Persons older than 55 years should have dilated eye examinations to determine their risk of developing advanced AMD. Those with extensive intermediate size drusen, at least 1 large druse, noncentral geographic atrophy in 1 or both eyes, or advanced AMD or vision loss due to AMD in 1 eye, and without contraindications such as smoking, should consider taking a supplement of antioxidants plus zinc such as that used in this study.
- Use of a high-dose formulation of vitamin C, vitamin E, and beta carotene in a relatively well-nourished older adult cohort had no apparent effect on the 7-year risk of development or progression of age-related lens opacities or visual acuity loss.

■ AGE-RELATED EYE DISEASE STUDY 2[3,6]

Purpose

1. To evaluate the effect of the two dietary xanthophylls (lutein and zeaxanthin) that accumulate in macula and two omega-3 long-chain polyunsaturated fatty acids (LCPUFAs), docosahexaenoic acid (DHA) and eicosapentaenoic acid (EPA), on progression to AMD and/or moderate vision loss in people at moderate-to high-risk for progression.
2. To evaluate the effects of eliminating beta-carotene from the original AREDS formulation on the development and progression of AMD.
3. To evaluate the effects of reducing zinc in the original AREDS formulation on the development and progression of AMD.
4. To contribute data for validation of the photographic AMD scales developed from the AREDS.

Background

The AREDS demonstrated beneficial effects of oral supplementation with antioxidant vitamins and minerals on the development of advanced AMD in persons with at least intermediate AMD (bilateral large drusen with or without pigment changes). Observational data suggest that other oral nutrient supplements might further reduce the risk of progression to advanced AMD.

Description
It was a multicenter, phase III, randomized, controlled clinical trial, 4,203 participants were enrolled at 82 clinical centers located in the United States. Enrolment concluded in June 2008 and the follow-up concluded in October 2012. All participants were randomly assigned to placebo ($n = 1,012$), L + Z (10 mg/2 mg; $n = 1,044$), ω-3 LCPUFAs [EPA + DHA (650 mg/350 mg); $n = 1069$], or the combination of L+Z and ω-3 LCPUFAs ($n = 1,078$). All participants were offered a secondary randomization to 1 of 4 variations of the original AREDS formulation keeping vitamins C (500 mg) and E (400 IU) and copper (2 mg) unchanged while varying zinc and β-carotene as follows: Zinc remains at the original level (80 mg), lower only zinc to 25 mg, omit β-carotene only, or lower zinc to 25 mg and omit β-carotene.

Inclusion Criteria
Persons aged 50–85 years with bilateral intermediate AMD or advanced AMD in one eye were included.

Study Measures
The main outcome measure was progression to advanced AMD determined by centralized grading of annual fundus photographs.

Results
- Baseline characteristics of participants were as follows: mean age 74 years, 57% female, 97% white, 7% current smokers, 19% with prior cardiovascular disease and 44% and 50% taking statin-class cholesterol lowering drugs and aspirin, respectively.
- Ocular characteristics include 59% with bilateral large drusen, 32% with advanced AMD in one eye and mean visual acuity of 20/32 in eyes without advanced AMD.
- During median follow-up of 5 years, 1,940 study eyes (1,608 participants) progressed to advanced AMD.
- Kaplan-Meier probabilities of progression to advanced AMD by 5 years were similar across all groups viz. 31% [493 eyes (406 participants)] for placebo, 29% [468 eyes (399 participants)] for L + Z, 31% [507 eyes (416 participants)] for DHA + EPA, and 30% [472 eyes (387 participants)] for L + Z + DHA + EPA.
- There was no apparent effect of beta carotene elimination or lower-dose zinc on progression to advanced AMD.
- More lung cancers were noted in former smokers in the beta carotene versus no beta carotene group [23 (2.0%) vs. 11 (0.9%), $p = 0.04$].

Conclusion
Addition of L + Z, DHA + EPA, or both to the AREDS formulation in primary analyses did not further reduce risk of progression to advanced AMD.

In view of potential increased incidence of lung cancer in former smokers, lutein + zeaxanthin could be an appropriate carotenoid substitute in the AREDS formulation.

■ COMPLICATIONS OF AGE-RELATED MACULAR DEGENERATION PREVENTION TRIAL (CAPT)[4,5]

Purpose

To determine whether application of low-intensity laser treatment of eyes with drusen in the macula can prevent later complications of AMD and thereby preserve visual function.

Background

Complications of AMD are the leading cause of severe vision loss among people aged 65 and over in the United States and many Western countries. Most, (approximately 90%), of this vision loss is due to the neovascular (or wet) form of AMD.

The first sign that an eye may develop AMD is the presence of drusen. Current data suggests that eyes with large drusen are at increased risk for developing the vision threatening complications of AMD. Since the 1970s investigators have reported consistently that laser photocoagulation causes a reduction in large drusen. However, results of the effects of laser treatment on preventing later complications of AMD have been less consistent and based on relatively small numbers of patients.

Further study into the ability of a treatment to prevent vision loss from the advanced forms of AMD would have profound public health implications. A treatment that could reduce the risk of developing neovascularization by 30% might reduce the risk of blindness from AMD by one half.

Description

The CAPT was a multicenter, prospective, randomized clinical trial. A total of 1,052 were enrolled at 22 clinical centers across the United States from May 1, 1999 to March 31, 2001. Eligible patients had one eye randomly assigned to laser treatment performed by a CAPT-certified ophthalmologist. The other eye was not treated. All patients were treated immediately after randomization and again at 12 months, dependent on clinical status. Initial laser treatment protocol specified 60 barely visible burns applied in a grid pattern within an annulus between 1,500 and 2,500 μm from the foveal center. At 12 months, eyes assigned to treatment that had sufficient drusen remaining were retreated with 30 burns by targeting drusen within an annulus between 1,000 and 2,000 μm from the foveal center.

All patients are followed via study visits and telephone calls for a minimum of 5 years. Study visit procedures included established tests of visual function conducted by examiners masked to the treatment assignment of each eye, a biomicroscopic examination by CAPT ophthalmologists, and photographs of each eye taken according to protocol and assessed by masked graders in a centralized photograph reading center.

Inclusion Criteria

Patients eligible for CAPT were either male or female, aged at least 50, vision in each eye 20/40 or better with at least 10 large (>125 μm) drusen in each eye.

Study Measures

The effectiveness of the treatment was assessed using the following criteria:
- Change in visual acuity (primary outcome measure of the study): Proportion of eyes at 5 years with loss of ≥3 lines of VA from baseline.
- Incidence of complications of AMD such as choroidal neovascularization (CNV), serous detachment of the pigment epithelium, and geographic atrophy (GA)
- Changes in contrast threshold and critical print size for reading
- Quality of life assessments for patients, using the Visual Function Questionnaire 25 (VFQ-25)—conducted at the time of enrolment and at 5 years.

Results

- At 5 years, 188 (20.5%) treated eyes and 188 (20.5%) observed eyes had VA scores ≥3 lines worse than at the initial visit ($p = 1.00$). Cumulative 5-year incidence rates for treated and observed eyes were 13.3% and 13.3% ($p = 0.95$) for CNV and 7.4% and 7.8% ($p = 0.64$) for GA, respectively. The contrast threshold doubled in 23.9% of treated eyes and in 20.5% of observed eyes ($p = 0.40$). The critical print size doubled in 29.6% of treated eyes and in 28.4% of observed eyes ($p = 0.70$). Seven treated eyes and 14 observed eyes had an adverse event of a ≥6-line loss in VA in the absence of late AMD or cataract.
- CNV developed in 141 observed eyes and 141 treated eyes, including 57 patients affected bilaterally. Statistically significant risk factors for CNV in the multivariate model for all eyes were older age [RR, 2.81 (95% CI, 1.33–5.94) for >79 years vs. 50-59 years], cigarette smoking [RR, 1.98 (95% CI, 1.16–3.39) for current vs. never], and focal hyperpigmentation [RR, 1.84 (95% CI, 1.22-2.76) for ≥250 μm vs. none]. Among eyes free of GA at baseline, endpoint GA developed in 61 observed eyes and in 58 treated eyes, including 29 patients affected bilaterally. Statistically significant risk factors for GA in the multivariate model for all eyes were older age [RR, 6.39 (95% CI, 1.64–24.9) for >79 years vs. 50-59 years], greater retinal area covered by drusen [RR, 5.10 (95% CI, 2.57-10.1) for ≥25% vs. <10%], retinal pigment epithelium (RPE) depigmentation [RR, 2.64 (95% CI, 1.26-5.53)], and focal hyperpigmentation [RR, 10.4 (95% CI, 4.51-24.0) for ≥250 μm vs. none].

Conclusion

- As applied in the CAPT, low-intensity laser treatment did not demonstrate a clinically significant benefit for vision in eyes of people with bilateral large drusen.
- Among CAPT participants, increased age and focal hyperpigmentation were risk factors for the development of CNV and for GA. Cigarette smoking was significantly associated with CNV only, whereas retinal area covered by drusen and RPE depigmentation were associated significantly with GA only.

Several studies have explored drugs targeting complement system for treatment of AMD especially geographic atrophy. Notable mentions include Lampalizumab, a humanized antigen binding fragment (Fab) targeting Complement Factor D, failed to reduce enlargement of geographic atrophy due to AMD in phase 3 trials CHROMA and SPECTRI despite a positive phase 2 trial MAHALO. Systemic Eculizumab, a humanized anti-C5 antibody failed to slow progression of geographic atrophy in phase 2 COMPLETE study.

Table 1: Summary of different clinical trials in age-related macular degeneration–IV.

Title	Purpose	No. of Patients	Inclusion criteria	Outcome measure	Result/Conclusion
AREDS (1992)	To determine clinical course, prognosis, and risk factors of AMD and cataract To evaluate effect of the two dietary xanthophylls and two omega-3 fatty acids (LCPUFAs), on progression to AMD and/or moderate vision loss in people at moderate to high risk for progression.	4,757	Extensive small drusen, intermediate drusen, large drusen, noncentral GA, or pigment abnormalities in one or both eyes, or advanced AMD or vision loss due to AMD in one eye. At least one eye had best-corrected visual acuity of 20/32 or better.	Increase from baseline in nuclear, cortical, or posterior subcapsular opacity grades or cataract surgery Moderate visual acuity loss from baseline	Patients with extensive intermediate sized drusen, at least one large druse, noncentral GA in one or both eyes, or advanced AMD or vision loss due to AMD in one eye should consider taking a supplement of antioxidants plus zinc Use of a high-dose formulations of vitamin C, E, and beta carotene in well-nourished older adult cohort had no apparent effect on the 7-year risk of development or progression of age-related lens opacities

Contd...

Contd...

Title	Purpose	No. of Patients	Inclusion criteria	Outcome measure	Result/Conclusion
AREDS-2 (2006)	To evaluate effect of the two dietary xanthophylls and two omega-3 fatty acids (LCPUFAs), on progression to AMD and/or moderate vision loss in people at moderate to high risk for progression	4,203	Persons aged 50–85 with bilateral intermediate AMD or advanced AMD in one eye	Progression to advanced AMD	Addition of L+Z, DHA + EPA, or both to the AREDS formulation did not further reduce risk of progression to advanced AMD. Lutein and Zeaxanthin could be an appropriate carotenoid substitute in the AREDS formulation in view of potential increased incidence of lung cancer in former smokers
CAPT (1999)	Low-intensity laser of eyes with drusen in the macula for preventing later complications of AMD	1,052	Male or female, aged at least 50, vision in each eye 20/40 or better with at least 10 large (>125 μm) drusen in each eye	Change in visual acuity and incidence of complications of AMD (CNV, GA)	Low-intensity laser treatment did not demonstrate a clinically significant benefit for vision. Risk factors for CNV and GA stated

(AMD: age-related macular degeneration; AREDS: Age-related Eye Disease Study; CAPT: Complications of Age-related Macular Degeneration Prevention Trial; CNV: choroidal neovascularization; DHA: docosahexaenoic acid; EPA: eicosapentaenoic acid; GA: geographic atrophy)

REFERENCES

1. Age-related Eye Disease Study Research Group. A randomized, placebo-controlled, clinical trial of high-dose supplementation with vitamins C and E, beta carotene, and zinc for age-related macular degeneration and vision loss: AREDS report no. 8. Arch Ophthalmol. 2001;119:1417-36.
2. Age-related Eye Disease Study Research Group. A randomized, placebo-controlled, clinical trial of high-dose supplementation with vitamins C and E and beta carotene for age-related cataract and vision loss: AREDS report no. 9. Arch Ophthalmol. 2001; 119:1439-52.
3. AREDS2 Research Group. The Age-related Eye Disease Study 2 (AREDS2): study design and baseline characteristics (AREDS2 report number 1). Ophthalmology. 2012;119:2282-9.
4. Complications of Age-related Macular Degeneration Prevention Trial Research Group: Laser treatment in patients with bilateral large drusen: the complications of age-related macular degeneration prevention trial. Ophthalmology. 2006; 113:1974-86.
5. Complications of Age-related Macular Degeneration Prevention Trial (CAPT) Research Group. Risk factors for choroidal neovascularization and geographic atrophy in the complications of age-related macular degeneration prevention trial. Ophthalmology. 2008;115:1474-1479.e1-6.
6. Age-related Eye Disease Study 2 Research Group. Lutein + zeaxanthin and omega-3 fatty acids for age-related macular degeneration: the Age-Related Eye Disease Study 2 (AREDS2) randomized clinical trial. JAMA. 2013;309(19):2005-15.

Clinical Trials in Retinal Detachment

Vinod Kumar, Neha Goel

■ SILICONE OIL STUDY[1-12]

Purpose

1. To compare, through a randomized, multicenter surgical trial, the postoperative tamponade effectiveness of intraocular silicone oil with that of an intraocular long-acting gas [initially sulfur hexafluoride (SF_6), later perfluoropropane (C_3F_8)] for the management of retinal detachment (RD) complicated by proliferative vitreoretinopathy (PVR), using vitrectomy and associated techniques.
2. To evaluate the ocular complications that result from the use of silicone oil and gas.

Background

The treatment of RD complicated by PVR remains controversial. Although some cases are managed successfully by pars plana vitrectomy (PPV) and with temporary tamponade provided by intraocular gas, others eventually redetach with this technique. Preliminary reports indicate improved anatomical success with prolonged liquid silicone-assisted tamponade, but the eventual visual outcome may be confounded by silicone-related complications, particularly glaucoma and keratopathy. The addition of hydraulic reattachment by simultaneous fluid/gas exchange to vitrectomy surgery has proved to be an important development. Although complications are few with these procedures, subsequent redetachment is frequent.

Description

Recruitment began in 1985, and was completed in 1991. Two groups of eyes were entered into the study: eyes that had not had a prior vitrectomy (Group 1) and those that had undergone previous vitrectomy outside the study (Group 2). A total of 151 eyes were randomized to receive either SF_6 gas or silicone oil (113 in Group 1 and 38 in Group 2). Four hundred and four eyes were randomized to receive either C_3F_8 gas or silicone oil (232 and 172 in Groups 1 and 2, respectively). At the time of study closeout (June 30, 1991), the National Eye Institute funded an extension of the Silicone Study to provide long-term follow-up in the cohort of eyes (randomized to silicone oil or long-acting gas) with attached maculas at the 36-months follow-up.

A critical element in the study was a standardized surgical procedure for PVR. The surgical procedure, intended to relieve retinal traction with vitrectomy techniques, was followed by assessment of the relief provided by an intraocular air tamponade. The eye was randomized to silicone oil or gas only after completion of the entire surgical procedure to eliminate investigator bias that might develop through knowledge of the treatment modality.

Patients were examined 5–14 days following the randomization and again at 1, 3, 6, 12, 18, 24, and 36 months after that date. Repeated surgery was permitted for either treatment modality. The Fundus Photograph Reading Center staff processed and analyzed photographs taken at all the clinics, graded the preoperative severity of PVR on the basis of baseline visit photographs, and confirmed the macular status at follow-up visits.

Inclusion Criteria

Eligibility criteria included but were not limited to PVR of Grade C-3 or greater according to the Retina Society Classification and visual acuity of light perception or better.

Study Measures

End points of the study were visual acuity of 5/200 or greater and macular reattachment for 6 months following the final surgical procedure. The successful outcomes and complication rates of the two modalities were compared.

Results

- *Results and implications for clinical practice outcomes comparing Group 1 versus Group 2:* Anatomic, vision results and prevalence of complications suggest that the differences in outcomes between Groups 1 (eyes that had not had a prior vitrectomy) and 2 (those that had undergone previous vitrectomy outside the study) were not as great as previously believed. Previous reports have stressed the perceived differences in pathologic anatomy and outcomes in eyes undergoing primary vitrectomy (Group 1 eyes) compared with eyes that have already failed at least one prior vitrectomy for PVR (Group 2 eyes). In those nonrandomized retrospective studies, Group 2 eyes have had poorer anatomic and visual results than Group 1 eyes.
- *IOP abnormalities:*[5] Chronically elevated IOP was found in 5% of the eyes; chronic hypotony was found in 24% of the eyes. Chronically elevated IOP was more prevalent in silicone oil eyes than in C_3F_8 gas eyes. Chronic hypotony was more prevalent in C_3F_8 gas eyes than in silicone oil eyes,

more prevalent in eyes with anatomical failure, and correlated with poor postoperative vision, corneal opacity, and RD. The presence of diffuse contraction of the retina anterior to the equator should alert the vitrectomy surgeon that the eye is likely to be hypotonous postoperatively.

- *Retinotomy in the Silicone Study:*[6] Eyes undergoing vitreous surgery for the first time for the treatment of PVR can be treated successfully in most instances by conventional techniques without the need for a relaxing retinotomy. Retinotomy may be required more frequently in patients undergoing repeat vitreous surgery for PVR.
- *Outcomes after silicone oil removal:*[7] Compared with the oil-retained eyes evaluated at a comparable time after silicone oil injection, oil-removed eyes at the examination before oil removal were more likely to have attached retinas, have visual acuity of 5/200, and not be hypotonous.
- *Corneal abnormalities in the Silicone Study:*[8] The Silicone Study was the first study to document that the postoperative incidence rates of corneal abnormalities are similar between oil and gas. The incidence of corneal abnormalities in eyes randomized to gas was higher than expected, and the incidence of corneal abnormalities in eyes randomized to silicone oil remained high despite the use of an inferior iridectomy. If rubeosis iridis or severe aqueous flare is present, preoperative treatment with intense topical and possibly periocular steroids might help to reduce preoperative and postoperative inflammation, which may mediate corneal damage.
- *Postoperative macular pucker in the Silicone Study:*[9] The 6-month point prevalence rate of postoperative macular pucker was 15%. The occurrence of macular pucker following successful surgery for RD complicated by severe PVR was not influenced by the choice of intraocular tamponade.
- *Prognosis using the Silicone Study Classification System:*[10] Identification of the anteroposterior extent of the PVR was prognostic of visual acuity and hypotony at 24 months. The joint knowledge of the location of PVR (using the Silicone Study classification system) and the tightness of the funnel for retinas with 9–12 clock hours involved by fixed folds (using the Retinal Study classification system) has prognostic utility for eyes presenting with anterior plus posterior PVR.
- *Comparison of outcome in anterior versus posterior PVR in the Silicone Study:*[11] Anterior PVR was more prevalent in these Silicone Study eyes than was posterior PVR and had a worse prognosis. Eyes with anterior PVR and clinically significant posterior PVR changes had a better visual prognosis if silicone oil rather than C_3F_8 gas was used.
- *Long-term outcome in the Silicone Study:*[12] No significant differences in the rates of complete retinal attachment, visual acuity greater than 5/200 or glaucoma were found between treatment groups. In contrast, gas-treated eyes had more hypotony. Success in the first operation for PVR was paramount in obtaining better visual results. Overall, surgery for PVR

had a high likelihood of retinal reattachment, and if anatomically and visually successful at 3 years, there is an excellent chance that the results will be maintained over a long-term.

■ SCLERAL BUCKLING VERSUS PRIMARY VITRECTOMY IN RHEGMATOGENOUS RETINAL DETACHMENTS (SPR) STUDY[13-17]

Purpose
To compare scleral buckling and primary vitrectomy in patients with rhegmatogenous retinal detachment (RRD).

Background
The treatment of patients with primary RRD has undergone considerable change over recent decades. In most centers, scleral buckling surgery (SBS) remains the method of choice in uncomplicated retinal situations, i.e., single breaks and/or a limited retinal detachment. In contrast, primary pars plana vitrectomy (PPPV) is indicated in complicated situations, i.e., vitreous hemorrhage/opacity, proliferative vitreoretinopathy (PVR), or breaks at the posterior pole. Despite these clear indications, there is a large group of RRDs with "medium severity" where the most appropriate operating method is controversial, and different surgeons use different techniques. It remains unclear whether better anatomical and functional results can be achieved in an uncomplicated RRD with primary vitrectomy than with scleral buckling. The SPR Study is designed to compare primary vitrectomy and scleral buckling techniques in these patients.

Of further interest is that the techniques used to perform primary vitrectomy vary significantly among as well as within the individual studies. For example, primary vitrectomy followed by additional scleral buckling was either never used at all, was performed in some or selected cases or was applied in all cases. It is unclear whether scleral buckling plus primary vitrectomy increases the success rate or adds further complications to the procedure. Further, four different types of tamponades have been used (air, SF_6, C_3F_8 and silicone oil). This stresses not only the great diversity of indications used for primary vitrectomy but also the differing opinions of experienced vitreoretinal surgeons regarding the technical details of the operating procedure.

Description
The SPR Study was a prospective, randomized, controlled multicenter clinical trial which addressed the question of whether SBS or PPPV are associated with a better functional and anatomical outcome in treating medium-severe RRDs.

Medium-severe RRD, as defined by the SPR study inclusion criteria, was characterized as primary RRD not treatable with a single 7.5 × 2.75 mm Silastic sponge. This included aphakic/pseudophakic patients with an unclear hole situation.

Due to differences in the preoperative pathological situations in phakic versus aphakic/pseudophakic patients as well as in their postoperative course, this study was divided into two separately conducted parallel trials: (1) the phakic subtrial and the (2) aphakic/pseudophakic subtrial. Between August 1998 and June 2003, 45 surgeons across 25 centers of 5 European countries recruited 681 patients for the SPR Study (416 for the phakic trial, 265 for the pseudophakic trial).

The scleral buckling procedure included use of silicone sponges and/or silicone encircling bands or a combination of both according to the surgeon's choice, treatment of retinal breaks using cryopexy, intraocular tamponade with injection of BSS, air or SF_6, drainage of subretinal fluid with a needle or using electrolysis (optional), puncture of the anterior chamber (optional). The primary vitrectomy procedure included standard three-port PPV, use of an encircling band based on the surgeon's decision (surgeons should apply their routine technique throughout the study, i.e., always use an additional encircling band or never), removal of the flap of the retinal tear to reduce persistent traction on the break (optional), use of PFCL (optional), treatment of the retinal break with cryotherapy or endolaser coagulation, intraocular tamponade with a 20–40% SF_6/air mixture (air, C_3F_8 or silicone oil not permitted as an initial tamponade), draining retinotomies if needed.

Every patient was examined at four scheduled follow-up visits: within the 1st week after surgery; at 8 weeks, 6 months, and 1 year after surgery. The primary outcome was assessed at 1 year.

Inclusion Criteria

Phakic trial:
1. Phakic
2. Clear break situation
3. Absence of intraocular operations

Simple cases, such as those with a single small retinal break or neighboring small breaks, and more complicated cases, such as those with giant retinal tears (>2 clock hours) or macular holes were excluded from this study. They also excluded patients with PVR grade B or C, patients with multiple breaks and localized detachment(s) and those with more than seven diopters of myopia.

Aphakic/pseudophakic subtrial:
1. Aphakia/pseudophakia (only cataract operations without any damage to the posterior capsule or zonular dialysis were permitted; secondary YAG laser capsulotomy could have been performed)
2. Unclear hole situation

3. One or more retinal holes which cannot be treated sufficiently with a single 7.5 × 2.75 mm Silastic sponge (e.g., large holes, multiple holes, multiple holes of varying anterior–posterior localization, massive traction)
4. Absence of breaks at or posterior to the vessel arcades.

Study Measures

The outcome of retinal detachment surgery was evaluated using the following six main endpoint criteria:
1. Change in visual acuity on ETDRS charts.
2. Postoperative occurrence of PVR grade B or C.
3. Retinal reattachment after one year without any retina-affecting reoperation. A "retina-affecting reoperation" is any manipulation that reattaches the retina or ensures its attachment (prophylaxis). "Retinal reattachment" refers to attachment of the retina central to the equator.
4. Retinal reattachment after 1 year (any kind of reoperation permitted).
5. Development of cataract in phakic eyes using the lens opacity classification system LOCS-III.
6. Number of retina-affecting reoperations.

Results

The SPR study involved 266 pseudophakic and 416 phakic patients who were randomized to undergo either scleral buckling surgery or primary vitrectomy with or without scleral buckling.

Phakic Trial

- At a 1-year follow-up, phakic patients who underwent scleral buckling achieved significantly greater improvements in final visual acuity than those who underwent primary vitrectomy. That is, in the 209 phakic patients in the scleral buckling group, mean visual acuity improved from 20/200 preoperatively to a final value of 20/40, a gain of seven lines, compared to an improvement from 20/200 to 20/63 in the primary vitrectomy group, a gain of only six lines.
- The only significant differences between the two treatment groups of phakic patients were in the rate of cataract progression and the rate of IOL implantation. Among primary vitrectomy patients, cataract progression occurred in 77.3% and cataract surgery was carried out in 58.0%, compared to cataract progression and surgery rates of 45.9% and 20.6%, respectively, in the scleral buckling group.
- The two groups of phakic patients were virtually the same in terms of their secondary endpoints. In the scleral buckling group and primary vitrectomy groups, the respective rates of redetachment were 26.3% and 26.6%, those of primary success were 63.6% and 61.8%, and those of final success were 95.7% and 94.7%. However, the rate of PVR was

slightly higher in the primary vitrectomy group (16.4%) than it was in the scleral buckling group (12.4%). In the 50.7% of phakic patients in the primary vitrectomy group who also underwent scleral buckling surgery, the rate of retinal redetachment was 29.5% and the rate of PVR was 21.9%. In the patients who did not undergo the additional procedure, the redetachment rate was slightly lower at 20.6% and the rate of PVR was considerably lower at 10.8%.

Aphakic/Pseudophakic Trial

- In pseudophakic patients, there was no significant difference between the groups in terms of functional outcome. Both groups gained six lines of visual acuity with vision improving from 20/200 to 20/63 in the scleral buckling group and from 20/200 to 20/50 in the primary vitrectomy group.
- However, regarding the secondary endpoints, the primary anatomical success rate (defined as retinal reattachment without any secondary retina affecting surgery) was significantly higher in the primary vitrectomy group at 72.0%, compared to 53.4% in the scleral buckling group. Moreover, the rate of retinal redetachment was 39.8% in the scleral buckling group, compared to 20.4% in the primary vitrectomy group. In pseudophakic patients, the addition of scleral buckling to primary vitrectomy appeared to greatly reduce the rate of retinal redetachment. In the 66.7% of the vitrectomy group who also underwent scleral buckling, the rate of redetachment was only 11.4%, compared to 40.9% in those without the additional scleral buckle. In addition, PVR occurred in only 11.4% of those who underwent vitrectomy and scleral buckling, compared to 22.7% of those who underwent vitrectomy alone.

Conclusion

In the subset of RRD patients as chosen in this study, there is a benefit of scleral buckling in phakic eyes with respect to BCVA improvement. No difference in BCVA was demonstrated in the pseudophakic trial; based on a better anatomical outcome, primary vitrectomy is recommended in these patients.

PNEUMATIC RETINOPEXY VERSUS VITRECTOMY FOR THE MANAGEMENT OF PRIMARY RHEGMATOGENOUS RETINAL DETACHMENT OUTCOMES RANDOMIZED TRIAL (PIVOT)[18]

Purpose

To compare outcomes of pneumatic retinopexy (PnR) versus pars plana vitrectomy (PPV) for the management of primary rhegmatogenous retinal detachment (RRD).

Background

The optimal surgery for RRD remains controversial in spite of all the advancements in the techniques and equipments. The use of PPV has become common all over the world due to revolution of technology. However PnR still offers the simplicity of procedure, less invasiveness and shorter recovery time. This study was meant to compare PnR with PPV for the repair of primary RRD.

Description

PIVOT was a single center prospective randomized controlled trial which assessed PnR versus PPV for primary RRD. The study participants were recruited between August 2012 and May 2016.

Inclusion Criteria

- Single retinal break or a group of breaks, no larger than one clock hours in a detached retina
- All breaks in detached retina to lie above the 8- and 4-O'clock meridians
- Any number, location and size of retinal breaks or lattice degeneration in an attached retina.

Exclusion Criteria

- Inferior breaks in detached retina
- Significant media opacity
- PVR grade B or worse
- Previous retinal detachment/PPV
- Age <18 years/mental incapacity
- Inability to read English Language
- Inability to maintain posture postoperatively
- Preexisting ocular diagnosis affecting visual outcome.

Study Measures

Macula on and macula off cases were operated within 24 and 72 hours, respectively. The minimum follow-up period was 1 year.
- The primary outcome was Early Treatment Diabetic Retinopathy Study (ETDRS) visual acuity (VA) at the end of 1 year.
- Secondary outcomes were
  - Subjective visual function (using 25-item National Eye Institute Visual Function Questionnaire),
  - Metamorphopsia score (M-CHARTS) and
  - Primary anatomic success (defined as complete retinal attachment with a single procedure, in the absence of a tamponade agent).

Results

176 patients were recruited between August 2012 and May 2016. Both the groups were similar at baseline. Seventy-seven patients (87.5%) in the PnR group and 73 patients (83%) in the PPV group completed the 1-year follow-up.

- The ETDRS VA in PnR group exceeded than those in PPV group at all-time points to 12 months. At 12 months, the difference was 4.9 letters (79.9 ± 10.4 letters vs. 75.0 ± 15.2 letters; $p = 0.024$). There was no evidence of difference in the effect of treatment group between those with macula-on versus macula-off status and those who were phakic versus pseudophakic.
- Composite 25-item National Eye Institute Visual Function Questionnaire scores were superior for PnR group at 3 and 6 months, but were comparable at 12 months.
- Vertical metamorphopsia scores were superior for the PnR group compared with the PPV group at 12 months. However, horizontal metamorphopsia did not reach statistical significance.
- Primary anatomic success at 12 months was achieved by 80.8% in PnR versus 93.2% in PPV group (p-0.045). 98.7% and 98.6% of patients in PnR and PPV groups, achieved secondary anatomic success.
- 65% of phakic patients in the PPV arm underwent cataract surgery in the study eye before 12 months versus 16% in the PnR group ($p < 0.001$).

Conclusion

Pneumatic retinopexy offers superior visual acuity, less vertical metamorphopsia, and reduced morbidity when compared with PPV and should be considered as first choice in patients fulfilling this study's criteria.

Clinical Trials in Retinal Detachment

Table 1: Summary of clinical trials in retinal detachment.

Title	Purpose	No. of patients	Inclusion criteria	Outcome measure	Result/Conclusion
• Silicone oil Study • 1985–91	Evaluate and compare silicone oil vs. long acting gas in RD with PVR	554	Proliferative vitreoretinopathy (PVR) of Grade C-3 or greater according to the Retina Society Classification and visual acuity (VA) of light perception or better	Visual acuity of 5/200 or greater and macular reattachment for 6 months	• No significant differences in the rates of complete retinal attachment, VA, corneal abnormalities or glaucoma were found between treatment groups. • Gas-treated eyes had more hypotony. • Anterior PVR was more prevalent than was posterior PVR and had a worse prognosis
• SPR – phakic subtrial • 1998–2003	Scleral buckling vs. primary vitrectomy in RRD	416	Phakic patient with clear break situation	Change in VA, postoperative development of PVR and cataract and retinal reattachment rate at 1 year	• SB achieved greater improvement in final VA than those who underwent primary PPV. • Cataract progression was more with PPV. • There is a benefit of SB in phakic eyes with respect to best-corrected visual acuity (BCVA) improvement
• SPR – pseudophakic subtrial • 1998–2003	Scleral buckling vs. primary vitrectomy in RRD	265	• Medium- severe RRD not treatable with a single 7.5 × 2.75 mm Silastic sponge, • Aphakic/pseudophakic patients with an unclear hole situation	Change in VA, postoperative development of PVR and cataract and retinal reattachment rate at 1 year	• No significant difference between the groups in terms of functional outcome. • Primary anatomical success rate was significantly higher in the primary PPV group compared to the SB group. • Primary vitrectomy is recommended in these patients
PIVOT	Pneumatic retinopexy vs. vitrectomy in RRD	176	Single retinal break or a group of breaks in less than one clock hours in superior detached retina	BCVA at one year and metamorphopsia	• BCVA at 1 year was better in pneumatic retinopexy group. • Metamorphosia was also less in pneumatic retinopexy group.

(PPV: pars plana vitrectomy; RRD: rhegmatogenous retinal detachment)

REFERENCES

1. Lean JS, Stern WH, Irvine AR, Azen SP, Silicone Study Group. Classification of proliferative vitreoretinopathy used in the silicone study. Ophthalmology. 1989;96:765-71.
2. Vitrectomy with silicone oil or sulfur hexafluoride gas in eyes with severe proliferative vitreoretinopathy: results of a randomized clinical trial. Silicone Study Report 1. Arch Ophthalmol. 1992;110:770-9.
3. Vitrectomy with silicone oil or perfluoropropane gas in eyes with severe proliferative vitreoretinopathy: results of a randomized clinical trial. Silicone Study Report 2. Arch Ophthalmol. 1992;110:780-92.
4. McCuen BW 2nd, Azen SP, Stern W, Lai MY, Lean JS, Linton KL, et al. Vitrectomy with silicone oil or perfluoropropane gas in eyes with severe proliferative vitreoretinopathy. Silicone Study Report 3. Retina. 1993;13:279-84.
5. Barr CC, Lai MY, Lean JS, Linton KL, Trese M, Abrams G, et al. Postoperative intraocular pressure abnormalities in the Silicone Study. Silicone Study Report 4. Ophthalmology. 1993;100:1629-35.
6. Blumenkranz MS, Azen SP, Aaberg T, Boone DC, Lewis H, Radtke N, et al. Relaxing retinotomy with silicone oil or long-acting gas in eyes with severe proliferative vitreoretinopathy. Silicone Study Report 5. The Silicone Study Group. Am J Ophthalmol 1993;116: 557-64.
7. Hutton WL, Azen SP, Blumenkranz MS, Lai MY, McCuen BW, Han DP, et al. The effects of silicone oil removal. Silicone Study Report 6. Arch Ophthalmol. 1994;112:778-85.
8. Abrams GW, Azen SP, Barr CC, Lai MY, Hutton WL, Trese MT, et al. The incidence of corneal abnormalities in the Silicone Study. Silicone Study Report 7. Arch Ophthalmol. 1995;113:764-9.
9. Cox MS, Azen SP, Barr CC, Linton KL, Diddie KR, Lai MY, et al. Macular pucker after successful surgery for proliferative vitreoretinopathy. Silicone Study Report 8. Ophthalmology. 1995;102:1884-91.
10. Lean J, Azen SP, Lopez PF, Qian D, Lai MY, McCuen B. The prognostic utility of the Silicone Study Classification System. Silicone Study Report 9. Silicone Study Group. Arch Ophthalmol. 1996;114:286-92.
11. Diddie KR, Azen SP, Freeman HM, Boone DC, Aaberg TM, Lewis H, et al. Anterior proliferative vitreoretinopathy in the silicone study. Silicone Study Report Number 10. Ophthalmology. 1996;103:1092-9.
12. Abrams GW, Azen SP, McCuen BW 2nd, Flynn HW Jr, Lai MY, Ryan SJ. Vitrectomy with silicone oil or long-acting gas in eyes with severe proliferative vitreoretinopathy: results of additional and long-term follow-up. Silicone Study report 11. Arch Ophthalmol 1997;115:335-44.
13. SPR Study Group. Scleral buckling versus primary vitrectomy in rhegmatogenous retinal detachment (SPR Study): design issues and implications. SPR Study report no. 1. Graefes Arch Clin Exp Ophthalmol. 2001;239:567-74.
14. SPR Study Group. Scleral buckling versus primary vitrectomy in rhegmatogenous retinal detachment study (SPR Study): recruitment list evaluation. Study report no. 2. Graefes Arch Clin Exp Ophthalmol. 2007;245:803-9.
15. SPR Study Group. Scleral buckling versus primary vitrectomy in rhegmatogenous retinal detachment: a prospective randomized multicenter clinical study. Ophthalmology. 2007;114:2142-54.
16. SPR Study Group. Scleral buckling versus primary vitrectomy in rhegmatogenous retinal detachment study (SPR Study): predictive factors for functional outcome. Study report no. 6. Graefes Arch Clin Exp Ophthalmol. 2011;249:1129-36.
17. SPR study investigators. Scleral buckling versus primary vitrectomy in rhegmatogenous retinal detachment study (SPR study): Risk assessment of anatomical outcome. SPR study report no.7. ActaOphthalmol. 2013;91(3):282-7.
18. Hillier RJ, Felfeli T, Berger AR, Wong DT, Altomare F, Dai D, et al. The pneumatic retinopexy versus vitrectomy for the management of primary rhegmatogenous retinal detachment outcomes randomized trial (PIVOT). Ophthalmology. 2019;126:531-9.

CHAPTER 13

Miscellaneous Clinical Trials: Endophthalmitis Vitrectomy Study

Vinod Kumar, Neha Goel

■ ENDOPHTHALMITIS VITRECTOMY STUDY (EVS)[1-7]

Purpose
1. To determine the role of initial pars plana vitrectomy in the management of postoperative bacterial endophthalmitis.
2. To determine the role of intravenous antibiotics in the management of bacterial endophthalmitis.
3. To determine which factors, other than treatment, predict outcome in postoperative bacterial endophthalmitis.

Background
Before the Endophthalmitis Vitrectomy Study (EVS), there were widely divergent opinions regarding the role of vitrectomy in endophthalmitis management, ranging from vitrectomy for all endophthalmitis cases to the use of vitrectomy for only the most severe cases with greater inflammation, worse visual acuity, and more rapid onset. Vitrectomy, which may help to manage endophthalmitis by removing infecting organisms and their toxins, had been shown to be of value in various animal models of endophthalmitis. However, human studies had not shown an advantage to vitrectomy with intraocular antibiotics compared with intraocular antibiotics alone.

The role of systemic antibiotics was also widely debated. Some centers advocated the use of systemic antibiotics, which usually meant hospitalization for 5 days or more with intravenous antibiotics, while others used solely intravitreal antibiotics. A study of eyes with similar expected visual outcomes randomized to different treatment regimens was needed to answer the major endophthalmitis treatment questions, and this was the goal of the EVS study.

Description
It was an investigator-initiated, multicenter, randomized clinical trial conducted from 1990 to 1995 in private and university-based retina-vitreous practices. A total of 420 patients who had clinical evidence of endophthalmitis within 6 weeks after cataract surgery or secondary intraocular lens (IOL) implantation were randomized according to a 2 × 2 factorial design to

one of two standard treatment strategies for the management of bacterial endophthalmitis.
- Eyes received either initial pars plana vitrectomy (VIT) with intravitreal antibiotics (Vancomycin 1 mg and Amikacin 0.4 mg), followed by re-tap and reinjection at 36–60 hours for eyes that did poorly as defined in the study or
- Initial anterior chamber and vitreous tap/biopsy (TAP) with injection of intravitreal antibiotics (Vancomycin 1 mg and Amikacin 0.4 mg), followed by vitrectomy and reinjection at 36–60 hours in eyes doing poorly.

In addition, all eyes were randomized to either treatment or no treatment with intravenous antibiotics (Ceftazidime and Amikacin).

Inclusion Criteria
- Clinical signs and symptoms of bacterial endophthalmitis in an eye that had cataract surgery or lens implantation within 6 weeks of onset of infection.
- The involved eye had to have either hypopyon or enough clouding of anterior chamber or vitreous media to obscure clear visualization of second-order arterioles.
- The involved eye had to have a cornea and anterior chamber clear enough to visualize some part of the iris, and clear enough to allow the possibility of pars plana vitrectomy.
- The eyes had to have a visual acuity of 20/50 or worse and light perception or better.

Exclusion Criteria
- Pre-existing eye disease that limited best-corrected visual acuity to 20/100 or worse before development of cataract
- Any other intraocular surgery before presentation (except for cataract extraction or lens implantation)
- Any treatment for endophthalmitis before presenting at the study center
- Any ocular or systemic condition that would prevent randomization to any of the study groups.

Study Measures
Study end points were:
1. Visual acuity, assessed by an Early Treatment Diabetic Retinopathy Study acuity chart.
2. Clarity of ocular media assessed both clinically and photographically.

Each patient's initial end point assessment occurred at 3 months, after which procedures to improve vision, such as late vitrectomy for nonclearing ocular media, were an option. The final outcome assessment occurred at 9 months.

Results

Immediate Vitrectomy

- In patients whose initial visual acuity was hand motions or better, there was no difference in visual outcome whether or not an immediate vitrectomy was performed.
- In patients with initial light perception-only vision, vitrectomy produced a threefold increase in the frequency of achieving 20/40 or better acuity (33% vs. 11%), approximately a twofold better chance of achieving 20/100 or better acuity (56% vs. 30%), and a 50% decrease in the frequency of severe visual loss (20% vs. 47%) over TAP ($p < 0.001$).

Systemic Antibiotics

There was no difference in final visual acuity or media clarity with or without the use of systemic antibiotics.

Microbiological Results

- Compared with the aqueous, undiluted vitreous produced a higher percentage of confirmed positive cultures. Thus the vitreous was a richer source of positive cultures and high colony counts than was the aqueous, either because it is more supportive of bacterial growth or because a somewhat larger inoculum of the vitreous than of aqueous could be obtained. Nevertheless, the aqueous and vitrectomy cassette fluid were the only source of a positive culture from the eye in 4.2% and 8.9% of eyes, respectively.[2]
- The overall rate of laboratory-confirmed infection was not statistically significantly higher in the vitrectomy group than in the tap or biopsy group. Vitrectomy, with culture of the vitrectomy cassette fluid, did not produce significantly more positive cultures than tap or biopsy material, and the procedure should not be performed to improve the microbiological yield.[2]
- A positive Gram stain from the aqueous or undiluted vitreous was highly predictive of a positive culture from the eye, but a negative Gram stain had little predictive value for the culture result. Thus the result of Gram stain should not determine the choice of antibiotic drugs in the treatment of endophthalmitis.[2]
- *Confirmed microbiologic growth* was demonstrated from intraocular specimens from 291 of 420 patients (69.3%). Gram-positive bacteria were isolated from 274 patients (94.2%) with confirmed growth and Gram-negative bacteria from 19 (6.5%). Two hundred twenty-six of the 323 isolates obtained (70.0%) were Gram-positive, coagulase-negative micrococci, 32 (9.9%) *Staphylococcus aureus*, 29 (9.0%) Streptococcus species, 7 (2.2%) Enterococcus species, 10 (3.1%) miscellaneous Gram-positive

species, and 19 (5.9%) Gram-negative species. All Gram-positive isolates tested were susceptible to Vancomycin. Seventeen Gram-negative isolates (89%) were susceptible to both Amikacin and Ceftazidime and two (11%) were resistant to both. Anterior chamber or secondary IOL implantations were associated with higher rates of infection with Gram-positives other than coagulase-negative micrococci than were posterior chamber IOL implantations ($p = 0.022$) or primary cataract extractions ($p = 0.024$).[3]

- *Eleven features of the initial clinical presentation were associated with significant differences in the microbiologic spectrum ($p <0.05$)*. Baseline factors correlating with higher rates of both Gram-negative and other Gram-positive isolates were: corneal infiltrate, cataract wound abnormalities, afferent pupillary defect, loss of red reflex, initial light perception-only vision, and symptom onset within 2 days of surgery. Gram-negative organisms did not grow in any eyes in which a retinal vessel could be visualized, and 61.9% of these eyes had equivocal or no growth. Diabetes mellitus was associated with a higher yield of Gram-positive, coagulase-negative micrococci. Eye pain was not a discriminator for culture results. The presenting characteristics of acute endophthalmitis after cataract surgery may be helpful in predicting the most likely culture results. Such predictions do not appear sufficiently strong to guide the initial empiric choice of intravitreal antibiotics.[4]

- *Visual prognosis was strongly associated with the type of infecting organism and gram stain positivity*. Rates of achieving final visual acuity of 20/100 or better for the more common isolates were as follows: gram-positive, coagulase-negative micrococci, 84%; *Staphylococcus aureus*, 50%; streptococci, 30%; enterococci, 14%; and Gram-negative organisms, 56%. A positive gram stain or infection with species other than gram-positive, coagulase-negative micrococci were significantly associated with poorer visual outcome ($p <0.001$ for species group comparisons). However, presenting visual acuity was more powerful than microbiologic factors in predicting visual outcome and favorable response to vitrectomy. Bacterial growth from the vitrectomy cassette specimen had prognostic significance equivalent to growth from other intraocular sources.[5]

- From all sites the most frequently isolated Coagulase-negative staphylococci were *Staphylococcus epidermidis* (81.9%) and *Staphylococcus lugdunensis* (5.9%). Where analysis was possible, eyelid isolates were indistinguishable from intraocular isolates in 71 (67.7%) of 105 comparisons. Non-*Staphylococcus epidermidis* Coagulase-negative staphylococci caused postoperative endophthalmitis in 5 patients. Four of the 5 had postoperative endophthalmitis caused by *Staphylococcus lugdunensis* and 1 by *Staphylococcus haemolyticus*. Coagulase-negative staphylococci from the patient's periocular skin flora play a significant role in causing intraocular infections, and non-*Staphylococcus epidermidis* Coagulase-negative staphylococci play a small but significant role.

These results reinforce the necessity to follow stringent surgical site preparation prior to eye surgery.[6]

Others

- Before the EVS, many retinal surgeons believed that the *rates of retinal detachment* would be much higher in eyes undergoing needle tap and vitrectomy biopsy. Retinal detachment occurred in 8.3% of subjects in the EVS.[6] The rates of retinal detachment were slightly higher in the vitreous tap and biopsy group (9.0% vs. 7.8%), but these differences between groups were not statistically significant ($p = 0.66$). The EVS confirmed that the occurrence of retinal detachment during endophthalmitis treatment was a poor prognostic sign, and often this subgroup of patients had the worst visual outcomes.

■ CONCLUSION

Omission of systemic antibiotic treatment can reduce toxic effects, costs, and length of hospital stay. Routine immediate vitrectomy is not necessary in patients with better than light perception vision at presentation but is of substantial benefit for those who have light perception-only vision.

■ LIMITATIONS

- Endophthalmitis Vitrectomy Study was performed when extracapsular cataract extraction (ECCE) was the common technique or cataract surgery. The results may not be directly applicable to today's surgeries which are performed via phacoemulsification through mainly clear corneal incisions.
- The EVS recommendations relate to acute-onset endophthalmitis following cataract surgery or secondary IOL implantation and may not be directly applied to other forms of endophthalmitis. For example, bleb-associated, traumatic, and endogenous types of endophthalmitis are more likely to be caused by organisms of greater virulence. In such cases, the benefits of vitrectomy may be greater because of the mechanical removal of bacteria and toxins from the eye.
- The systemic antibiotics used in EVS were Amikacin and Ceftazidime. The study made no recommendations regarding treatment with additional antimicrobial agents (e.g., systemic fluoroquinolones) or systemic antimicrobial agents for other types of endophthalmitis (e.g., chronic, bleb-associated, traumatic, fungal, and endogenous).
- Potential study subjects with significant opacification of the anterior chamber or without light perception were excluded from the EVS. Because these eyes with more severe infection or involving more virulent organisms were excluded from the EVS, the effect might have shifted the EVS outcomes to more favorable results.

Table 1: Summary of Endophthalmitis Vitrectomy Study (EVS).

Title	Purpose	Inclusion criteria	No. of patients	Outcome measure	Follow-up	Results	Conclusion
EVS 1990–1995	Role of early PPV vs. intravitreal antibiotics and intravenous antibiotics in postoperative endophthalmitis	Patients with endophthalmitis following cataract surgery or IOL implantation with VA <20/50 and > light perception (LP)	420	Visual acuity (VA) by ETDRS chart and media clarity	3 and 9 months	VA was better with PPV in patients with LP vision Results were comparable when initial vision was HM or better Intravenous antibiotics did not affect outcome	Immediate vitrectomy is not necessary in patients with better than light perception vision at presentation while results are better with PPV in patients in whom VA is light perception only

(ETDRS: Early Treatment Diabetic Retinopathy Study; PPV: pars plana vitrectomy)

REFERENCES

1. Results of the Endophthalmitis Vitrectomy Study. A randomized trial of immediate vitrectomy and of intravenous antibiotics for the treatment of postoperative bacterial endophthalmitis. Endophthalmitis Vitrectomy Study Group. Arch Ophthalmol. 1995;113:1479-96.
2. Barza M, Pavan PR, Doft BH, Wisniewski SR, Wilson LA, Han DP, et al. Evaluation of microbiological diagnostic techniques in postoperative endophthalmitis in the Endophthalmitis Vitrectomy Study. Arch Ophthalmol. 1997;115:1142-50.
3. Han DP, Wisniewski SR, Wilson LA, Barza M, Vine AK, Doft BH, et al. Spectrum and susceptibilities of microbiologic isolates in the Endophthalmitis Vitrectomy Study. Am J Ophthalmol. 1996; 122:1-17.
4. Johnson MW, Doft BH, Kelsey SF, Barza M, Wilson LA, Barr CC, et al. The Endophthalmitis Vitrectomy Study. Relationship between clinical presentation and microbiologic spectrum. Ophthalmology. 1997;104:261-72.
5. Microbiologic factors and visual outcome in the endophthalmitis vitrectomy study. Am J Ophthalmol. 1996;122:830-46.
6. Bannerman TL, Rhoden DL, McAllister SK, Miller JM, Wilson LA. The source of coagulase-negative staphylococci in the Endophthalmitis Vitrectomy Study. a comparison of eyelid and intraocular isolates using pulsed-field gel electrophoresis. Arch Ophthalmol. 1997;115:357-61.
7. Doft BM, Kelsey SK, Wisniewski SR. Endophthalmitis Vitrectomy Study Group. Retinal detachment in the Endophthalmitis Vitrectomy Study. Arch Ophthalmol. 2000;118:1661-5.

Clinical Trials in Retinopathy of Prematurity

Pooja Shah, Neha Goel

CRYOTHERAPY FOR RETINOPATHY OF PREMATURITY (CRYO-ROP)[1-4]

Purpose

1. To determine the safety and efficacy of trans-scleral cryotherapy of the peripheral retina in certain low birth weight infants with retinopathy of prematurity (ROP) for reducing blindness from ROP.
2. To determine the long-term outcome for eyes that had severe ("threshold") ROP, both with and without cryotherapy.

Background

Retinopathy of prematurity is a disease of the eyes of prematurely born infants in which the retinal blood vessels increase in number and branch excessively, sometimes leading to hemorrhage or scarring. In most infants who develop ROP, the disease spontaneously subsides, permitting development of normal vision. But other infants who progress to a severe form of ROP are in danger of becoming permanently blind. Before the establishment of this study in 1985, more than 500 infants annually were blinded by ROP in the United States alone. As techniques of managing smaller and less mature preterm infants continue to improve, it is expected that the number of infants at risk for blindness will continue to increase.

More than 40 years ago, the National Institutes of Health sponsored a clinical trial that showed that if premature babies are given oxygen only as needed, the number of infants who develop ROP drops dramatically. Subsequently, hospitals cut back on giving excessive oxygen routinely to premature babies. But, with improvements in neonatal care over the last three decades, the number of babies at risk has increased as survival rates for smaller premature infants improve. The lower the birth weight, the higher is the incidence and severity of ROP.

Description

The multicenter trial of cryotherapy for ROP enrolled more than 4,000 premature infants (1986–1988) who weighed no more than 1,250 g at birth.

This category of infants has the greatest risk of developing ROP. Twenty-three centers collaborated in this prospectively designed study.

The eyes of the infants enrolled in the study were examined at predetermined intervals while the subjects were still in the intensive care nursery. Patients' examinations began 4–6 weeks from birth. The eyes were examined by an ophthalmologist using a binocular indirect ophthalmoscope after pupillary dilation. The natural history of the condition of each infant's retina was recorded.

When examination disclosed the severe form of ROP (threshold ROP) in both eyes, and the parents gave informed consent, one of the infant's eyes was randomly selected to receive cryotherapy. Cryotherapy was lightly applied to the avascular zone between the ridge of ROP and the ora serrata, in an average of about 50 separate spots.

Inclusion Criteria

Premature infants of either gender who were eligible for the natural history study had weighed less than 1,251 g at birth and had survived the first 28 days of life. They had no major ocular or systemic congenital anomalies. Infants who met these criteria and also had a *threshold level of ROP* [defined as stage 3+ of the International Classification of Retinopathy of Prematurity occupying five or more contiguous or eight cumulative 30 degree sectors (clock hours) of stage 3 ROP in zone I or II in the presence of plus disease] could be referred for examination to determine eligibility for entry to the cryotherapy trial.

Study Measures

Outcome of the therapy was assessed at 3 months and 12 months following randomization, by means of masked readings of fundus photographs (neither the trained photograph readers who evaluated the pictures from both eyes nor the specially trained vision testers knew which eyes had received cryotherapy). *Adverse outcome* was defined as retinal detachment, macular fold, or retrolental mass.

The 12-month examination also measured visual function with preferential-looking techniques. Such measurements allowed correlations between fundus photographs and visual function and a comparison of visual function for treated versus control eyes.

Additional assessments of visual acuity and retinal status have been made approximately each year through age 10, with a final examination at age 15 for patients in the randomized trial of cryotherapy who did not have bilateral total retinal detachment and blindness.

Results

This study registered 9,751 infants with birth weights less than 1,251 g at 23 study centers. Of these infants, 4,099 were systematically examined. The defined threshold severity of ROP developed in 291 infants.

1. Cryotherapy was performed in half the eligible eyes of the 291 infants. 12 months after randomization, the results of masked grading of fundus photographs of the posterior pole indicated an unfavorable outcome in 25.7% of the eyes that had received cryotherapy and in 47.4% of the control eyes. Masked Teller Acuity Card assessment of grating acuity indicated an unfavorable functional outcome in 35% of the treated eyes, compared with 56.3% of the control eyes. Although the surgery was stressful, no major complications occurred during or following treatment. Physicians' diagnoses and the unbiased photograph gradings were statistically similar.
2. At *3½ years* following randomization, functional outcome was evaluated by masked assessment of visual acuity (using only the letters H, O, T, and V) and of grating acuity (using the Teller Acuity Card procedure). Structural outcome was evaluated by the physician's assessment of ROP residua in the posterior pole. All three outcome measures showed a reduction of unfavorable outcomes in treated versus control eyes: 46.6% versus 57.5% ($p < 0.01$) for letter acuity, 52.4% versus 65.6% ($p < 0.001$) for grating acuity, and 26.1% versus 45.4% ($p < 0.001$) for posterior pole status.[1]
3. At *5½ years* following randomization, Snellen visual acuity was measured by masked testers. Again, structural outcome was evaluated by the physician's assessment of ROP residua in the posterior pole. Both visual acuity and fundus structure continued to show fewer unfavorable outcomes in treated versus control eyes: 47.1% versus 61.7% ($p < 0.005$) for visual acuity, and 26.9% versus 45.4% ($p < 0.001$) for fundus status. Detailed analysis of visual acuity outcomes for all eyes revealed that while fewer treated eyes (31.5%) than control eyes (47.7%) were blind ($p < 0.001$), there was a slight trend toward fewer eyes with a visual acuity of 20/40 or better in the treated (12.6%) versus control (16.7%) groups ($p = 0.19$).[2]
4. Findings from the *10-year* examination showed fewer unfavorable outcomes for both visual acuity and structure in treated versus untreated eyes. For distance visual acuity, 44.4% of treated eyes had unfavorable outcomes versus 62.1% of control eyes ($p < 0.001$). Similarly, for near visual acuity, 42.5% of treated eyes versus 61.6% of control eyes had unfavorable outcomes ($p < 0.001$). The fundus status results showed that 27.2% of treated eyes versus 47.9% of control eyes had unfavorable outcomes ($p < 0.001$). Eyes that received cryotherapy were at least as likely as control eyes to have 20/40 or better visual acuity.

The examination at age 10 included measurement of contrast sensitivity and visual fields. Results of *contrast sensitivity* testing demonstrated no evidence of adverse treatment effects in eyes that received cryotherapy: 39.7% of treated eyes had unfavorable outcomes versus 59.3% of control eyes ($p < 0.001$). The findings for *visual field testing* with Goldmann perimetry showed a visual field area that was 25% larger in treated eyes versus untreated eyes, when blind eyes were included and assigned a score of 0. When blind eyes were excluded, visual field area was 5% smaller for treated eyes than for untreated eyes, indicating that cryotherapy slightly reduces the visual field area in eyes with severe ROP. This small reduction in visual field area in treated eyes is minor when compared with the much greater risk that an eye will be blind without treatment. However, this and any other possible adverse side effects are important considerations in determining whether to treat milder cases of ROP that have a relatively good prognosis for vision without treatment.[3]

5. At age *15 years,* unfavorable ocular structure was posterior retinal fold or worse judged by study-certified ophthalmologists. Unfavorable distance visual acuity was 20/200 or worse measured by study-certified testers using Early Treatment of Diabetic Retinopathy Study recognition acuity charts. 30% of treated eyes and 51.9% of control eyes ($p <0.001$) had unfavorable structural outcomes. Between 10 and 15 years of age, new retinal folds, detachments, or obscuring of the view of the posterior pole occurred in 4.5% of treated and 7.7% of control eyes. Unfavorable visual acuity outcomes were found in 44.7% of treated and 64.3% of control eyes ($p <0.001$).[4]

Conclusion

- Cryotherapy reduces the risk of unfavorable retinal (by approximately one-half) and functional outcome from threshold ROP.
- Results at 3½ years and 5½ years following randomization continue to support the long-term efficacy and safety of cryotherapy in the treatment of severe ROP. However, the data show preliminary evidence of a possible adverse effect of this treatment on visual acuity.
- At 10 years, eyes that had received cryotherapy were much less likely than control eyes to be blind. A previous trend for a higher proportion of sighted control eyes than sighted treated eyes to show acuity in the normal range was not confirmed. The results show long-term value from cryotherapy in preserving visual acuity in eyes with threshold ROP.
- The benefit of cryotherapy for treatment of threshold ROP, for both structure and visual function, was maintained across 15 years of follow-up. New retinal detachments, even in eyes with relatively good structural findings at age 10 years, suggest value in long-term, regular follow-up of eyes that experience threshold ROP.

EARLY TREATMENT FOR RETINOPATHY OF PREMATURITY STUDY (ETROP)[5-10]

Purpose

To test the hypothesis that earlier treatment [early treatment (ET)] in carefully selected cases will result in an overall better visual outcome than treatment at the conventional CRYO-ROP threshold point in the disease [conventional management (CM)].

Background

Two concerns emerged from the CRYO-ROP extensive study on the natural history of ROP and treatment of threshold ROP. The first of these was failure of peripheral retinal ablation to eliminate all, or nearly all cases, of retinal detachment due to ROP. In the CRYO-ROP Study, while treatment at threshold results in approximately a 50% reduction in the rate of retinal detachment, 26% of eyes with threshold disease in zone II and 78% of eyes with zone I threshold disease had an unfavorable structural outcome despite treatment. The second concern was that most children who developed threshold ROP disease had visual acuity worse than 20/40 even if the eye had a favorable structural outcome.

Since no other treatment had been shown to be effective in preventing blindness from ROP, retinal ablation remains the treatment of choice. The ETROP Study tested whether decreases the probability of an unfavorable structural outcome as well as determined whether earlier treatment was more effective than treatment at threshold in improving functional (visual acuity) outcome following ROP.

Recognizing that a substantial number of eyes undergo spontaneous resolution of ROP, eyes were randomized to early treatment only when high risk for an unfavorable visual acuity outcome was identified. High-risk was determined using a risk model analysis program (RM-ROP$_2$) based on longitudinal natural history data obtained from the CRYO-ROP study. This model integrated risk factors to assign a risk of progression to blindness without treatment. These factors included birth weight, gestational age, ethnicity, singleton/multiple status, outborn status, zone on first examination, severity of ROP and rate of progression of ROP.

Description

A total of 317 infants with birth weights less than 1,251 g and birth dates between 2000 and 2002 were enrolled at 26 participating centers.

Earlier treatment was defined as retinal ablation administered to the avascular retina when an eye reached *high-risk prethreshold ROP*. If at least one eye reached prethreshold ROP, the infant's demographic and ROP information was entered into the RM-ROP$_2$ risk model. If the risk of progression to an unfavorable outcome in the absence of treatment was calculated to be ≥15% ("high-risk" prethreshold), randomization occurred. Eyes with <15% risk were termed "low-risk" and were followed every 2–4 days for at least 2 weeks until the ROP regressed, or the risk progressed to ≥15%. If both eyes were eligible for randomization, one eye was assigned at random to earlier treatment with ablative therapy within 48 hours of the first diagnosis of high-risk prethreshold ROP. The fellow eye served as the control and was managed conventionally, which meant that it was observed either until it reached threshold and was treated or until the ROP regressed without progressing to threshold. In cases where only one eye had reached high-risk prethreshold ROP, that eye was randomized to treatment within 48 hours or to serve as a conventionally managed control, receiving treatment only if the ROP progressed to threshold severity.

Treatment was generally laser therapy, but cryotherapy was allowed.

Functional outcome consisted of visual acuity outcome (monocular grating acuity) that was measured by masked observers after wearing best correction using the Teller Acuity Card Procedure (used previously in the CRYO-ROP study) at 9 months corrected age. The visual acuity outcome was divided into four categories of functional response: normal, defined as greater than or equal to 3.70 cycles per degree; below normal, defined as 1.85 to less than 3.70 cycles per degree; poor, if less than 1.85 cycles per degree but measurable with one of the standard acuity cards (not the LV card); and blind/low vision (NLP, LP only, or LV only). These functional outcome categories of grating acuity results were further grouped into "favorable" (normal and below normal) and "unfavorable" (poor and blind/low vision) designations.

Structural outcome was documented with a dilated fundus examination at 6 months and 9 months corrected age by study-certified examiners. At the 9-month examination, a developmental questionnaire [Denver developmental screening test (DDST)] was conducted. At 6 months, an unfavorable outcome was defined as: (1) a posterior retinal fold involving the macula, (2) a retinal detachment involving the macula, or (3) retrolental tissue or "mass" obscuring the view of the posterior pole. If an infant required a vitrectomy or scleral buckle, the 6-month examination was conducted prior to the surgery. At the 9-month examination, eyes that had received a vitrectomy or scleral buckle were classified for study purposes as having an unfavorable structural outcome.

Inclusion Criteria

Infants <1,251 g birth weight born at participating centers and/or examined by 42 days of life were eligible. The early treatment trial required that an infant have prethreshold ROP. *Prethreshold ROP* indicated any Zone I ROP; or Zone II stage 2 with plus disease, or stage 3; or Zone II with less than 5 contiguous or 8 cumulative clock hours of stage 3 ROP with plus disease. Infants in whom either eye had developed threshold ROP prior to randomization were excluded from the study.

Study Measures

The functional outcome of each randomized eye at 9 months corrected age was evaluated by assessment of monocular grating acuity (Primary outcome).

The structural outcome was documented with a dilated fundus examination at 6 months and 9 months corrected age (Secondary outcome).

Results

At the 26 clinical sites, 828 infants whose parents had given consent for systematic follow-up of ROP were identified as having prethreshold disease in one or both eyes. Among these, there were 401 infants that were enrolled into the randomized trial. Infants with bilateral high-risk prethreshold ROP ($n = 317$) had one eye randomized to early treatment with the fellow eye managed conventionally (control eye). In asymmetric cases ($n = 84$), the eye with high-risk prethreshold ROP was randomized to early treatment or conventional management. 329 infants, who had prethreshold ROP that was judged to be low-risk, were followed as clinically indicated.

The mean birth weight was 703 g and the mean gestational age was 25.3 weeks. The average age at high-risk prethreshold treatment was 35.2 weeks postmenstrual age (SD, 2.3; range, 30.6–42.1 weeks) and 10.0 weeks chronological age (SD, 2.0). The average age for treatment of eyes in the conventionally managed group that went on to threshold was 37.0 weeks postmenstrual age (SD, 2.5; range, 31.9–46.6 weeks) and 11.9 weeks chronological age (SD, 2.2). Only one eye received cryotherapy at threshold ROP as the primary treatment for ROP, with the others receiving laser retinal ablation. Some eyes received supplementary cryotherapy at the time of the initial treatment.

1. *Grating acuity results* showed a reduction in unfavorable visual acuity outcomes with earlier treatment, from 19.8 to 14.3% ($p < 0.005$). Results from the 33 infants with bilateral disease in whom there were discordant outcomes in the two eyes provide even stronger evidence of a beneficial effect of treatment at high-risk prethreshold ROP ($p < 0.005$). Although differences were not statistically significant in smaller categories, there were more high-risk prethreshold treated eyes than conventionally managed eyes that had grating acuity in the normal range for age ($p = 0.38$). In addition, fewer eyes randomized to high-risk prethreshold treatment than conventionally managed eyes were designated as blind or low vision ($p = 0.07$).
2. Unfavorable *structural outcomes* were reduced from 15.6 to 9.0% ($p < 0.001$) at 9 months. As is the case for grating acuity outcome, results from infants with bilateral disease in whom there were discordant outcomes in the two eyes provide strong evidence of a beneficial effect of treatment at high-risk prethreshold.
3. 6-month structural outcome data were also collected for low-risk prethreshold eyes (determined by the RM-ROP$_2$ program to have a <15% risk for an unfavorable outcome). Among this group of 329 infants, 51 (15.5%) had at least one eye that progressed to the conventional threshold

for treatment and was treated accordingly. An unfavorable outcome occurred in only 1.3% of the 302 low-risk prethreshold eyes for which 6-month structural outcome data were available.

4. Whereas the rates of ophthalmologic complications were similar among the two treatment arms, infants in the high-risk prethreshold treatment group were more likely to experience systemic complications of apnea, bradycardia, or reintubation following earlier treatment than with treatment at conventional threshold, perhaps due to the earlier average postmenstrual age at which treatment was conducted. There was no mortality or known permanent morbidity attributed to treatment in either group.

5. Further analysis supported retinal ablative therapy for eyes with *type I ROP*, defined as zone I, any stage ROP with plus disease; zone I, stage 3 ROP without plus disease; or zone II, stage 2 or 3 with plus disease. The analysis supported a "wait and watch" approach to *type II ROP*, defined as zone I, stage 1 and 2 without plus disease, or zone II, stage 3 without plus disease. These eyes should be considered for treatment only if they progress to type I ROP or threshold.

6. *6-year results*[7-10]

    i. Analysis of grating visual acuity results (measured using Teller acuity cards) and ETDRS visual acuity results for all study participants with high-risk prethreshold ROP showed no statistically significant overall benefit of ET. When the results were analyzed according to a clinical algorithm (high-risk types 1 and 2 prethreshold ROP), a benefit was seen in type 1 eyes undergoing ET, but not in type 2 eyes.[7,8]

    ii. Visual field extent (measured using white-sphere kinetic perimetry along the superotemporal, inferotemporal, inferonasal, and superonasal meridian) was 0.1–3.7° larger in ET eyes when blind eyes were assigned a score of 0°. When data were examined from eyes of participants with 1 sighted ET eye and 1 sighted CM eye, ET eyes showed a small (1.3–3.1°) reduction, which was statistically significant only along the superonasal meridian ($p = 0.005$). In bilaterally sighted children, visual field extent was not significantly reduced for high-risk type 1 ET eyes (-0.9–1.8°). However, in ET eyes with high-risk type 2 disease, visual field extent was significantly smaller compared with that of CM eyes [3.6–8.7° superonasal field ($p = 0.003$); inferonasal field ($p < 0.001$)].[9]

    iii. Among the 342 children evaluated at 6 years, the prevalence of strabismus was 42.2%. Even with favorable acuity scores in both eyes, the prevalence of strabismus was 25.4%, and with favorable structural outcomes in both eyes the prevalence of strabismus was 34.2%. Of children categorized as visually impaired as the result of either ocular or cerebral causes, 80% were strabismic at the 6-year examination. Of 103 study participants who were strabismic at 9 months, 77 (74.8%)

remained so at 6 years. Most strabismus was constant at both the 9-month (62.7%) and the 6-year examination (72.3%). After multiple logistic regression analysis, risk factors for strabismus were abnormal fixation behavior in one or both eyes ($p < 0.001$), history of amblyopia ($p < 0.003$), unfavorable structural outcome in one or both eyes ($p = 0.025$), and history of anisometropia ($p = 0.04$). Strabismus surgery was performed for 53 children. By 6 years, the cumulative prevalence of strabismus was 59.4%.[10]

Conclusion

- Early treatment of high-risk prethreshold ROP significantly reduced unfavorable outcomes in both primary (functional) and secondary (structural) measures. Early treatment for type 1 high-risk prethreshold eyes improved visual acuity outcomes at 6 years of age. Early treatment for type 2 high-risk prethreshold eyes did not. Early treatment preserves peripheral vision, with only a small reduction of visual field extent.
- It is possible to identify characteristics of ROP that predict which eyes are most likely to benefit from early peripheral retinal ablation. A clinical algorithm was developed to identify for early treatment eyes with prethreshold ROP that are at highest risk for retinal detachment and blindness, while minimizing treatment of prethreshold eyes likely to show spontaneous regression of ROP. The use of this algorithm (Type I or Type II ROP) circumvents the need for computer-based calculation of low risk or high-risk, as was used in this study.
- Most children with a history of high-risk prethreshold ROP develop strabismus at some time during the first 6 years of life.

BEVACIZUMAB ELIMINATES THE ANGIOGENIC THREAT OF RETINOPATHY OF PREMATURITY (BEAT-ROP)[11]

Purpose

To determine whether intravitreal injections of an anti-vascular endothelial growth factor (VEGF) will reduce the incidence of blindness by suppressing the neovascular phase of ROP compared to a control group receiving conventional laser therapy. The purpose of this study was thus to determine the efficacy of intravitreal bevacizumab in the treatment of ROP and compare it with conventional laser in vision threatening ROP.

Background

Peripheral retinal ablation with conventional (confluent) laser therapy is destructive, causes complications, and does not prevent all vision loss, especially in cases of ROP affecting zone I of the eye. A major ocular side effect, especially in infants with zone I ROP, is clinically significant loss of visual field. Case series in which patients were treated with VEGF inhibitors suggest that these agents may be useful in treating ROP. Bevacizumab is an inexpensive drug that can be rapidly administered at the bedside by any ophthalmologist. In contrast, conventional laser therapy is laborious and requires special training to administer, as well as expensive equipment, endotracheal intubation, and a location designated for the use of lasers.

Description

This was a prospective, controlled, randomized, stratified, multicenter trial to assess intravitreal bevacizumab monotherapy for zone I or zone II posterior stage 3+ (i.e., stage 3 with plus disease) ROP. This study enrolled confirmed cases of vision threatening ROP (between ETROP and CRYO-ROP) which have definite plus disease. This was done because of the controversy regarding determining plus disease and the increasing concern that many infants are being treated whose ROP would spontaneously regress. 150 infants (total sample of 300 eyes) were enrolled from 2008 to 2010.

Infants were randomly assigned to receive intravitreal bevacizumab (Avastin, 0.625 mg in 0.025 mL of solution) or conventional laser therapy (diode laser applied to the avascular peripheral retina anterior to the vascularized posterior retina), bilaterally. There was no intent to give additional doses unless there was a recurrence of vision threatening stage 3 ROP with plus disease since the disease is self-limited by completion of vascularization. Infants, rather than eyes, were randomly assigned to the study groups because VEGF circulates in the blood, and recurrence in one eye could therefore affect the contralateral eye, and because substantial inflammation after conventional laser therapy in one eye and little inflammation after intravitreal bevacizumab therapy in the other eye could result in irreversible deprivation amblyopia in the eye that underwent conventional laser therapy.

Clinical response and any evidence of ocular toxicities will be documented by RetCam retinal images taken preinjection, 1 week and 1 month post injection, and at 6 months of age (54 weeks postmenstrual age, window of 50–70 weeks postmenstrual age) (primary outcome) and at 12 months of age (80 weeks postmenstrual age) (window of 75–100 weeks PMA) (structural documentation). RetCam fluorescein angiograms will be taken when possible to document structural outcomes in greater detail. Any evidence of systemic toxicities will be documented by appropriate clinical and laboratory tests.

Inclusion Criteria

The following infants were included in the study:
- Infants who have been screened by the AAO, AAP, and the AAPOS guidelines (≤1,500 grams at birth and ≤30 weeks gestation) beginning at 4 weeks' chronologic age or 31 weeks' postmenstrual age, whichever was later, who develop Stage 3+ ROP in zone I or posterior zone II.
- Informed consent from a parent or guardian.

The following infants were excluded from the study:
- Infants who have a congenital systemic anomaly or have a congenital ocular abnormality.
- Infants who cannot be treated by conventional laser therapy because of problems with media clarity. Generally, blind external cryotherapy would be utilized as an initial therapy and the infant would be excluded from the study even if the media clear subsequently.
- Informed consent from a parent or guardian refused. This will mean that an infant automatically will receive laser therapy. Bevacizumab (Avastin®) treatment cannot be given outside of the protocol. No data will be used from an infant without informed consent.

Study Measures

The primary ocular outcome measure was an unfavorable outcome, defined as recurrence of neovascularization in one or both eyes arising from the retinal vessels and requiring re-treatment (in either eye) before the infant reached 54 weeks postmenstrual age (window of 50-70 weeks).

Secondary outcome measures were determination of visual acuity, visual field, refraction, motility examination or any other ocular parameter related to severe ROP.

Results

- A total of 150 infants with stage 3+ ROP were enrolled—67 infants with zone I disease and 83 infants with zone II posterior disease. A total of 75 infants were randomly assigned to undergo intravitreal bevacizumab monotherapy, and 75 to conventional laser therapy.
- 143 infants survived to 54 weeks' postmenstrual age, and the 7 infants who died were not included in the primary-outcome analyses.
- ROP recurred in 4 infants in the bevacizumab group [6 of 140 eyes (4%)] and 19 infants in the laser-therapy group [32 of 146 eyes (22%), $p = 0.002$]. The rate of recurrence (primary outcome) for zone I and posterior zone II combined was significantly higher with conventional laser therapy than with intravitreal bevacizumab [26% (19 of 73 infants) vs. 6% (4 of 70 infants); odds ratio with bevacizumab, 0.17; 95% confidence interval (CI), 0.05-0.53; $p = 0.002$].
- The rate of recurrence with zone I disease alone was significantly higher with conventional laser therapy than with intravitreal bevacizumab [42% (14 of 33 infants) vs. 6% (2 of 31 infants); odds ratio with bevacizumab, 0.09; 95% CI, 0.02-0.43; $p = 0.003$].
- The rate of recurrence with zone II posterior disease alone did not differ significantly between the laser-therapy group and the bevacizumab group [12% (5 of 40 infants) and 5% (2 of 39 infants); odds ratio with bevacizumab, 0.39; 95% CI, 0.07-2.11; $p = 0.27$].

Conclusion

Intravitreal bevacizumab monotherapy, as compared with conventional laser therapy, in infants with stage 3+ retinopathy of prematurity showed a significant benefit for zone I but not zone II disease. Development of peripheral retinal vessels continued after treatment with intravitreal bevacizumab, but conventional laser therapy led to permanent destruction of the peripheral retina. This trial was too small to assess safety.

■ SUPPLEMENTAL THERAPEUTIC OXYGEN FOR PRETHRESHOLD RETINOPATHY OF PREMATURITY (STOP-ROP)[12]

Purpose

To test the efficacy, safety, and costs of providing supplemental oxygen in moderately severe ROP (prethreshold ROP).

Background

More than 80% of infants who develop ROP heal the retinal neovascularization spontaneously, while only the minority progress to severe stages. While the use of cryo- or laser ablation of peripheral retina during the severe stages of ROP reduces the proportion of infants who progress to retinal detachments, less destructive treatment would be desirable. Apparently, the normal physiologic control of retinal vascular growth is usually enough to control ROP. This observation led to basic studies on the control of normal and abnormal retinal vascularization that has identified tissue oxygen levels as important in the control of vessel growth. Combined with the observation of marginally low oxygen levels in the sickest of premature infants during their long convalescence from lung disease, an idea emerged. The hypothesis was that marginally low blood oxygen levels could interfere with control of retinal neovascularization—the low levels further stimulating the vessel overgrowth. When that proved true in animal studies, the reverse experiment was tested and showed that raising the oxygen slightly over normal was enough to improve the retinopathy in its convalescent stages. Therefore, the STOP-ROP clinical trial was designed to test the hypothesis that supplemental oxygen in moderately severe (prethreshold) ROP would reduce the proportion of eyes that would progress to severe (threshold) levels of ROP.

Description

Infants who developed moderately severe ROP were recruited to participate in STOP-ROP. To make it possible to detect a reduction in progression to threshold ROP from 30% to 20%, 880 infants were planned to be enrolled.

A total of 649 infants were enrolled from 30 centers over 5 years; recruitment was completed on March 31, 1999.

Following informed consent, eligible infants were randomized to oxygen administration with continuous saturation monitoring at conventional levels (target pulse oximetry, 89–94% saturation) versus supplemental levels (target pulse oximetry, 96–99% saturation). Pulse oximetry was monitored continuously, and feedback to the bedside nurses was provided in a variety of formats on a laptop computer screen. Compliance with study targets was recorded systematically. Exact severity of ROP was confirmed by two independent, masked ophthalmologists at study entry and again if severe ROP (threshold) occurred. Infants remained on study-assigned oxygen saturation ranges for at least 2 weeks and until both eyes reached study end points.

Weekly examinations of the infants by study-certified, masked ophthalmologists were carried out. All infants received a final follow-up examination to confirm retinal status and pediatric end points at 3 months following their expected full-term due date (usually 5–6 months following birth).

Inclusion Criteria

Newborns with prethreshold ROP in one or both eyes were eligible.

Study Measures

An adverse end point was progression to threshold ROP (with referral for possible ablative therapy). A favorable end point was regression of the ROP into zone 3 for at least two examinations, or complete retinal vascularization. The pediatric end points of rate of growth, cardiopulmonary stability, and achievement of early motor milestones were measured as secondary end points.

Results

A total of 649 infants were enrolled of which 325 received conventional oxygen supplementation (89–94% pulse oximetry saturation) and 324 received supplemental oxygen (96–99% pulse oximetry saturation). 597 (92%) infants attained known ophthalmic endpoints, and 600 (92%) completed the ophthalmic 3-month assessment.
- Use of supplemental oxygen did not cause additional progression of prethreshold ROP but also did not significantly reduce the number of infants requiring peripheral retinal ablative surgery.
- A subgroup analysis suggested a benefit of supplemental oxygen among infants who have prethreshold ROP without plus disease, but this finding requires additional study.

- Supplemental oxygen increased the risk of adverse pulmonary events including pneumonia and/or exacerbations of chronic lung disease and the need for oxygen, diuretics, and hospitalization at 3 months of corrected age.

Conclusion

Although the relative risk/benefit of supplemental oxygen for each infant must be individually considered, clinicians need no longer be concerned that supplemental oxygen, as used in this study, will worsen active prethreshold ROP.

HIGH OXYGEN PERCENTAGE IN RETINOPATHY OF PREMATURITY STUDY (HOPE-ROP)[13]

Purpose

To determine the rate of progression from prethreshold to threshold ROP in infants excluded from STOP-ROP because their median arterial oxygen saturation by pulse oximetry (SpO_2) values were >94% in room air at the time of prethreshold diagnosis and to compare them with infants who were enrolled in STOP-ROP and had median SpO_2 ≤94% in room air.

Description

Fifteen of the 30 centers that participated in STOP-ROP elected to participate in the HOPE-ROP from January 1996 to March 1999. Infants were followed prospectively from the time prethreshold ROP was diagnosed until ROP either progressed to threshold in at least 1 study eye (adverse outcome) or resolved (favorable outcome).

Inclusion Criteria

Newborns with prethreshold ROP in one or both eyes were eligible.

Study Measures

An adverse end point was progression to threshold ROP (with referral for possible ablative therapy). A favorable end point was regression of the ROP into zone 3 for at least two examinations, or complete retinal vascularization. The pediatric end points of rate of growth, cardiopulmonary stability, and achievement of early motor milestones were measured as secondary end points.

Results

A total of 136 HOPE-ROP infants were compared with 229 STOP-ROP infants enrolled during the same time period from the same 15 hospitals. HOPE-ROP infants were of greater gestational age at birth (26.2 ± 1.8 vs. 25.2 ± 1.4 weeks) and greater postmenstrual age at the time of prethreshold ROP diagnosis (36.7 ± 2.5 vs. 35.4 ± 2.5 weeks). HOPE-ROP infants progressed to threshold ROP 25% of the time compared with 46% of STOP-ROP infants. After gestational age, race, postmenstrual age at prethreshold diagnosis, zone 1 disease, and plus disease at prethreshold diagnosis were controlled for, logistic regression analysis showed that HOPE-ROP infants progressed from prethreshold to threshold ROP less often than STOP-ROP infants (odds ratio: 0.607; 95% CI: 0.359–1.026).

Conclusion

The mechanisms that result in better ROP outcome for HOPE-ROP versus STOP-ROP are not fully understood. It seems that an infant's SpO_2 value at the time of prethreshold diagnosis is a prognostic indicator for which infants may progress to severe ROP. When other known prognostic indicators are factored in, the SpO_2 is of borderline significance.

EFFECTS OF LIGHT REDUCTION ON RETINOPATHY OF PREMATURITY (LIGHT-ROP)[14]

Purpose

To evaluate the effect of ambient light reduction on the incidence of ROP.

Background

The investigators hypothesize that reducing the amount of light that reaches the eyes of preterm infants may be effective in preventing ROP. Although previous reports on the use of light reduction to the eyes of preterm infants in the nursery have produced conflicting results, there are sufficient reasons to believe that this strategy may be effective in reducing the incidence and severity of ROP. These reasons center on the role of light in the production of destructive free radicals. Supplemental oxygen produces the same free radicals, and the two mechanisms may be additive.

Description

In this masked, controlled study, infants weighing less than 1,251 g at birth were prospectively randomized within 24 hours of birth to wear goggles or not to wear goggles. Goggles contain 97% near neutral density filters and were worn until the infant reached either 31 weeks gestational age or 4 weeks postnatal age, whichever was longer. The goggled and nongoggled infants were exposed to the same ambient light conditions within any given Study Center.

The study recruited approximately 400 infants (1995–1997), equally divided into goggle-wearing and control group. Since randomization must occur within 24 hours of birth, the investigators anticipated a mortality rate of between 10 and 20% of enrollees prior to outcome.

Eyes of all infants were examined on a prescribed schedule by certified examiners to determine the incidence of any confirmed ROP until either ROP regression or normal full retinal vascularization was established. A final examination occurred at adjusted age 6 months.

Inclusion Criteria

Premature infants weighing less than 1,251 g at birth and having a gestational age of less than 31 weeks were eligible for randomization. Patients with major congenital anomalies were excluded.

Study Measures

The primary objective was to answer the following question: Does light reduction to the eyes of extremely low birth-weight infants decrease the incidence of any confirmed ROP (at least 3 contiguous clock hours, any stage, any zone)? The primary end points were therefore ROP or full vascularization.

The secondary objective was to evaluate the following question: Does light reduction to the eyes of extremely low birth weight infants decrease the incidence of more severe ROP (prethreshold ROP—the secondary end point)?

Results

There were 188 infants in the group that wore goggles and 173 in the control group who survived and were available for follow-up. The mean birth weights were 906 g (1.99 pounds) in the goggles group and 914 g (2.01 pounds) in the control group. The mean gestational ages were 27.4 weeks and 27.2 weeks, respectively. The mean ambient-light level adjacent to the infants' faces was 399 lux (lumens per square meter) for the goggles group and 447 lux for the control group. ROP was diagnosed in 102 infants (54%) in the goggles group and 100 (58%) in the control group (relative risk, 0.9; 95% CI, 0.8–1.1; $p = 0.50$).

Conclusion

A reduction in the ambient-light exposure does not alter the incidence of ROP.

■ PHOTOGRAPHIC SCREENING FOR RETINOPATHY OF PREMATURITY STUDY (PHOTO-ROP)[15]

Purpose

To evaluate the utility of remote digital fundus imaging as compared to indirect ophthalmoscopy to screen for ROP.

Background

The standard method for diagnosis of ROP has been bedside indirect ophthalmoscopy for both routine clinical care and clinical trials. One limitation to this approach is that the examiner's interpretation of fundus findings is presumed to be correct without opportunity for review. The reading-center paradigm has become the gold standard for the conduct of ophthalmic clinical trials. To date, however, all large ROP trials have gathered data by requiring examiners to draw the retinal findings as noted during the clinical examination. The task of screening all at-risk infants for ROP poses manpower challenges. Many physicians do not perform ROP screening for fear of litigation. Experience with extreme prematurity may be limited. This combination of factors has fuelled interest in a telemedicine approach to ROP screening.

Description

It was a prospective, multicenter, masked, and Internet-based clinical trial. Consecutive infants from each of the six study centers were enrolled from February 1, 2001 to February 1, 2002. The last infant was imaged on May 30, 2002. The target number of infants was 50, and 62 were enrolled. Of those enrolled, 51 infants (102 eyes) were considered eligible.

Examinations began at 31 weeks postmenstrual age or 4 weeks postnatal age, whichever was later. Both eyes of all infants were imaged with a panoramic fundus imaging system, the RetCam-120 (Clarity Medical, Pleasanton, CA), followed by indirect ophthalmoscopic fundus examination. A standard set of six images per eye were captured from each infant in each exam session for each eye (iris and disc images, followed by images of temporal, nasal, superior, and inferior retinal fields). Images were transmitted via Internet to the Reading Center for interpretation by masked graders. Clinical interpretations based on indirect ophthalmoscopy were recorded for comparison with the Reading Center determinations. Examinations were performed weekly for 10 weeks or until an infant was discharged from the hospital.

For the purposes of this study, the Reading Center established a definition of *clinically significant ROP (CSROP)* representing five descriptions of ROP seen on digital fundus images sufficiently severe to warrant onsite examination by an ophthalmologist experienced in ROP:

1. Zone 1, any ROP, without vascular dilation or tortuosity.
2. Zone II, stage 2, with up to one quadrant of vascular dilation and tortuosity.
3. Zone II, stage 3, with up to one quadrant of vascular dilation and tortuosity.
4. Any vascular dilation and tortuosity noted in eyes for which ridge characteristics were not interpretable (not imaged or poor image quality).
5. Any ROP noted in eyes for which disc features (plus disease) were not interpretable (not imaged or poor image quality).

Inclusion Criteria

Premature infants <31 weeks postmenstrual age at birth and <1,000 g birth weight were eligible.

Study Measures

Sensitivity, specificity, positive and negative predictive values of Reading Center image interpretations were compared to clinical impressions based on bedside indirect ophthalmoscopy with the bedside examination determination as the "gold standard".

Results

Mean weekly examinations per infant (±SD) were 5.73 ± 3.22 (median 7; range 2–10).

- Three hundred image sets (3,836 images) were acquired for remote reading at the Reading Center. Ninety two percent (293/300) of the image sets were interpretable, i.e., one or more of the images in the set could be used to score zone, stage, and plus disease with confidence for a given eye. Uninterpretable image sets were typically a consequence of—(1) inadequate dilation limiting adequate illumination of the retina or casting an obstructing shadow, (2) dark fundus pigmentation with poor image contrast, (3) vitreous haze due to extreme prematurity, or some combination of one or more of these features.
- A single clear wide-angle image of the posterior pole was often adequate to determine the presence of CSROP or ETROP. The CSROP or ETROP criterion most scored on a single image of the posterior pole was plus disease. When images were of poorer quality (with regard to lighting, focus, clarity, field, or any combination thereof) the entire image set was used to make a determination as to the ROP status of the eye.
- Using the ROP diagnosis from the indirect ophthalmoscopic examinations as the reference standard, CSROP developed in 57.8% (59/102 eyes) with 22% (13/59 eyes) progressing further to ETROP Type I prethreshold ROP. In the 22.03% (13/59; seven right and six left) of eyes with CSROP that progressed to ETROP Type I, the mean interval to progression was 25.72 days (26.43 days for right and 25 days for left).
- Using onsite indirect ophthalmoscopic diagnosis as the reference standard, CSROP was identified by digital images with a sensitivity of 92% (94% right eyes and 89% left eyes) and specificity of 37.21% (40% right eyes and 35% left eyes), and ETROP prethreshold Type I with a sensitivity of 92% (86% right eyes and 100% left eyes) and specificity of 67.39% (67% right eyes and 68% left eyes).

- When image quality was high (i.e., excluding CSROP 4 and CSROP 5) there was no statistically significant difference in timing of diagnosis of CSROP or ETROP Type I between the Reading Center and Clinical Centers.

Conclusion

Remote interpretation of digital fundus images is a useful adjunct to conventional bedside ROP screening by indirect ophthalmoscopy. Diagnostic sensitivity in this study was excellent. It was highly unlikely that severe ROP would be missed when image quality was high. Differences between the two screening approaches in timing of diagnosis of CSROP and ETROP were not statistically significant. Remote digital fundus imaging as deployed in this study is unlikely to supplant bedside ophthalmoscopic examination due to limitations in diagnostic sensitivity, specificity, and accuracy when image quality is poor.

RANIBIZUMAB VERSUS LASER THERAPY FOR THE TREATMENT OF VERY LOW BIRTH WEIGHT INFANTS WITH RETINOPATHY OF PREMATURITY (RAINBOW): AN OPEN-LABEL RANDOMIZED CONTROLLED TRIAL[16]

Purpose

To evaluate the efficacy and safety of intravitreal ranibizumab compared with laser therapy in treatment of ROP.

Background

BEAT-ROP study paved way for use of antivascular endothelial growth factor agents for treatment of retinopathy of prematurity (ROP). To address the limited literature on ocular efficacy, the appropriate drug and dose, the need for retreatment, and the possibility of long-term systemic effects, RAINBOW trial was designed.

Description

This was a randomized, open-label, superiority multicenter, three-arm, parallel group trial was done in 87 neonatal and ophthalmic centers in 26 countries, one of them was India. 225 very low birthweight (<1,500 g) preterm babies with bilateral ROP zone I stage 1+, 2+, 3, or 3+, or zone II stage 3+, or aggressive posterior ROP (AP-ROP) (2015-2017) were randomized to receive a single bilateral intravitreal dose of RBZ 0.2 mg ($n = 74$) or RBZ 0.1 mg ($n = 77$), or laser therapy ($n = 74$).

Study Measures

The primary outcome was survival with no active retinopathy, no unfavorable structural outcomes, or need for a different treatment modality at or before 24 weeks.

Results

- ROP was present in zone I in 86 (38%) infants and in zone II in 138 (61%) infants. Most infants had stage 3+ disease, 135 (60%) in zone II and 37 (16%) in zone I. AP-ROP was present in 30 (13%) of 225 infants, 29 of whom had zone I disease.
- 214 infants were assessed for the primary outcome ($n = 70$, $n = 76$, $n = 68$, respectively). Seven were withdrawn before treatment ($n = 1$, $n = 1$, $n = 5$, respectively) and 17 did not complete follow-up to 24 weeks, including four deaths in each group.
- Treatment success occurred in 56 (80%) infants receiving RBZ 0.2 mg compared with 57 (75%) infants receiving RBZ 0.1 mg and 45 (66%) infants after laser therapy. Overall, treatment success was higher for all three groups in zone II than in zone I.
- The odds ratio for treatment success compared to laser therapy was higher for RBZ 0.2 mg [2.19 (95% CI 0.99–4.82, $p = 0.051$)] then RBZ 0.1 mg [1.57 (95% CI 0.76-3.26)]. Odds ratio for RBZ 0.2 mg compared to 0.1 mg was 1.35 (95% CI 0.61–2.98).
- Full peripheral vascularization assessed by indirect ophthalmoscopy occurred by day 169 in 28 (38%) infants in the ranibizumab 0.2 mg group and 21 (27%) infants in the ranibizumab 0.1 mg group.
- Unfavorable structural outcomes were least following ranibizumab 0.2 mg ($n = 1$), compared with ranibizumab 0.1 mg ($n = 5$) and laser therapy ($n = 7$).
- Death, serious adverse events (AEs), and nonserious systemic AEs and ocular adverse events were evenly distributed among the three groups. There was no clear evidence of plasma VEGF suppression or of differences between the three treatment groups.

Conclusion

Ranibizumab 0.2 mg might be superior to laser therapy for treatment of ROP with fewer unfavorable ocular outcomes than laser therapy and with an acceptable 24-week safety profile.

Table 1: Summary of clinical trials in the field of retinopathy of prematurity.

Title	Purpose	No. of patients	Inclusion criteria	Outcome measure	Result/Conclusion
CRYO-ROP (1986)	Safety and efficacy of trans-scleral cryotherapy in infants with ROP	291	Premature infants weighing <1,251 g at birth and had survived the first 28 days of life with threshold ROP	Fundus photo and VA at 1 year of age	• Cryotherapy reduces the risk of unfavorable retinal and functional outcome (by half) from threshold ROP • The benefit of cryotherapy was maintained across 15 years of follow-up
ET-ROP (2000)	Early versus conventional timing of treatment in ROP	317	Infants <1,251 g birth weight, examined by 42 days of life and with prethreshold ROP	Functional (primary) and structural (secondary) outcome at 9 months	• Early treatment of ROP significantly reduced unfavorable outcomes in both primary and secondary measures • Retinal ablative laser therapy for type I ROP; wait and watch for type II ROP
BEAT-ROP (2008)	Efficacy of intravitreal bevacizumab in ROP and compare it with conventional laser in ROP	150	Infants ≤1500 g at birth and ≤30 weeks gestation who develop Stage 3+ ROP in zone I or posterior zone II	Recurrence of neovascularization in one or both eyes requiring re-treatment before 54 weeks postmenstrual age	• Intravitreal bevacizumab monotherapy, compared with conventional laser therapy showed a benefit for zone I but not zone II disease • Trial was too small to assess safety
RAINBOW (2019)	Intravitreal Ranibizumab (0.2 mg, 0.1 mg) versus laser therapy for ROP	225	Very low birth weight preterm babies with bilateral ROP zone I stage 1+, 2+, 3, or 3+, or zone II stage 3+, or APROP	Survival with no active retinopathy, no unfavorable structural outcomes, or need for a different treatment modality at or before 24 weeks	Intravitreal Ranibizumab 0.2 mg might be superior to laser therapy

Contd...

Contd...

Title	Purpose	No. of patients	Inclusion criteria	Outcome measure	Result/Conclusion
HOPE-ROP (1996)	Rate of progression from prethreshold to threshold ROP in infants excluded from STOP-ROP	136	Newborns with prethreshold ROP in one or both eyes	• Adverse end point was progression to threshold ROP • Favorable end point was regression of the ROP into zone 3 or complete retinal vascularization	HOPE-ROP infants progressed from prethreshold to threshold ROP less often than STOP-ROP infants
LIGHT-ROP (1995)	Effect of ambient light reduction on the incidence of ROP	400	Premature infants weighing <1,251 g at birth and having a gestational age of <31 weeks	Development of ROP or full vascularization	Reduction in the ambient-light exposure does not alter the incidence of ROP
PHOTO-ROP (2000)	Digital fundus imaging compared to indirect ophthalmoscopy to screen for ROP	51	Premature infants <31 weeks postmenstrual age at birth and <1,000 g birthweight	Sensitivity, specificity, positive and negative predictive values of reading center image interpretations compared to clinical impressions based on bedside indirect ophthalmoscopy	• Remote digital fundus imaging is unlikely to supplant bedside ophthalmoscopy due to limitations in diagnostic sensitivity, specificity, and accuracy when image quality is poor • However fundus imaging is useful adjunct to indirect ophthalmoscopy especially when image quality is good
STOP-ROP (1994)	Supplemental oxygen in moderately severe ROP (prethreshold ROP)	649	Newborns with prethreshold ROP in one or both eyes	• Adverse end point was progression to threshold ROP • Favorable end point was regression of the ROP into zone 3 or complete retinal vascularization	• Supplemental oxygen did not cause additional progression of prethreshold ROP but also did not significantly reduce the need of peripheral retinal ablative surgery • Supplemental oxygen increased the risk of adverse pulmonary events

REFERENCES

1. Cryotherapy for Retinopathy of Prematurity Cooperative Group. Multicenter Trial of Cryotherapy for Retinopathy of Prematurity: 3½ year outcome—structure and function. Arch Ophthalmol. 1993;111:339-44.
2. Cryotherapy for Retinopathy of Prematurity Cooperative Group. Multicenter Trial of Cryotherapy for Retinopathy of Prematurity: Snellen acuity and structural outcome at 5½ years. Arch Ophthalmol. 1996;114:417-24.
3. Cryotherapy for Retinopathy of Prematurity Cooperative Group. Multicenter trial of cryotherapy for retinopathy of prematurity: Ophthalmological outcomes at 10 years. Arch Ophthalmol. 2001;119:1110-8.
4. Cryotherapy for Retinopathy of Prematurity Cooperative Group. 15-year outcomes following threshold retinopathy of prematurity: final results from the multicenter trial of cryotherapy for retinopathy of prematurity. Arch Ophthalmol. 2005;123:311-8.
5. Early Treatment for Retinopathy of Prematurity Cooperative Group. Multicenter trial of Early Treatment for Retinopathy of Prematurity: study design. Contr Clin Trials. 2004;25:311-25.
6. Early Treatment for Retinopathy of Prematurity Cooperative Group. Revised indications for the treatment of retinopathy of prematurity: results of the early treatment for retinopathy of prematurity randomized trial. Arch Ophthalmol. 2003;121:1684-94.
7. Early Treatment for Retinopathy of Prematurity Cooperative Group. Grating visual acuity results in the early treatment for retinopathy of prematurity study. Arch Ophthalmol. 2011;129:840-6.
8. Early Treatment for Retinopathy of Prematurity Cooperative Group. Final visual acuity results in the early treatment for retinopathy of prematurity study. Arch Ophthalmol. 2010;128:663-71.
9. Early Treatment for Retinopathy of Prematurity Cooperative Group. Visual field extent at 6 years of age in children who had high-risk prethreshold retinopathy of prematurity. Arch Ophthalmol. 2011;129:127-32.
10. Early Treatment for Retinopathy of Prematurity Cooperative Group. Prevalence and course of strabismus through age 6 years in participants of the Early Treatment for Retinopathy of Prematurity randomized trial. J AAPOS. 2011;15:536-40.
11. BEAT-ROP Cooperative Group: Efficacy of intravitreal bevacizumab for stage 3+ retinopathy of prematurity. N Engl J Med. 2011;364:603-15.
12. The STOP-ROP Multicenter Study Group. Supplemental Therapeutic Oxygen for Prethreshold Retinopathy of Prematurity (STOP-ROP). A randomized, controlled trial. I: Primary outcomes. Pediatrics. 2000;105: 295-310.
13. HOPE-ROP Multicenter Group. High Oxygen Percentage in Retinopathy of Prematurity study: Retinopathy of prematurity outcome in infants with prethreshold retinopathy of prematurity and oxygen saturation >94% in room air: the high oxygen percentage in retinopathy of prematurity study. Pediatrics. 2002;110:540-4.
14. Light Reduction in Retinopathy of Prematurity Cooperative Group. Lack of Efficacy of Light Reduction in Preventing Retinopathy of Prematurity. N Engl J Med. 1998;338:1572-6.
15. Photographic Screening for Retinopathy of Prematurity (Photo-ROP) Cooperative Group. The Photographic Screening for Retinopathy of Prematurity Study (Photo-ROP): study design and baseline characteristics of enrolled patients. Retina. 2006;26: S4-10.
16. Stahl A, Lepore D, Fielder A, Fleck B, Reynolds Chiang MF, et al. Ranibizumab versus laser therapy for the treatment of very low birthweight infants with retinopathy of prematurity (RAINBOW): an open-label randomised controlled trial. Lancet. 2019;394(10208):1551-9.

Miscellaneous Clinical Trials: Infant Aphakia Treatment Study

Neha Goel, Sonali Gupta

■ INFANT APHAKIA TREATMENT STUDY (IATS)[1-3]

Purpose

1. To compare the use of contact lenses (CLs) and intraocular lenses (IOLs) for the optical correction of unilateral aphakia during infancy.
2. To compare the occurrence of postoperative complications and the degree of parental stress between the two treatments.

Background

Intraocular lenses are now a commonly accepted treatment for cataracts in older children and are used increasingly in younger children and infants. IOLs are superior to contact lenses in that they more closely replicate the optics of the crystalline lens, do not require daily ongoing care, and ensure at least a partial optical correction at all times. The simplicity and improved visual outcome of an IOL correction may make caring for a child with a unilateral congenital cataract less stressful for parents. However, contact lenses remain the accepted treatment for children under 1 year of age due to concerns about the long-term safety of IOLs, higher frequency of postoperative complications and the potential for a large myopic shift developing in these eyes as they grow. Contact lenses provide excellent visual results in infants treated for bilateral congenital cataracts; however, two-thirds of infants treated with contact lenses for unilateral congenital cataracts remain legally blind in their aphakic eye. These poor visual outcomes are usually ascribed to competition from the sound eye and poor compliance with patching and contact lens wear regimens (poor cooperation while inserting and removing the lenses, the high costs of contact lenses, problems with lens loss, the difficulty of fitting the steep corneas of infants and the risk of bacterial keratitis).

Data from a pilot study and the literature suggest that superior visual results can be obtained if an IOL is used to correct unilateral aphakia during infancy, but these eyes will experience more complications. This clinical trial aims to determine if the higher rate of complications with IOLs is offset by improved visual outcome and decreased parenting stress.

Description

In a randomized, multicenter (12 sites) clinical trial, 114 infants with unilateral congenital cataracts were assigned to undergo cataract surgery with or without IOL implantation between 1 and 6 months of age. Enrolment began December 23, 2004, and was completed January 16, 2009.

Cataract surgery was performed in a standardized fashion by a surgeon who had been certified for the study. Surgery consisted of a lensectomy, posterior capsulotomy, and anterior vitrectomy. Infants were randomized at the time of surgery to one of two treatment groups. Infants randomized to the IOL group had an IOL implanted into the capsular bag. The IOL power was determined based on the Holladay 1 formula targeting an 8 D undercorrection for infants 4–6 weeks of age and a 6 D undercorrection for infants older than 6 weeks. Spectacles were subsequently used to correct the residual refractive errors. Within a week after cataract surgery, patients randomized to the contact lens group were fitted with a soft (Bausch and Lomb, Rochester, NY) or a rigid gas permeable (RGP) contact lens with a 2.0 D overcorrection to provide a near point correction. If an accurate refraction could not be obtained, a +32 D contact lens was dispensed. Both groups received the same patching therapy and follow-up.

Follow-up examinations were performed by an Infant Aphakia Treatment Study (IATS) certified investigator at 1 day, 1 week, 1 month, and 3 months following cataract surgery. Thereafter, follow-up examinations were performed at 3-month (± 2 weeks) intervals. When the child reached 4 years of age, follow-up examinations were performed at 4, 4¼, 4½ and 5 years of age. Examinations included an assessment of: visual acuity, the anterior segments and pupils, the degree of refractive error and ocular alignment. In addition, the fit of the contact lens was assessed by a contact lens specialist.

The Parenting Stress Index (PSI) and the Ocular Treatment Index (OTI) were administered to parents 3 months after surgery, at the first visit following the grating acuity assessment and at 4.25 years of age.

Inclusion Criteria

The major eligibility criteria for enrolment included the following:
- Visually significant unilateral congenital cataract (central opacity ≥3 mm in size).
- Cataract surgery performed when the patient is 28–210 days of age and at least 41 postconceptional weeks.

Children with cataract acquired due to trauma, or as a side effect of radiation or medical therapy, any other ocular or systemic condition affecting visual acuity or visual potential or history of any previous intraocular surgery were excluded.

Study Measures

The primary outcome measure was visual acuity measured at 12 months (grating acuity) and 4.5 years (HOTV visual acuity) of age. The secondary outcome measures were complications and parenting stress, in the time frame of 12 months to 5 years of age.

Other secondary outcomes assessed at 4.5 years included: stereopsis, pachymetry, keratometry, tonometry and eye movements. Secondary outcomes measured at 5 years of age included: ocular motility and alignment, optical biometry, non-contact specular microscopy, tonometry, and keratometry.

Results

- The median age at the time of cataract surgery was 1.8 months. Fifty patients were 4–6 weeks of age at the time of enrolment; 32, 7 weeks to 3 months of age; and the remaining 32, more than 3 to less than 7 months of age. Fifty-seven children were randomized to each treatment group. Eyes with cataracts had shorter axial lengths and steeper corneas on average than the fellow eyes.
- Grating acuity at 1 year of age:[2] The median logMAR visual acuity was not significantly different between the treated eyes in the 2 groups (contact lens group, 0.80; IOL group, 0.97; $P = 0.19$). More patients in the IOL group underwent 1 or more additional intraocular operations than patients in the contact lens group (63% vs. 12%; $P < 0.001$). Most of these additional operations were performed to clear lens reproliferation and pupillary membranes from the visual axis.
- Glaucoma related adverse events at 1 year of age[3]: Of these 114 patients, 10 (9%) developed glaucoma and 4 (4%) had glaucoma suspect, for a total of 14 patients (12%) with a glaucoma-related adverse event in the treated eye through the first year of follow-up. Of the 57 patients who underwent lensectomy and anterior vitrectomy, 5 (9%) developed a glaucoma-related adverse event; of the 57 patients who underwent an IOL, 9 (16%) developed a glaucoma-related adverse event. The odds of developing a glaucoma-related adverse event were 3.1 times higher for a child with persistent fetal vasculature and 1.6 times higher for each month of age younger at cataract surgery.

■ CONCLUSION

- There was no statistically significant difference in grating visual acuity at age 1 year between the IOL and contact lens groups; however, additional intraocular operations were performed more frequently in the IOL group. Until longer-term follow-up data are available, caution should be exercised when performing IOL implantation in children aged 6 months

or younger given the higher incidence of adverse events and the absence of an improved short-term visual outcome compared with contact lens use.
- Modern surgical techniques do not eliminate the early development of glaucoma following congenital cataract surgery with or without an IOL implant. Younger patients with or without persistent fetal vasculature seem more likely to develop a glaucoma-related adverse event in the first year of follow-up. Vigilance for the early development of glaucoma is needed following congenital cataract surgery, especially when surgery is performed during early infancy or for a child with persistent fetal vasculature.

Table 1: Summary of Infant Aphakia Treatment Study (IATS).

Title	Purpose	No. of patients	Inclusion criteria	Outcome measure	Conclusion
IATS 2004–2009	Compare contact lenses and IOLs for the optical correction of unilateral aphakia during infancy	114	Visually significant unilateral congenital cataract with surgery performed at 28–210 days of age	VA at 12 months and 4.5 years of age	No difference in visual acuity at age 1 year between the IOL and contact lens groups Higher incidence of adverse events when performing IOL implantation in children aged <6 months

(IOLs: intraocular lenses; VA: visual acuity)

REFERENCES

1. Infant Aphakia Treatment Study Group. The infant aphakia treatment study: design and clinical measures at enrollment. Arch Ophthalmol. 2010;128:21-7.
2. Infant Aphakia Treatment Study Group. A randomized clinical trial comparing contact lens with intraocular lens correction of monocular aphakia during infancy: grating acuity and adverse events at age 1 year. Arch Ophthalmol. 2010;128:810-8.
3. Infant Aphakia Treatment Study Group. Glaucoma-related adverse events in the Infant Aphakia Treatment Study: 1-year results. Arch Ophthalmol. 2012;130:300-5.

Clinical Trials in Amblyopia: Pediatric Eye Disease Investigator Group (PEDIG) Studies

Sumit Monga, Neha Goel

INTRODUCTION

Amblyopia is the most common cause of monocular visual impairment in children and young adults. Most cases are associated with strabismus, usually esotropia in infancy or early childhood. Less frequently the cause is anisometropia, a combination of strabismus and anisometropia, or visual deprivation. Until recently, most published studies on amblyopia treatment were retrospective reviews of large numbers of patients. Much of the information gained in the past few years has been from studies conducted by the Pediatric Eye Disease Investigator Group (PEDIG), a network of community and university based ophthalmologists and optometrists operating in over one hundred sites. PEDIG studies are funded by the National Eye Institute, and the data coordinating center is located at the JAEB Center for Health Research in Tampa, Florida.

Pediatric Eye Disease Investigator Group studies use a standard visual acuity testing protocol. For children less than age 7, HOTV letters are presented individually with surround bars to account for the crowding phenomenon in amblyopia (single-surround HOTV optotypes), and older children use the electronic Early Treatment Diabetic Retinopathy Study (ETDRS) vision test.

AMBLYOPIA TREATMENT STUDY (ATS)-1[1,2]

Purpose

- To compare patching and atropine as treatments for moderate amblyopia (20/40–20/100 in the amblyopic eye) in children 3 to <7 years old
- To develop estimates of the success rates of treatment
- To identify factors that may be associated with successful treatment.

Background

Occlusion therapy with patching of the sound eye has been the mainstay of amblyopia treatment despite the lack of meaningful data demonstrating its superiority compared with other modalities. Opinions vary on the number of hours of patching per day that should be prescribed. Compliance is often cited as a major problem because of patients' dislike of occlusion owing to skin irritation and visual, social, and psychological reasons. The success of occlusion therapy is reported to be dependent on compliance.

Although less widely prescribed, pharmacologic penalization is an alternative to occlusion therapy for amblyopia. This method involves the instillation of a long-acting topical cycloplegic agent, such as atropine sulfate, into the sound eye. The cycloplegia prevents accommodation, blurring the sound eye at near fixation. When the sound eye is hyperopic, the penalization effect is potentially augmented if less than full plus spectacle correction is prescribed for the cyclopleged sound eye, effectively blurring its vision at both near and distance fixation. Pharmacologic penalization has generally been advocated only for mild and moderate amblyopia (20/100 or better) because the blurring effect on the sound eye may be insufficient when visual acuity in the amblyopic eye is worse than 20/100. Clinical experience has found that pharmacologic penalization has a high acceptability to patients and parents, and consequently high rates of compliance.

Description

In a randomized multicenter clinical trial (47 clinical sites), 419 children aged 3–7 years with amblyopia and visual acuity in the range of 20/40–20/100 were assigned to receive either patching or atropine for 6 months. Between 6 months and 2 years, treatment was at the discretion of the investigator.

Patching Protocol

- The initial patching time was a minimum of 6 hours per day (maximum, all waking hours)
- If criteria for successful treatment were met, patching time could be reduced but needed to be at least 7 hours per week as long as the visual acuity in the amblyopic eye was 1 or more lines worse than that in the sound eye
- If the visual acuity in the two eyes became equal, patching could be discontinued
- If criteria for successful treatment were not met by the 16-week visit, and patching time had been less than 12 hours per day, patching time was increased to 12 or more hours per day for 2 months prior to the 6-month outcome examination.

Adhesive skin patches provided by the study were used unless there was skin allergy or irritation nonresponsive to both local treatment with a skin emollient and a change in the brand of patch, in which case a spectacle occluder could be prescribed.

Atropine Protocol

At enrollment, patients were prescribed 1 drop per day of atropine sulfate 1%. Sunglasses were also provided, with the advice that they be worn with a hat when the child was in sunlight. Daily atropine use was continued unless the visual acuity in the amblyopic eye met criteria for successful treatment, in which case (at the investigator's discretion) the frequency could be reduced to a minimum of 2 times a week and could be discontinued if the acuities became equal in the two eyes. For patients with hyperopia in the sound eye, if the amblyopic eye was not successfully treated by the 16-week visit, the spectacle lens was reduced to Plano for 2 months prior to the 6-month outcome examination. If an allergy to atropine developed, topical homatropine 5% could be substituted instead. Protocol-specified follow-up visits were conducted after a period of 5 ± 2 weeks, 16 ± 2 weeks, and 26 ± 1 weeks (primary outcome). At baseline and each protocol-specified visit, visual acuity was measured in both eyes using the ATS visual acuity testing protocol administered by a study-certified vision tester. The test was administered either on the Baylor Video Acuity Tester or the Electronic Visual Acuity Tester. At the 5-week visit, a questionnaire designed to assess the effect of amblyopia treatment on the child and parent (*Amblyopia Treatment Index*) was completed by the parent. The questionnaire consisted of 18 items, each scored from 1 to 5, with 5 representing the most difficult. Three subscales measured the adverse effects of treatment (8 items), difficulties with compliance (5 items), and social stigma of treatment (3 items). Items were summed to compute each subscale score, and then scaled to a common range from 1 to 5. At the 6-month outcome examination, visual acuity testing of the amblyopic eye was conducted by a tester masked to the patient's treatment group. Outcome examination testing also included the measurement of visual acuity in the sound eye and assessment of ocular alignment using a simultaneous prism and cover test at distance and near fixation.

A patient was considered to be successfully treated with regard to the protocol when the amblyopic eye's visual acuity was 20/30 or better or had improved 3 or more lines from baseline.

Inclusion Criteria

Eligibility criteria for the trial included:
- Age younger than 7 years
- Visual acuity in the amblyopic eye from 20/40–20/100
- The presence or history of an amblyogenic factor meeting study-specified criteria for strabismus or anisometropia
- Visual acuity in the sound eye of 20/40 or better
- Inter eye acuity difference of 3 or more logarithm of the minimum angle of resolution (logMAR) lines
- Wearing of optimal spectacle correction for a minimum of 4 weeks at the time of enrollment.

Study Measures

Visual acuity in the amblyopic eye after 6 months was the primary efficacy outcome measure, and acuity in the sound eye was the primary safety outcome measure.

Results

- Visual acuity in the amblyopic eye improved in both groups (improvement from baseline to 6 months was 3.16 lines in the patching group and 2.84 lines in the atropine group). At 2 years follow-up, improvement from baseline to 6 months was 3.7 lines in the patching group and 3.6 lines in the atropine group
- Improvement was initially faster in the patching group, but after 6 months, the difference in visual acuity between treatment groups was small and clinically inconsequential (mean difference at 6 months, 0.034 logMAR units; 95% confidence interval, 0.005–0.064 logMAR units).
- The 6-month acuity was 20/30 or better in the amblyopic eye and/or improved from baseline by 3 or more lines in 79% of the patching group and 74% of the atropine group. This increased to 86% and 84% respectively at 2 years follow-up.
- The effect of treatment was similar in subgroups based on age (<5 years old, ≥5 years old), cause of amblyopia (strabismus, anisometropia, combined), baseline visual acuity in the amblyopic eye (20/80–20/100, 20/40–20/60).
- Both treatments were well-tolerated, although atropine had a slightly higher degree of acceptability on a parental questionnaire.
- More patients in the atropine group than in the patching group had reduced acuity in the sound eye at 6 months, but this did not persist with further follow-up. Some cases were due to improper refractive correction; in other cases there was likely residual cycloplegia from atropine not having been discontinued.
- In both treatment groups, at the end of 2 years, the mean amblyopic eye acuity was approximately 20/32, 1.8 lines worse than the mean sound eye acuity, which was approximately 20/20.

Conclusion

Atropine or patching for 6 months followed by best clinical care until 2 years produced similar improvement of moderate amblyopia in children between 3 and 7 years of age at enrollment. However, on average the amblyopic eye acuity was still approximately 2 lines worse than the sound eye.

AMBLYOPIA TREATMENT STUDY (ATS)—2A, 2B, 2C[3-5]

Occlusion therapy with patching of the sound eye has been the mainstay of amblyopia treatment. However, opinions vary on the number of hours of daily patching that should be prescribed, ranging from as little as 1 or 2 hours, to 24 hours per day. No prior study has provided conclusive data on the optimal number of patching hours.

Amblyopia Treatment Study—2A[3]

Purpose

To compare full-time patching (all hours or all but 1 hour per day) to 6 hours of patching per day, as prescribed treatments for severe amblyopia (20/100–20/400) in children younger than 7 years.

Description

In a prospective, randomized multicenter clinical trial (32 sites), 175 children younger than 7 years with amblyopia and visual acuity in the range of 20/100–20/400 were assigned either to full-time patching or to 6 hours of patching per day, each combined with at least 1 hour of near-visual activities during patching.

The assigned patching regimen was used for the 4-month study duration, with the following exceptions: (1) if the acuity in the amblyopic eye improved to be the same as or 1 line worse than the acuity in the sound eye, patching could be continued at the initial number of hours or could be decreased at investigator discretion, provided it was at least 7 hours per week, and (2) if the acuity in the amblyopic eye became better than the acuity in the sound eye or if reverse amblyopia was considered by the investigator to have developed, then treatment could be continued, reduced, or stopped at investigator discretion.

Protocol-specified follow-up visits were conducted at 5 ± 1 weeks and 17 ± 1 weeks. At baseline and at each protocol-specified visit, visual acuity was measured in both eyes using the ATS visual acuity testing protocol, administered by a study-certified vision examiner using an electronic visual acuity tester.

At the 5-week visit, a questionnaire designed to assess the impact of the amblyopia treatment on the quality of life of the child and parent (Amblyopia Treatment Index) was completed by the parent.

At the 4-month outcome examination, visual acuity testing was conducted by a study-certified vision tester who was masked to the patient's treatment group. Additional testing done at this visit included assessment of ocular alignment with a simultaneous prism and cover test and measurement of stereoacuity with the Titmus Test (fly only), Randot Stereo Tests and Randot Preschool Stereoacuity Test.

Inclusion Criteria

Eligibility criteria for the trial included:
- Age younger than 7 years
- Visual acuity in the amblyopic eye from 20/100 to 20/400
- The presence or history of an amblyogenic factor meeting study-specified criteria for strabismus or anisometropia

- Visual acuity in the sound eye of 20/40 or better
- Inter eye acuity difference of 3 or more logMAR lines
- The wearing of optimal spectacle correction for a minimum of 4 weeks at the time of enrollment.

Study Measures
Visual acuity in the amblyopic eye after 4 months.

Results
Visual acuity in the amblyopic eye improved a similar amount in both groups. The improvement in the amblyopic eye acuity from baseline to 4 months averaged 4.8 lines in the 6-hour group and 4.7 lines in the full-time group ($p = 0.45$).

Conclusion
Six hours of prescribed daily patching produces an improvement in visual acuity that is of similar rate and magnitude to the improvement produced by prescribed full-time patching in treating severe amblyopia in children 3 to less than 7 years of age. Prescribing fewer hours of daily patching may ease the implementation of patching therapy and monitoring of compliance for some parents.

Amblyopia Treatment Study-2B[4]

Purpose
To compare 2 hours versus 6 hours of daily patching as treatments for moderate amblyopia (20/40 20/80) in children younger than 7 years.

Description
In a prospective, randomized multicenter clinical trial (35 sites), 189 children younger than 7 years with amblyopia and visual acuity in the range of 20/40–20/80 were assigned to receive either 2 hours or 6 hours of daily patching combined with at least 1 hour per day of near visual activities during patching.

The patching regimen, follow-up visits and protocol at each visit was similar to that of ATS—2A.

Inclusion Criteria
Eligibility criteria for the trial included:
- Age younger than 7 years
- Visual acuity in the amblyopic eye from 20/100 to 20/400
- The presence or history of an amblyogenic factor meeting study-specified criteria for strabismus or anisometropia

- Visual acuity in the sound eye of 20/40 or better
- Inter eye acuity difference of 3 or more logMAR lines
- The wearing of optimal spectacle correction for a minimum of 4 weeks at the time of enrollment.

Study Measures
Visual acuity in the amblyopic eye after 4 months.

Results
Visual acuity in the amblyopic eye improved a similar amount in both groups. The improvement in the visual acuity of the amblyopic eye from baseline to 4 months averaged 2.40 lines in each group ($p = 0.98$). The 4-month visual acuity was at least 20/32 and/or improved from baseline by 3 or more lines in 62% of patients in each group ($p > 0.99$).

Conclusion
When combined with prescribing 1 hour of near visual activities, 2 hours of daily patching produces an improvement in visual acuity that is of similar magnitude to the improvement produced by 6 hours of daily patching in treating moderate amblyopia in children aged 3–7 years. A shorter duration of patching may ease the implementation of patching therapy and monitoring compliance for some parents.

Amblyopia Treatment Study-2C[5]

Purpose
To conduct a prospective study of children who had been successfully treated for amblyopia and for whom treatment was to be stopped to estimate the risk of amblyopia recurrence during the following year.

Description
In a prospective, observational study, 156 children with successfully treated anisometropic or strabismic amblyopia (145 completed follow-up) were enrolled at 30 clinical sites. Patients were followed off treatment for 52 weeks to assess recurrence of amblyopia, defined as a 2 or more logMAR level reduction of visual acuity from enrollment, confirmed by a second examination. Recurrence was also considered to have occurred if treatment was restarted because of a nonreplicated 2 or more logMAR level reduction of visual acuity.

Protocol-specified follow-up visits were conducted at 5 ± 1 weeks, 13 ± 2 weeks, 26 ± 2 weeks, and 52 ± 2 weeks. At baseline and at each protocol-specified visit, visual acuity was measured in each eye using the ATS visual acuity testing protocol administered by a study certified vision examiner using the electronic visual acuity tester.

Inclusion Criteria

Eligibility criteria for the trial included children who were younger than 8 years of age and who received continuous amblyopia treatment for the previous 3 months (prescribed at least 2 hours of daily patching or prescribed at least one drop of atropine per week) and who had improved at least 3 logMAR levels during the period of continuous treatment.

Results

- Recurrence occurred in 35 (24%) of 145 cases (95% confidence interval 17-32%) and was similar in patients who stopped patching (25%) and in patients who stopped atropine (21%).
- Recurrence occurred throughout the 52-week follow-up, but recurrences occurred more frequently during the first 13 weeks after cessation of treatment.
- In patients treated with moderately intense patching (6-8 hours per day), recurrence was more common (11 of 26; 42%) when treatment was not reduced prior to cessation than when treatment was reduced to 2 hours per day prior to cessation (3 of 22; 14%, odds ratio 4.4, 95% confidence interval 1.0-18.7).

Conclusion

- Approximately one-fourth of successfully treated amblyopic children experience a recurrence within the first year of treatment.
- Follow-up through at least 1 year is needed, but follow-up visits during the first 3 months after stopping treatment might allow detection and retreatment of the majority of recurrences that occur during the first year.
- For patients treated with 6 or more hours of daily patching, the risk of recurrence is greater when patching is stopped abruptly rather than when it is reduced to 2 hours per day prior to cessation. A randomized clinical trial of no weaning versus weaning in successfully-treated amblyopia is warranted to confirm these observational findings.

AMBLYOPIA TREATMENT STUDY-3[6]

Purpose

- To evaluate the effectiveness of treatment of amblyopia in children aged 7-17 years.
- To determine the frequency of recidivism of successfully-treated amblyopia in children 7-17 years.

Background

Although there is consensus that amblyopia can be treated effectively in young children, many eye care professionals believe that treatment beyond a certain age is ineffective. Some believe that a treatment response is unlikely after the age of 6 or 7 years, while others consider age 9 or 10 years to be the upper age limit for successful treatment. The American Academy of Ophthalmology Preferred Practice Pattern for amblyopia recommends treatment up to age 10 years. The opinion that amblyopia treatment is ineffective in older children may have arisen because the age of 6-7 years is thought to be the end of the "critical period" for visual development in humans. This belief, however, is not based on adequate prospectively collected data. In fact, there are numerous reports, primarily retrospective case series, of older children and adults with amblyopia responding to treatment with patching.

Description

In a prospective, randomized multicenter clinical trial (49 sites), 507 children aged 7-17 years with amblyopia and visual acuity in the range of 20/40-20/400 were provided with optical correction and then randomized to a:
- Treatment group (2-6 hours per day of prescribed patching combined with near visual activities for all patients plus atropine sulfate for children aged 7-12 years) or an
- Optical correction group (optical correction alone).

Baseline testing included—(1) Visual acuity, measured in each eye with the patient wearing optimal correction by a study-certified vision tester using the electronic ETDRS testing procedure, (2) assessment of binocularity with the Titmus test (fly only) and the Randot Preschool Stereoacuity Test, (3) measurement of ocular alignment with a simultaneous prism and cover test at distance and near fixation (modified Krimsky test used if fixation poor), (4) cycloplegic refraction, (5) ocular examination including pupillary dilation, and (6) assessment of eccentric fixation with a direct ophthalmoscope.

Follow-up visits occurred every 6 weeks until criteria were met to classify the patient as a responder or nonresponder.

Patients whose amblyopic eye acuity improved 10 or more letters (≥2 lines) by 24 weeks were considered responders.

The observation phase consisted of visits at 13 weeks, 26 weeks, and 52 weeks after treatment discontinuation. Visual acuity was assessed at each visit. Recurrence was defined as visual acuity 10 or more letters worse than visual acuity at treatment discontinuation.

Inclusion Criteria

Eligibility criteria for the trial included:
- Age 7-17 years
- Visual acuity in the amblyopic eye from 20/40 to 20/400

- The presence or history of an amblyogenic factor meeting study-specified criteria for strabismus or anisometropia
- No more than 6 diopters (D) of myopia in the amblyopic eye
- Best-corrected sound eye acuity of 20/25 or better
- No more than 1 month of amblyopia treatment in the last 6 months, and no amblyopia treatment (other than spectacles) in the last month.

Study Measures

The primary outcome was the proportion of patients in each group classified as a responder. A patient was classified as a responder if the amblyopic eye acuity was 10 or more letters (2 lines) better than the baseline acuity on the testing conducted by the masked examiner at the 6-week, 12-week, 18-week, or 24-week visit. By the 24-week visit, if the amblyopic eye acuity had not improved 10 or more letters, then the patient was classified as a nonresponder. A patient could also be classified as a nonresponder at an earlier visit if there was no improvement (0 letters) from the prior follow-up visit or minimal improvement from baseline (defined at the 6-week visit as 0-letter improvement from baseline, at the 12-week visit as <3-letter improvement from baseline, and at the 18-week visit as <5-letter improvement from baseline).

Results

In the 7–12-years-old ($n = 404$), 53% of the treatment group were responders compared with 25% of the optical correction group ($p < 0.001$).
- In the 13–17-years-old ($n = 103$), the responder rates were 25% and 23%, respectively, overall (adjusted $p = 0.22$) but 47% and 20%, respectively, among patients not previously treated with patching and/or atropine for amblyopia (adjusted $p = 0.03$).
- Most patients, including responders, were left with a residual visual acuity deficit.

Conclusion

- Amblyopia improves with optical correction alone in about one-fourth of patients aged 7–17 years, although most patients who are initially treated with optical correction alone will require additional treatment for amblyopia.
- For patients aged 7–12 years, prescribing 2–6 hours per day of patching with near visual activities and atropine can improve visual acuity even if the amblyopia has been previously treated.
- For patients 13–17 years, prescribing patching 2–6 hours per day with near visual activities may improve visual acuity when amblyopia has not been previously treated but appears to be of little benefit if amblyopia was previously treated with patching.

- It is not yet known whether visual acuity improvement will be sustained once treatment is discontinued; therefore, conclusions regarding the long-term benefit of treatment and the development of treatment recommendations for amblyopia in children 7 years and older await the results of a follow-up study.

AMBLYOPIA TREATMENT STUDY-4[7]

Purpose
- To compare daily versus weekend atropine (2 days) as prescribed treatments for moderate amblyopia (20/40–20/80) in children 3 to <7 years old
- To determine the maximum amount of improvement that could be achieved with these atropine schedules.

Description
In a prospective, randomized multicenter clinical trial (30 sites), 168 children younger than 7 years with amblyopia in the range of 20/40–20/80 associated with strabismus, anisometropia, or both were randomized either to daily atropine or to weekend atropine for 4 months. Partial responders were continued on the randomized treatment until no further improvement was noted. For patients in the daily atropine group, if the amblyopic eye acuity improved to be the same as or better than the sound eye acuity, atropine could be decreased to no less than twice per week.

At enrollment and at each follow-up visit, visual acuity was measured in each eye by a study-certified vision tester using single-surrounded HOTV optotypes on an electronic visual acuity tester. Additional baseline testing included (1) a cycloplegic refraction; (2) an ocular examination; (3) measurement of ocular alignment with a simultaneous prism and cover test at distance and near fixation; (4) assessment of binocularity with the Titmus Test (fly only), the Randot Suppression Test and the Randot Preschool Stereoacuity Test; and (5) measurement of near visual acuity in each eye before cycloplegia and in the sound eye after cycloplegia. Follow-up visits were performed at 5 weeks and 17 weeks within a specified 2-week time window. At the 5-week visit, a questionnaire designed to assess the impact of the pharmacologic amblyopia treatment on the quality of life of the child and family (Amblyopia Treatment Index) was completed by the parent.

At the 17-week (4-month) outcome examination, visual acuity testing was conducted by a study-certified vision tester who was masked as to the patient's treatment group. After the 17-week visit, atropine was discontinued, and the patient returned 2–4 weeks later to assess the sound eye acuity, near acuity in each eye, ocular alignment and binocularity (referred to as the sound eye outcome visit).

Inclusion Criteria
Eligibility criteria for the trial included:
- Age <7 years
- Visual acuity in the amblyopic eye from 20/40 to 20/80
- The presence or history of an amblyogenic factor meeting study-specified criteria for strabismus or anisometropia
- Visual acuity in the sound eye of 20/40 or better
- Inter eye acuity difference of 3 or more logMAR lines
- The wearing of optimal spectacle correction for a minimum of 4 weeks at the time of enrollment.
- No amblyopia treatment in the past month and no more than 1 month of amblyopia treatment in the past 6 months.

Children with myopia greater than 6.00 D in the amblyopic eye, myopia greater than 0.50 D in the sound eye, or Down syndrome were excluded.

Study Measures
Visual acuity in the amblyopic eye after 4 months was the primary outcome. Maximum visual acuity improvement was the secondary outcome measure.

Results
The improvement in visual acuity of the amblyopic eye from baseline to 4 months averaged 2.3 lines in each group. The visual acuity of the amblyopic eye at study completion was either (1) at least 20/25 or (2) better than or equal to that of the sound eye in 39 children (47%) in the daily group and 45 children (53%) in the weekend group. The visual acuity of the sound eye at the end of follow-up was reduced by 2 lines in one patient in each group. Stereoacuity outcomes were similar in the 2 groups.

Conclusion
Weekend atropine provides an improvement in visual acuity of a magnitude similar to that of the improvement provided by daily atropine in treating moderate amblyopia in children 3–7 years old.

AMBLYOPIA TREATMENT STUDY-5(1)[8]

Purpose
To evaluate the effectiveness of refractive error alone, in treatment of untreated anisometropic amblyopia, in the age group 3 to <7 years old.

Background
Although there have been reports that refractive correction alone results in improved vision in anisometropic amblyopia, 2–7 it is generally held that the majority of cases will need additional treatment because refractive correction

alone will not be sufficient to completely treat the amblyopia. Thus, patching or pharmacological treatment is often prescribed simultaneously or soon after the refractive correction is provided. PEDIG conducted a prospective study of the treatment of untreated anisometropic amblyopia in children 3 to <7 years old with spectacle correction alone. The objectives were to determine (1) the incidence of resolution of amblyopia, (2) the time course of visual acuity improvement, and (3) factors associated with resolution of amblyopia with spectacles alone.

Participants
84 children 3 to <7 years old with untreated anisometropic amblyopia ranging from 6/12 to 6/75.

Methods
Optimal refractive correction was provided, and visual acuity at baseline and at 5-week intervals until visual acuity stabilized or amblyopia resolved.

Main Outcome Measure
Maximum improvement in best corrected visual acuity (BCVA) in the amblyopic eye and proportion of children whose amblyopia resolved (interocular difference of </ ≥1 one line) with refractive correction, alone.

Results
Amblyopia improved with optical correction by ≥2 lines in 77% and resolved in 27% of the patients. Improvement took up to 30 weeks for stabilization criteria to be met.

Conclusion
Refractive correction alone improves visual acuity in many cases and results in resolution of amblyopia in at-least one-third of 3 to <7 years old children with untreated anisometropic amblyopia.

AMBLYOPIA TREATMENT STUDY-5(2)[9]

Purpose
To evaluate effectiveness of 2 hours of daily patching (combined with 1 hour of concurrent near visual activities) versus control group of spectacle wear alone for the treatment of moderate to severe amblyopia in children 3–7 years old.

Background
Despite expert opinion and experimental evidence that amblyopia improves with patching, some authors had questioned whether there is benefit to

patching, because few studies have included an untreated control group. Although results from randomized clinical trials comparing patching with control have been reported, no study has been published to date that has done all of the following: (1) clearly defined amblyopia at enrollment, (2) incorporated a prolonged spectacles run-in phase with criteria for determining when maximum improvement has occurred, and (3) included a no-patching control group. To address the question of whether patching improves amblyopia after a period of refractive correction, we conducted a randomized clinical trial to compare the effect of 2 hours of daily patching combined with 1 hour of near activities versus a control group in children age 3-7 years old with amblyopia caused by strabismus, anisometropia or both.

Participants
180 children (3-7 years old) with BCVA amblyopic eye (visual acuity) of 6/12-6/120 associated with strabismus, anisometropia or both, who had worn optimal refractive correction for at least 16 weeks or for two consecutive visits without improvement.

Interventions
Randomization either to 2 hours of daily patching with 1 hour of near visual activities or to spectacles alone. Patients were continued on the randomized treatment (or no treatment) until no further improvement was noted.

Methods
Visual acuity was measured at baseline and 5 weeks interval, until visual acuity stabilized or amblyopia resolved.

Main Outcome Measure
Best corrected visual acuity in the amblyopic eye after 5 weeks.

Results
Improvement in visual acuity of the amblyopic eye from baseline to 5 weeks averaged 1.1 lines in the patching group and 0.5 lines in the control group ($p = 0.006$), and improvement from baseline to best measured visual acuity at any visit averaged 2.2 lines in the patching group and 1.3 lines in the control group ($p < 0.001$). There was no significant interaction between treatment group and baseline visual acuity ($p = 0.07$), gender ($p = 0.07$), race ($p = 0.30$), age at randomization ($p = 0.14$), prior amblyopia treatment ($p = 0.80$), participation in the spectacle phase of the study ($p = 0.22$), or cause of amblyopia (strabismus >5 prism diopters or anisometropia/microtropia, $p = 0.16$) on the outcome visual acuity in the amblyopic eye.

Conclusion

After a period of treatment with spectacles, 2 hours of daily patching, combined with 1 hour of near visual activity, modestly improves moderate to severe amblyopia in children 3-7 years old. Although not designed to determine the magnitude of benefit from patching, this trial provides conclusive evidence that occlusion of the sound eye improves amblyopia from strabismus, anisometropia or both.

■ AMBLYOPIA TREATMENT STUDY-6[10]

Purpose

To determine whether performing near activities, while patching for amblyopia, and enhances improvement in visual acuity.

Background

Near visual activities are often prescribed during patching for amblyopia based on the assumption that those activities stimulate the visual system. A number of uncontrolled case series have suggested a benefit to prescribing near activities, but the question has not been rigorously studied. In recent randomized clinical trials comparing patching regimes for amblyopia conducted by the PEDIG, near activities were incorporated into each of the prescribed treatment regimes. Most children completing these studies showed significant improvement of visual acuity, but it was unknown whether concurrent near activities enhanced the effect of patching.

Design

Randomized clinical trial.

Participants

425 children, 3 to <7 years old, with amblyopia (20/40-20/400) due to anisometropia, strabismus or both, and which persisted after treatment with spectacles.

Methods

Children were randomized to 2 hours of patching per day with near activities or 2 hours of patching per day with distance activities. Instruction sheets describing common near and distance activities were given to the parents. Study visits were scheduled at 2, 5, 8, and 17 weeks. In weeks without a visit, weekly telephone calls were made to the parent to monitor and encourage compliance, during the first 8 weeks.

Main Outcome Measure

Masked assessment of visual acuity by isolated crowded HOTV optotypes at 8 weeks.

Results

At 8 weeks, improvement in amblyopic eye visual acuity averaged 2.6 lines in the distance activities group and 2.5 lines in the near activities group (mean difference in acuity between groups, adjusted for baseline acuity, 0.0 lines; 95% confidence interval, -0.3 to 0.3). The two groups also appeared statistically similar at the 2-week, 5-week, and 17-week visits. At the 17-week examination, children with severe amblyopia improved a mean of 3.7 lines with 2 hours of daily patching.

Conclusion

Performing common near activities does not improve visual acuity outcome when treating anisometropic, strabismic or combined amblyopia with 2 hours of daily patching. Children with severe amblyopia may respond to 2 hours of daily patching.

AMBLYOPIA TREATMENT STUDY 7[11]

Purpose

To determine the amount and time course of binocular visual acuity improvement during treatment of bilateral refractive amblyopia in children age 3 to <10 years old.

Background

Bilateral refractive amblyopia can develop in children with large amounts of uncorrected hypermetropia and/or astigmatism in both eyes. Treatment consists of prescribing the appropriate refractive correction with the possible addition of occlusion or pharmacologic penalization if asymmetric visual acuity is present after correction is provided. The prevalence of bilateral amblyopia at the time of entry into school was estimated in one study to be 0.5%. The presumed mechanism of bilateral refractive amblyopia is pattern vision deprivation. Abnormal binocular interaction with suppression may also contribute in those cases with concomitant strabismus. There are few published studies of treatment for bilateral amblyopia. Most have been limited by small numbers of subjects and short follow-up times. To address these limitations, a prospective cohort study to determine the amount and time course of binocular visual acuity improvement during usual treatment of previously untreated bilateral refractive amblyopia.

Design

Prospective, multicenter, noncomparative intervention.

Methods

113 children (mean age = 5.1 years) with previously untreated bilateral refractive amblyopia were enrolled at 27 community- and university-based sites and were provided optimal spectacle correction. Bilateral refractive amblyopia was defined as 20/40–20/400 best-corrected binocular acuity in the presence of ≥4.00 D hypermetropia by spherical equivalent and/or ≥2.00 D astigmatism in each eye. Best-corrected binocular and monocular visual acuities were measured at baseline and at 5, 13, 26, and 52 weeks. The primary study outcome was binocular acuity at 1 year.

Results

Mean binocular visual acuity improved from 0.50 logMAR (20/63) at baseline to 0.11 logMAR (20/25) at 1 year [mean improvement 3.9 lines, 95% confidence interval (CI) = 3.5–4.2]. Mean improvement at 1 year for the 84 children with baseline binocular acuity of 20/40–20/80 was 3.4 lines (95% CI = 3.2–3.7) and for the 16 children with baseline binocular acuity of 20/100–20/320 was 6.3 lines (95% CI = 5.1–7.5). The cumulative probability of binocular acuity of 20/25 or better was 21% at 5 weeks, 46% at 13 weeks, 59% at 26 weeks, and 74% at 52 weeks.

Conclusion

Treatment of bilateral refractive amblyopia with spectacle correction improves binocular visual acuity in children age 3 to <10 years old, with most improving to 20/25 or better within 1 year.

AMBLYOPIA TREATMENT STUDY-8[12]

Objective

To compare weekend atropine augmented by a plano lens for the sound eye with weekend atropine alone for moderate amblyopia in children 3 to <7 years old.

Background

Pharmacological penalization of the sound eye with atropine had gained increased use as an alternative to patching. For patients whose sound eyes are optically corrected for distance, atropine results in blur of the sound eye at near only. In patients with hypermetropia, distance vision also will be blurred when the hypermetropic refractive error is left uncorrected or undercorrected.

Methods

In a multicenter clinical trial, 180 children with moderate amblyopia (20/40-20/100) were randomized to weekend atropine augmented by a plano lens or weekend atropine alone.

Main Outcome Measure

Masked assessment of amblyopic eye visual acuity using the ATS HOTV testing protocol at 18 weeks.

Results

At 18 weeks, amblyopic eye improvement averaged 2.8 lines in the atropine plus plano lens group and 2.4 lines in the atropine alone group (mean difference between groups adjusted for baseline acuity 0.3 lines; 95% confidence interval, -0.2 to 0.8). Amblyopic eye acuity was 20/25 or better in 24 (29%) patients in the atropine-only group and 35 (40%) patients in the atropine plus plano lens group ($p = 0.03$). More patients in the atropine plus plano lens group had reduced sound eye acuity at 18 weeks; however, there were no cases of persistent reverse amblyopia.

Conclusion

As an initial treatment for moderate amblyopia, the augmentation of weekend atropine with a plano lens does not substantially improve amblyopic eye acuity when compared with atropine alone.

■ AMBLYOPIA TREATMENT STUDY 9(1)[13]

Purpose

Patching with atropine eye drops in the treatment of moderate amblyopia (visual acuity, 6/12-6/30) in children aged 7-12 years.

Background

To explore the effectiveness of amblyopia treatment in children 7 years and older, the PEDIG previously conducted a randomized trial of 507 subjects aged 7-17 years with amblyopic eye visual acuity ranging from 20/40 to 20/400. The previous study was one of the first randomized clinical trials of treatment in older children with amblyopia. Therefore, that study was designed to combine patching and atropine for 7-12 years old, to maximize the chance of finding a treatment effect, if such an effect existed. Once treatment of older children had been found to have merit, most clinicians did not initiate amblyopia treatment by combining patching and atropine. The researchers, therefore, designed the present randomized clinical trial to compare these two therapies in 7-12 years old with amblyopia caused by anisometropia and/or strabismus.

Participants
193 children with amblyopia were assigned to receive weekend atropine or patching of the sound eye 2 hours per day.

Main Outcome Measure
Visual acuity in the amblyopic eye at 17 weeks.

Results
At 17 weeks, visual acuity had improved from baseline by an average of 7.6 letters in the atropine group and 8.6 letters in the patching group. Visual acuity of amblyopic eye was 6/7.5 or better in 17% of the atropine group and 24% of the patching group.

Conclusion
Treatment with atropine or patching led to similar degrees of improvement among 7-12 years old, with moderate amblyopia. About 1 in 5 achieves 20/25 or better visual acuity in the amblyopic eye.

■ AMBLYOPIA TREATMENT STUDY 9 (2)[14]

Purpose
To determine the effectiveness of weekend atropine for severe amblyopia from strabismus, anisometropia, or both combined among children 3-12 years of age.

Background
Atropine eye drops, when administered to the sound eye, have been found to improve the visual acuity of eyes with moderate amblyopia. PEDIG had recently completed two clinical trials in which we enrolled children aged 3-12 years with moderate amblyopia (visual acuity 20/40-20/100 in the amblyopic eye). In each of these studies, we also enrolled otherwise eligible subjects who had severe amblyopia (20/125-20/400) to explore the effectiveness of weekend atropine treatment for severe amblyopia. The purpose of this study was to provide those results for severe amblyopia.

Participants
The researchers enrolled children into two prospective, randomized multicenter clinical trials of amblyopia therapy. Herein we report the results

for severe amblyopia, 20/125-20/400. In trial 1, 60 children 3-6 years of age (mean, 4.4 years) were randomized to weekend atropine plus a plano lens or weekend atropine plus full spectacle correction for the sound eye. In trial 2, 40 children 7-12 years of age (mean, 9.3 years) were randomized to weekend atropine or 2 hours of daily patching. The visual acuity outcome was assessed at 18 weeks in trial 1 and 17 weeks in trial 2.

Main Outcome Measure
Visual acuity in the amblyopic eye at 17 weeks.

Results
In trial 1, visual acuity improved by an average of 4.5 lines in the atropine plus correction group (95% CI, 3.2-5.8 lines) and 5.1 lines in the atropine plus plano lens group (95% CI, 3.7-6.4 lines). In trial 2, visual acuity improved by an average of 1.5 lines in the atropine group (95% CI, 0.5-2.5 lines) and 1.8 lines in the patching group (95% CI, 1.1-2.6 lines).

Conclusion
Weekend atropine can improve visual acuity in children 3-12 years of age with severe amblyopia. Improvement may be greater in younger children.

■ AMBLYOPIA TREATMENT STUDY 10[15]

Purpose
To determine whether visual acuity improvement with Bangerter filters is similar to improvement with patching as initial therapy for children with moderate amblyopia.

Background
Although patching and atropine are well established as effective treatments for amblyopia. Bangerter filters or foils placed on the spectacle lens of the fellow eye have also been used. These transparent filters, available since the 1960s, were designed as a method to modulate the degree of deprivation from occlusion, by producing diffuse image defocus that degrades the fellow eye visual acuity to predicted levels. Bangerter filters have been used mostly as secondary treatment after either patching or atropine. The potential advantages of using Bangerter filters compared with patching include the ability to change the density of the filter to modulate the degree of deprivation, the possibility of better compliance because the filter is applied to the glasses and not the skin, the possibility of higher parental and child acceptance because the filter is not readily apparent to casual observers, and the possibility that the filter may be less disruptive to

binocular function. Potential disadvantages of the filters are that glasses must always be worn properly during treatment; peeking around the filters is relatively easy, and the filters may not uniformly degrade visual acuity to the predicted level reported by the manufacturer. The researchers designed a randomized trial to determine whether visual acuity improvement with Bangerter filters was similar to daily patching when initiating therapy for moderate amblyopia in children ages 3-10 years.

Design
Randomized, clinical trial.

Participants
The researchers enrolled 186 children, 3-10 years old, with moderate amblyopia (20/40-20/80).

Methods
Children were randomly assigned to receive either daily patching or to use a Bangerter filter on the spectacle lens in front of the fellow eye. Study visits were scheduled at 6, 12, 18, and 24 weeks.

Main Outcome Measures
Visual acuity in amblyopic eyes at 24 weeks.

Results
At 24 weeks, amblyopic eye improvement averaged 1.9 lines in the Bangerter group and 2.3 lines in the patching group (difference in mean visual acuities between groups adjusted for baseline acuity 0.38 line). The upper limit of one sided 95% confidence interval was 0.76 line, which slightly exceeded a respecified noninferiority limit of 0.75 line. Similar percentages of subjects in each group improved 3 lines (Bangerter group 38% vs. patching group 35%; $p = 0.61$) or had 20/25 amblyopic eye acuity (36% vs. 31%, respectively; $p = 0.86$). There was a lower treatment burden in the Bangerter group as measured with the Amblyopia Treatment Index. With Bangerter filters, neither a fixation switch to the amblyopic eye nor induced blurring in the fellow eye to worse than that of the amblyopic eye was required for visual acuity improvement.

Conclusion
Because the average difference in visual acuity improvement between Bangerter filters and patching was less than half a line, and there was lower burden of treatment on the child and family, Bangerter filter treatment is a reasonable option to consider for initial treatment of moderate amblyopia.

AMBLYOPIA TREATMENT STUDY 11[16]

Purpose
Randomized trial to evaluate combined patching and atropine for residual amblyopia in 3 to <10 years age group.

Background
Many children fail to achieve normal visual acuity after treatment for amblyopia. This remaining deficit may be called residual amblyopia. The researchers conducted a randomized trial to determine whether an intensive final push with combined patching and atropine can improve visual acuity in children with residual amblyopia.

Participant
55 children, 3 to <10 years old, with either strabismic or anisometropic amblyopia, BCVA of 20/32–20/63, interocular acuity difference greater than or equal to 2 lines, and no improvement in amblyopic eye acuity between two consecutive visits at least 6 weeks apart. Before enrollment, eligible subjects had no improvement with 6 hours daily patching or daily atropine. Intensive treatment group had 6 hours of prescribed daily patching combined with daily atropine; weaning group had 4 weeks of reduced treatment, then stopped. Amblyopic eye visual acuity improved similarly in both groups, an average of 0.56 lines in the intensive group. Condition of power analysis indicating that the study was unlikely to find a statistically significant benefit. Intensive final push of combined treatment with patching and daily atropine did not produce a better visual acuity outcome after 10 weeks.

The study was stopped on recommendation of the data and safety monitoring committee due to slow recruitment.

AMBLYOPIA TREATMENT STUDY 12[17]

Purpose
Pediatric Eye Disease Investigator Group conducted a pilot randomized clinical trial of office-based active vision therapy for the treatment of childhood amblyopia to determine the feasibility of conducting a full-scale randomized clinical trial.

Background
Vision therapy for amblyopia consists of a sequence of visual activities prescribed to facilitate the effects of refractive correction and occlusion by directly treating other aspects of visual function such as accommodation, eye movements, and suppression. There is a clinical impression that active

vision therapy can not only expedite visual acuity improvement, but may also reduce the likelihood of amblyopia recurrence/regression, especially for anisometropic amblyopia. Vision therapy for amblyopia is often administered in the office on a weekly basis by a therapist under the supervision of an eye care provider, and supplemented by similar therapy procedures prescribed to be completed at home to reinforce visual skills. The effectiveness of vision therapy for amblyopia treatment had not been evaluated in randomized clinical trials.

Methods

A training and certification program and manual of procedures were developed to certify therapists to administer a standardized vision therapy program in ophthalmology and optometry offices consisting of weekly visits for 16 weeks. Nineteen children, 7 to less than 13 years of age, with amblyopia (20/40-20/100) were randomly assigned to receive either 2 hours of daily patching with active vision therapy or 2 hours of daily patching with placebo vision therapy.

Results

Therapists in diverse practice settings were successfully trained and certified to perform standardized vision therapy in strict adherence with protocol. Subjects completed 85% of required weekly in-office vision therapy visits. Eligibility criteria based on age, visual acuity and stereoacuity used to identify children receiving standardized vision therapy resulted in insufficient recruitment as this criteria rendered high proportion of subjects screened as ineligible for receiving standardized vision therapy. There were difficulties in retrieving adherence data for the computerized home therapy procedures.

Conclusion

This study demonstrated that a 16-week treatment trial of vision therapy was feasible with respect to maintaining protocol adherence; however, recruitment under the proposed eligibility criteria, necessitated by the standardized approach to vision therapy, was not successful.

The study was terminated prematurely, due to difficulty in recruitment under the proposed eligibility criteria.

AMBLYOPIA TREATMENT STUDY 13[18]

Purpose

Visual acuity improvement in children with strabismic and combined strabismic-anisometropic amblyopia treated with optical correction, alone.

Background

Patching and atropine penalization have been considered the cornerstone of amblyopia treatment, with spectacle correction considered an adjunct rather than a primary treatment. Nevertheless, recent studies of children with anisometropic amblyopia have found spectacle correction alone often results in significant improvement in amblyopic eye visual acuity beyond that found from the immediate optical correction of refractive error. While similar observations have been reported for children with strabismic and combined-mechanism (strabismic-anisometropic) amblyopia, these studies had small numbers of subjects and did not report eye alignment before and after refractive correction. The present study was designed to quantify the visual acuity improvement in children 3 to <7 years of age with strabismic or combined-mechanism amblyopia treated with spectacle correction alone. In addition, we sought to explore the time course of improvement and factors associated with visual acuity improvement, particularly changes in ocular alignment.

Participants

146 children, 3 to <7 years old, with previously untreated strabismic amblyopia or combined mechanism amblyopia.

Methods

Optical treatment was provided as spectacles that were worn for the first at the baseline visit. Visual acuity measured at baseline and every 9 weeks thereafter until no further improvement in visual acuity. Ocular alignment was assessed at each visit.

Main Outcome Measure

Visual acuity, 18 weeks after baseline.

Results

Mean 2.6 lines improvement. 75% improved 2 or more lines and 54% improved 3 or more lines. Amblyopia resolution occurred in 32% of patients. Treatment effect was greater for strabismic amblyopia than for combined mechanism amblyopia.

Conclusion

Consideration should be given to prescribing refractive correction as the sole initial treatment for children with strabismic or combined mechanism amblyopia, before initiating other therapies.

AMBLYOPIA TREATMENT STUDY 14[18]

Purpose

Pilot study to evaluate levodopa as treatment for residual amblyopia in 8–17 years old. At the time of enrollment, subjects were required to have been treated with at least 2 hours per day of daily patching, with stable visual acuity.

Background

Prior studies have evaluated levodopa as an adjunct to occlusion therapy in the treatment of amblyopia. Improvement in visual acuity after completion of a course of levodopa has been reported; however, regression has occurred in several studies after stopping the medication. 4–6 reported side effects of levodopa included nausea, headache, fatigue, mood changes, emesis, dizziness, dry mouth, decreased appetite, and nightmares. In preparation for conducting a phase 3 randomized trial, PEDIG conducted a prospective randomized pilot study to provide a preliminary assessment of the efficacy and safety of two doses of levodopa combined with daily ocular occlusion therapy of the fellow eye in older.

Methods

The study intervention consisted of continuing 2 hours of daily patching plus the addition of levodopa in one of two doses randomly assigned with equal probability (0.51 or 0.76 mg/kg/tid, referred to as lower dose and higher dose, respectively). The lower dose has been used in most prior studies. The study medication was administered for 8 weeks with one additional week for tapering of treatment. Levodopa was prepared in capsules combined with carbidopa 0.17 mg/kg/tid. Carbidopa was combined with levodopa to reduce side-effects associated with levodopa alone. Follow-up visits occurred at 4 ± 1 weeks from randomization, 9 ± 1 weeks from starting levodopa treatment as the primary outcome, and 10 ± 2 weeks after stopping levodopa treatment. The assigned levodopa/carbidopa dose was continued until 1 week prior to the 9-week visit, when it was tapered over 1 week. Following the 9-week visit, patching alone was continued for 10 ± 2 weeks. At each visit, visual acuity was measured using the E-ETDRS method.

Information about adverse effects of treatment was solicited during phone calls conducted after 1, 2, and 6 weeks and at each visit during treatment. An adverse event was defined as any untoward medical occurrence in a study subject, and reported even if considered unrelated to the study treatment. Subjects and study personnel were masked to treatment assignment.

Results

The mean improvement in amblyopic eye in 9 weeks primary outcome visit was +4 (± 4) letters in the 16 subjects in the lower dose group and + 6 (± 6) letters in the 17 subjects in the higher dose group. An improvement of 10 or more letters noted in 2 (13%) in low dose, and 5 (29%) in high dose group at 9 weeks. Fellow eye improved 1 letter in high dose and 0 letter in low dose group.

Conclusion

The results suggested that levodopa/carbidopa therapy for residual amblyopia in older children and teenagers is well-tolerated and may improve visual acuity. There was a suggestion of partial regression of the improvement in visual acuity after treatment was discontinued. No serious adverse effects were noted. Headache and nausea were infrequent. Without a patching-only control group, no conclusions about the efficacy, safety, or frequency of side effects associated with this treatment can be made. A placebo controlled trial is necessary to determine whether levodopa can successfully augment occlusion therapy in the treatment of amblyopia.

AMBLYOPIA TREATMENT STUDY 15[19]

Purpose

After treatment with refractive correction and patching, some patients have residual amblyopia resulting from strabismus or anisometropia. We conducted a clinical trial to evaluate the effectiveness of increasing prescribed daily patching from 2 to 6 hours in children with stable residual amblyopia.

Background

Partly on the basis of previous randomized amblyopia treatment trials performed by the PEDIG, many practitioners prescribe an initial dose of 2 hours daily patching of the fellow eye if strabismic or anisometropic amblyopia does not resolve with spectacles alone. Although many children are successfully treated with this regimen, some fail to attain normal visual acuity in the amblyopic eye. When improvement with initial patching therapy stops and amblyopia is still present, treatment options include maintaining the same treatment and dose, increasing the intensity of the same treatment, switching to another treatment, or combining different treatment modalities. Many clinicians will choose to increase the patching dosage, but it is unknown whether this approach is effective. Our aim was to determine whether increasing prescribed patching dosage improves amblyopic eye visual acuity in children aged 3 to <8 years with apparently stable residual amblyopia after prescribed initial treatment with 2 hours of daily patching.

Design

Prospective, randomized, multicenter clinical trial.

Participants

A total of 169 children aged 3 to <8 years (mean, 5.9 years) with stable residual amblyopia (20/32–20/160) after 2 hours of daily patching for at least 12 weeks.

Intervention

Random assignment to continue 2 hours of daily patching or increase patching time to an average of 6 hours/day.

Main Outcome Measures

Best-corrected visual acuity in the amblyopic eye after 10 weeks.

Results

Baseline visual acuity was 0.44 logMAR (20/50). 10 weeks after randomization, amblyopic eye visual acuity had improved an average of 1.2 lines in the 6-hour group and 0.5 line in the 2-hour group (difference in mean visual acuity adjusted for acuity at randomization = 0.6 line; 95% confidence interval, 0.3–1.0; p = 0.002). Improvement of 2 or more lines occurred in 40% of participants patched for 6 hours versus 18% of those who continued to patch for 2 hours (p = 0.003).

Conclusion

When amblyopic eye visual acuity stops improving with 2 hours of daily patching, increasing the daily patching dosage to 6 hours results in more improvement in visual acuity after 10 weeks compared with continuing 2 hours daily.

■ AMBLYOPIA TREATMENT STUDY 16[20]

Purpose

Augmenting atropine treatment for amblyopia in 3 to <8 years old, 20/50–20/400, with plano lens to the sound eye.

Background

When improvement with initial atropine treatment ceases and amblyopia is still present, treatment options include continuing the same treatment, switching to another treatment, such as patching, and combining different treatment modalities. Most children with amblyopia have a hyperopic refractive error, and for these children another approach for subsequent therapy is to augment atropine with optical blur of the fellow eye by reducing the hyperopic correction or replacing it with a plano lens. The researchers conducted a randomized trial to determine whether addition of a plano lens to atropine treatment for the fellow eye improves amblyopic-eye visual acuity in 3-8-years old children with clinically stable residual amblyopia following prescribed initial treatment with at least 12 weeks of daily or weekend atropine. Some children have residual amblyopia after treatment with atropine eye drops for amblyopia due to strabismus and/or anisometropia. A randomized clinical trial was conducted to evaluate the effectiveness of augmenting the effect of atropine by changing the lens over the fellow eye to Plano in children with residual amblyopia.

Methods
A total of 73 children 3 to <8 years of age (mean, 5.8 years) with stable residual amblyopia (range, 20/32–20/160, mean 20/63 + 1) were enrolled after at least 12 weeks of atropine treatment of the fellow eye. Participants were randomly assigned to continuing weekend atropine alone or wearing a plano lens over the fellow eye (while continuing atropine). The primary outcome was assessed at 10 weeks, and participants were followed until improvement ceased.

Results
At the 10-week primary outcome visit, amblyopic-eye visual acuity had improved an average of 1.1 lines with the plano lens and 0.6 lines with atropine only (difference adjusted for baseline visual acuity = + 0.5 line; 95% CI, −0.1 to +1.2). At the primary outcome or later visit when the best-measured visual acuity was observed, the mean amblyopic-eye improvement from baseline was 1.9 lines with the plano lens and 0.8 lines with atropine only.

Conclusion
When amblyopic-eye visual acuity stops improving with atropine treatment, there may be a small benefit to augmenting atropine therapy with a plano lens over the fellow eye. However, the effect was not statistically significant, and the large confidence interval raises the possibility of no benefit or a benefit larger than we observed. A larger study would be necessary to get a more precise estimate of the treatment effect.

AMBLYOPIA TREATMENT STUDY 17[21]

Purpose
To assess the efficacy and short-term safety of levodopa as adjunctive treatment to patching for amblyopia.

Background
Prior studies had evaluated levodopa as an adjunct to occlusion therapy in the treatment of amblyopia. Improvement in visual acuity after completion of a course of levodopa has been reported; however, regression has occurred

in several studies after stopping the medication. Reported side-effects of levodopa were mild. They have included nausea, headache, fatigue, mood changes, emesis, dizziness, dry mouth, decreased appetite, and nightmares. In preparation for conducting a phase 3 randomized trial, the researchers conducted a prospective randomized pilot study to provide a preliminary assessment of the efficacy and safety of two doses of levodopa combined with daily ocular occlusion therapy of the fellow eye in older children and teenagers with residual amblyopia from strabismus, anisometropia, or both combined.

Design
Randomized, placebo-controlled trial.

Participants
One hundred thirty-nine children 7–12 years of age with residual amblyopia resulting from strabismus, anisometropia or both combined (20/50–20/400) following patching.

Methods
Participants were randomly assigned (using a permutated block design stratified by site and by baseline visual acuity) in a 2:1 ratio to three times per day use of oral levodopa 0.76 mg/kg with carbidopa 0.17 mg/kg (subsequently referred to as "Levodopa") or oral placebo. Carbidopa is added to levodopa to reduce peripheral side-effects. All participants had 2 hours of daily patching (of fellow eye) prescribed and took oral medication for 16 weeks, with a 4-day taper of the oral medication prior to the primary outcome examination 2 weeks later (at 18 weeks). A central pharmacy compounded the study medication based upon body weight. Levodopa and placebo were placed in identical gelatin capsules.

Main Outcome Measures
Mean change in best-corrected amblyopic-eye visual acuity at 18 weeks.

Results
At 18 weeks, amblyopic-eye visual acuity improved from randomization by an average of 5.2 letters in the levodopa group and 3.8 letters in the placebo group (difference adjusted for baseline visual acuity = +1.4 letters, 1-sided $p = 0.06$; 2-sided 95% confidence interval = −0.4 to +3.3 letters). No serious adverse effects from levodopa were reported during treatment.

Conclusion
For children 7–12 years of age with residual amblyopia following patching therapy, oral levodopa while continuing to patch 2 hours per day does not

produce a clinically or statistically meaningful improvement in visual acuity compared with placebo and patching.

■ AMBLYOPIA TREATMENT STUDY 18[22]

Purpose

To compare visual acuity improvement in teenagers with amblyopia treated with a binocular iPad® game versus part-time patching.

Background

Amblyopia treatment has been historically considered less effective in older children and adults, 1–5 but there is now emerging evidence that a binocular approach to the treatment of amblyopia can improve amblyopic eye visual acuity for adults with strabismic, anisometropic, and mixed mechanism amblyopia, and possibly at a greater rate than patching treatment. To achieve a binocular percept, dichoptic displays have been used to present high-contrast images to the amblyopic eye and low-contrast images to the fellow eye in order to overcome binocular suppression commonly found in amblyopia. This type of binocular treatment has recently been adapted to an iPad (Apple Inc.) device such that the treatment can be prescribed for home use. The purpose of this randomized clinical trial was to compare the improvement in amblyopic eye visual acuity after 16 weeks of home-based treatment with binocular game play on an iPad device prescribed for 1 hour a day versus patching prescribed for 2 hours a day, in teenagers aged 13 to <17 years with amblyopic eye visual acuities of 20/40–20/200.

Methods

One hundred participants aged 13 to <17 years (mean 14.3 years) with amblyopia (20/40–20/200, mean ~20/63) resulting from strabismus, anisometropia, or both were enrolled into a randomized clinical trial. Participants were randomly assigned to treatment for 16 weeks of either a binocular iPad game prescribed for 1 hour per day ($n = 40$) or patching of the fellow eye prescribed for 2 hours per day ($n = 60$). The main outcome measure was change in amblyopic eye visual acuity from baseline to 16 weeks.

Results

Mean amblyopic eye visual acuity improved from baseline by 3.5 letters (2-sided 95% confidence interval (CI): 1.3–5.7 letters) in the binocular group and by 6.5 letters (2-sided 95% CI: 4.4–8.5 letters) in the patching group. After adjusting for baseline visual acuity, the difference between the binocular and patching groups was −2.7 letters (95% CI: −5.7 to 0.3 letters, $p = 0.082$) or 0.5 lines, favoring patching. In the binocular group, treatment adherence data from the iPad device indicated only 13% of participants completed >75% of prescribed treatment.

Conclusion

In teenagers aged 13 to <17 years, improvement in amblyopic eye visual acuity with the binocular iPad game used in this study was not found to be better than patching, and was possibly worse. Nevertheless, it remains unclear whether the minimal treatment response to binocular treatment was due to poor treatment adherence or lack of treatment effect.

■ AMBLYOPIA TREATMENT STUDY 18[23]

Purpose

To compare visual acuity improvement in children with amblyopia treated with a binocular iPad® game versus part-time patching.

Background

A binocular approach to treating anisometropic and strabismic amblyopia has recently been advocated, without patching, atropine drops, or Bangerter filters applied to the fellow eye. In such binocular therapy, images are presented dichoptically, with high-contrast images presented to the amblyopic eye and low-contrast images to the fellow eye, to achieve a binocular percept. Recently, this binocular treatment has been adapted to an iPad® device as a "falling blocks" game, which uses red-green anaglyphic glasses. Initial studies have yielded promising results, suggesting that a larger randomized clinical trial is warranted. The purpose of the present randomized clinical trial was to establish whether treatment of amblyopia with a binocular iPad game (prescribed 1 hour per day for 16 weeks) was not substantially worse (noninferior) than treatment with patching of the fellow eye (prescribed 2 hours per day) in children age 5 to <13 years, with 20/40–20/200 amblyopic-eye visual acuity.

Design

Randomized, noninferiority clinical trial.

Setting

Multicenter, community and institutional practices.

Participants

385 participants 5 to <13 years of age (mean 8.5 years) with amblyopia (20/40–20/200, mean 20/63) resulting from strabismus, anisometropia, or both.

Interventions

Participants were randomly assigned to either 16 weeks of a binocular iPad game, prescribed for 1 hour a day ($n = 190$, binocular group) or patching of the fellow eye prescribed for 2 hours a day ($n = 195$, patching group). Study follow-up visits were scheduled at 4, 8, 12, and 16 weeks.

Main Outcome Measure

Change in amblyopic-eye visual acuity from baseline to 16 weeks.

Results

At 16 weeks, mean amblyopic-eye visual acuity improved 1.05 lines (2-sided 95% confidence interval (CI): 0.85–1.24 lines) in the binocular group and 1.35 lines (2-sided 95% CI: 1.17–1.54 lines) in the patching group, with an adjusted treatment group difference of 0.31 lines favoring patching (upper limit of the 1-sided 95% CI 0.53 lines). This upper limit exceeded the prespecified noninferiority limit of 0.5 lines. Only 22% of participants randomized to the binocular game performed >75% of the prescribed treatment (median 46%, interquartile range 20–72%). In younger participants age 5 to <7 years old, without prior amblyopia treatment, amblyopic-eye visual acuity improved 2.5 ± 1.5 lines in the binocular group and 2.8 ± 0.8 in the patching group. Adverse effects (including diplopia) were uncommon and of similar frequency between groups.

Conclusion and Relevance

In children 5 to <13 years of age, amblyopic-eye visual acuity improved with binocular game play and with patching, particularly in younger children age 5 to <7 years without prior amblyopia treatment. Although the primary noninferiority analysis was indeterminate, a posthoc analysis suggested visual acuity improvement with this particular binocular iPad treatment was not as good as with 2 hours of prescribed daily patching.

■ AMBLYOPIA TREATMENT STUDY 19[24]

Purpose

To compare visual acuity improvement in teenagers with amblyopia treated with a binocular iPad game versus part-time patching.

Background

Amblyopia treatment has been historically considered less effective in older children and adults, but there is now emerging evidence that a binocular approach to the treatment of amblyopia can improve amblyopic eye visual acuity for adults with strabismic, anisometropic, and mixed mechanism amblyopia, and possibly at a greater rate than patching treatment. To achieve a binocular percept, dichoptic displays have been used to present high contrast images to the amblyopic eye and low-contrast images to the fellow eye in order to overcome binocular suppression commonly found in amblyopia. This type of binocular treatment has recently been adapted to an iPad (Apple Inc.) device such that the treatment can be prescribed for home use.

The purpose of this randomized clinical trial was to compare the improvement in amblyopic eye visual acuity after 16 weeks of home-based treatment with binocular game play on an iPad device prescribed for 1 hour a day versus patching prescribed for 2 hours a day, in teenagers aged 13 to <17 years with amblyopic eye visual acuities of 20/40–20/200.

Methods

One hundred participants aged 13 to <17 years (mean 14.3 years) with amblyopia (20/40–20/200, mean ~20/63) resulting from strabismus, anisometropia, or both were enrolled into a randomized clinical trial. Participants were randomly assigned to treatment for 16 weeks of either a binocular iPad game prescribed for 1 hour per day ($n = 40$) or patching of the fellow eye prescribed for 2 hours per day ($n = 60$). The main outcome measure was change in amblyopic eye visual acuity from baseline to 16 weeks.

Results

Mean amblyopic eye visual acuity improved from baseline by 3.5 letters (2-sided 95% confidence interval (CI): 1.3 to 5.7 letters) in the binocular group and by 6.5 letters (2-sided 95% CI: 4.4 to 8.5 letters) in the patching group. After adjusting for baseline visual acuity, the difference between the binocular and patching groups was –2.7 letters (95% CI: –5.7 to 0.3 letters, $p = 0.082$) or 0.5 lines, favoring patching. In the binocular group, treatment adherence data from the iPad device indicated only 13% of participants completed >75% of prescribed treatment.

Conclusion

In teenagers aged 13 to <17 years, improvement in amblyopic eye visual acuity with the binocular iPad game used in this study was not found to be better than patching, and was possibly worse. Nevertheless, it remains unclear whether the minimal treatment response to binocular treatment was due to poor treatment adherence or lack of treatment effect.

■ AMBLYOPIA TREATMENT STUDY 20[25]

Purpose

To compare visual acuity improvement in children aged 7–12 years with amblyopia treated with a binocular iPad game plus continued spectacle correction versus continued spectacle correction alone.

Background
Small case series and single-center randomized trials have been supportive of dichoptic binocular treatment for amblyopia (henceforth referred to as "binocular treatment") as an intervention for anisometropic, strabismic, or combined-mechanism amblyopia that does not rely on patching or penalization. Results from 2 recent large multicenter randomized clinical trials using a falling-blocks binocular game played on handheld devices found less improvement in amblyopic-eye visual acuity with binocular treatment than with part-time patching or no greater improvement than a nonbinocular control game treatment. In both of these previous randomized clinical trials, poor adherence was blamed for failure to find a greater effect. A new binocular game ("Dig Rush") has become available that may be more engaging than the falling-blocks game and for which a pilot study found better adherence and evidence of effectiveness among amblyopic children aged 4-9 years. The researchers conducted a multicenter randomized clinical trial to compare amblyopic-eye visual acuity improvement between treatment with the Dig Rush binocular game plus spectacle wear (if needed) and treatment with continued spectacle wear alone (if needed), in children aged 7-12 years.

Design
Multicenter randomized clinical trial.

Participants
One hundred thirty-eight participants aged 7-12 years with amblyopia (33-72 letters, i.e., approximately 20/200-20/40) resulting from strabismus, anisometropia, or both. Participants were required to have at least 16 weeks of optical treatment in spectacles if needed or demonstrate no improvement in amblyopic eye visual acuity for at least 8 weeks prior to enrollment.

Methods
Eligible participants (mean age 9.6 years, mean baseline visual acuity of 59.6 letters, history of prior amblyopia treatment other than spectacles in 96%) were randomly assigned to treatment for 8 weeks with the dichoptic binocular Dig Rush iPad game (prescribed for 1 hour per day 5 days per week) plus spectacle wear if needed ($n = 69$) or continued spectacle correction alone if needed ($n = 69$).

Main Outcome Measures
Change in amblyopic-eye visual acuity from baseline to 4 weeks, assessed by a masked examiner.

Results

At 4 weeks, mean amblyopic-eye visual acuity letter score improved from baseline by 1.3 [2-sided 95% confidence interval (CI): 0.1e2.6; 0.026 logMAR] with binocular treatment and by 1.7 (2-sided 95% CI: 0.4e3.0; 0.034 logMAR) with continued spectacle correction alone. After adjustment for baseline visual acuity, the letter score difference between groups (binocular minus control) was -0.3 (95% CI: -2.2 to 1.5, $p = 0.71$, difference of -0.006 logMAR). No difference in letter scores was observed between groups when the analysis was repeated after 8 weeks of treatment (adjusted mean: -0.1, 98.3% CI: -2.4 to 2.1). For the binocular group, adherence data from the iPad indicated that slightly more than half of the participants (58% and 56%) completed >75% of prescribed treatment by the 4- and 8-week visits, respectively.

Conclusion

In children aged 7–12 years who have received previous treatment for amblyopia other than spectacles, there was no benefit to visual acuity or stereoacuity from 4 or 8 weeks of treatment with the dichoptic binocular Dig Rush iPad game.

Table 1: Summary of amblyopia treatment studies [Pediatric Eye Disease Investigators' Group (PEDIG studies)]: Common outcome measure—vision in the amblyopic eye.

Title/Year	Purpose	Inclusion criteria	No. of patients	Follow-up	Results	Conclusion
ATS-1 1999–2001	Patching versus atropine	• 3 to <7 years • Moderate amblyopia (20/40–20/100)	419	6 months (2 years)	Both groups had similar improvement	Atropine had slightly better acceptability on a parental questionnaire
ATS-2A 2001–03	Full-time patching versus 6 hours of patching	• 3 to <7 years • Severe amblyopia (20/100–20/400)	175	4 months	Both groups had similar improvement	Fewer hours of daily patching may improve compliance
ATS-2B 2001–02	2 hours versus 6 hours of daily patching	• 3 to <7 years • Moderate amblyopia (20/40–20/80)	189	4 months	Both groups had similar improvement	Fewer hours of daily patching may improve compliance
ATS-2C 2001–02	Recurrence after successful amblyopia treatment	• <8 years • Amblyopia treatment for last 3 months	156	52 weeks	Recurrence (2 or more logMAR level reduction of visual acuity) in one-fourth, maximum in first 3 months after stopping treatment	Weaning (to 2 hours/day) rather than stopping patching abruptly, may reduce risk of recurrence
ATS-3 2002–04	Optical correction + patching versus optical correction alone	• 7–17 years • Amblyopia (20/40–20/400)	507	24 weeks	Amblyopia improves with optical correction alone in one-fourth patients	Amblyopia treatment improves visual acuity in patients 7–12 years, even if amblyopia has been previously treated. In 13–17 year olds, it is of benefit only if previously untreated

Contd...

Contd...

Title/Year	Purpose	Inclusion criteria	No. of patients	Follow-up	Results	Conclusion
ATS-4 2002–03	Daily versus weekend atropine	• 3 to <7 years • Moderate amblyopia (20/40–20/80)	168	4 months	Both groups had similar improvement	Weekend atropine similar to daily atropine
ATS 5(1) 2006	Refractive error alone for anisometropic amblyopia	• 3 to <7 years • Amblyopia ranging from 6/12 to 6/75	84	5 weekly	Amblyopia improved with optical correction in 77% of the patients and resolved in 27%	With glasses alone, resolution of amblyopia can occur in at least one-third of patients
ATS 5 (2) 2006	2 hours of daily patching (with near activities) with a control group of spectacle wear alone (if needed) for treatment of amblyopia	• 3 to 7 years old • 20/40–20/400	180	5 weeks	Amblyopic eye vision improved by around 1.1 lines in the patching group and 0.5 lines in the control group ($p = 0.006$)	2 hours of daily patching combined with 1 hour of near visual activities modestly improves moderate to severe amblyopia
ATS 6 2007–8	Additional benefit of near activities, along-with patching therapy	• 3 to <7 years old • Amblyopia (20/40–20/400)	425	8 weeks	• At 8 weeks, improvement in amblyopic eye visual acuity averaged 2.6 lines in the distance • Activities group and 2.5 lines in the near activities group	Performing common near activities does not improve visual acuity outcome when treating anisometropic, strabismic or combined amblyopia with 2 hours of daily patching

Contd...

Clinical Trials in Amblyopia

Contd...

Title/Year	Purpose	Inclusion criteria	No. of patients	Follow-up	Results	Conclusion
ATS 7 2007	Amount and time course of binocular visual acuity improvement during treatment of bilateral refractive amblyopia in 3 to <10 years of age	• 33 to <10 years of age • 220/40–20/400	113	1 year	• Mean binocular visual acuity improved from 0.50 logMAR (20/63) at baseline to 0.11 LogMAR (20/25) at 1 year	Treatment of bilateral refractive amblyopia with spectacle correction improves binocular visual acuity in children age 3 to <10 years old
ATS 8 2008–9	To compare weekend atropine augmented by a plano lens for the sound eye with weekend atropine alone for moderate amblyopia in children 3 to <7 years old	• 3 to <7 years old • 20/40–20/100	180	18 weeks	• Amblyopic eye acuity was 20/25 or better in 24 (29%) patients in the atropine-only group and 35 (40%) patients in the atropine plus Plano lens group ($p = 0.03$)	As an initial treatment for moderate amblyopia, the augmentation of weekend atropine with a plano lens does not substantially improve amblyopic eye acuity when compared with atropine alone
ATS 9(1) 2008	Patching with atropine eye drops in the treatment of moderate amblyopia (visual acuity, 6/12–6/30) in children aged 7–12 years	• 7–12 years • 6/12–6/30	193	17 weeks	Visual acuity of amblyopic eye was 6/7.5 or better in 17% of the atropine group and 24% of the patching group	Treatment with atropine or patching led to similar degrees of improvement among 7–12 year old, with moderate amblyopia

Contd...

Contd...

Title/Year	Purpose	Inclusion criteria	No. of patients	Follow-up	Results	Conclusion
ATS 9(2) 2008–9	Patching with atropine eye drops in the treatment of severe amblyopia (visual acuity, 20/125–20/400) in children aged 3–12 years	• 3–6 years (trial 1) • 7–12 years (trial 2)	100	17 weeks	*Trial 1*: 4.5 lines improvement in Atropine + glass, versus. 5.1 lines in Atropine + Plano lens group. *Trial 2*: 1.5 lines improvement in Atropine group versus 1.8 lines in patching group	Weekend atropine can improve vision in severe amblyopes (3–12 years). Improvement is greater for younger children
ATS 10 2010	Bangerter foil as a treatment alternative for moderate amblyopia	• 3–10 years • 20/40–20/80	186	24 weeks	Similar improvement in 2 groups (Bangerter group 38% vs. patching group 35%; $p = 0.61$) or had $>= 20/25$ amblyopic eye acuity (36% vs. 31%, respectively; $p = 0.86$)	Bangerter filter treatment is a reasonable option to consider for initial treatment of moderate amblyopia
ATS 11 2011	Randomized trial to evaluate combined patching and atropine for residual amblyopia in 3 to <10 year age group	• 3–10 year • 20/32–20/63	55	10 weeks	Intensive final push of combined treatment with patching and daily atropine did not produce a better visual acuity outcome	The study was stopped on recommendation of the data and safety monitoring committee due to slow recruitment

Contd...

Contd...

Title/Year	Purpose	Inclusion criteria	No. of patients	Follow-up	Results	Conclusion
ATS 12 2013	A randomized trial comparing patching with active vision therapy to patching with control vision therapy as treatment for amblyopia in children 7 to <13 year old	• 7–13 years old • 6/12–6/60	19	16 weeks	Inconclusive	The terminated prematurely, due to difficulty in recruitment under the proposed eligibility criteria
ATS13 2012	Visual acuity improvement in children with strabismic and combined strabismic-anisometropic amblyopia treated with optical correction, alone	3 to <7 years old	146	18 weeks	Amblyopia resolution occurred in 32% of patients. Treatment effect was greater for strabismic amblyopia than for combined mechanism amblyopia	Consideration should be given to prescribing refractive correction as the sole initial treatment for children with strabismic or combined amblyopia
ATS14 2010	To assess the efficacy and short-term safety of levodopa as adjunctive treatment to patching for amblyopia	• 7–12 years • 20/50–20/400	139	18 weeks	Amblyopic-eye visual acuity improved from randomization by an average of 5.2 letters in the levodopa group and 3.8 letters in the placebo group	Oral levodopa while continuing to patch 2 hours per day does not produce a clinically or statistically meaningful improvement in visual acuity compared with placebo and patching

Contd...

Contd...

Title/Year	Purpose	Inclusion criteria	No. of patients	Follow-up	Results	Conclusion
ATS15 2013	Clinical trial to evaluate the effectiveness of increasing prescribed daily patching from 2–6 hours in children with stable residual amblyopia	• 3 to <8 years • 20/32–20/160	169	10 weeks	Improvement of 2 or more lines occurred in 40% of participants patched for 6 hours versus 18% of those who continued to patch for 2 hours (p = 0.003)	When amblyopic eye visual acuity stops improving with 2 hours of patching, increasing the number of hours helps
ATS 16 2015	Effect of Atropine augmentation with plano lens to sound eye, in cases of residual amblyopia	• 3–8 years • Residual amblyopia (20/32–20/160)	73	10 weeks	1.1 line improvement with plano lens; 0.6 line improvement with atropine alone (not statistically significant)	Small benefit of adding plano lens to sound eye, if amblyopia does not improve by atropine alone
ATS 17 2015	Efficacy and short term safety of levodopa as adjunct to patching for amblyopia	• 7–12 years • 20/50–20/400 amblyopia	139	18 weeks	Average of 5.2 letters in levodopa group, versus 3.8 letters in placebo group. No gross side-effects of levo-dopa	May consider levodopa as adjunct to patching in cases of residual amblyopia (7–12 years)
ATS 18 2016	Effectiveness of binocular iPad game versus part time patching, for amblyopia	• 5–13 years • 20/40–20/200 amblyopia	385	16 weeks	Mean versus improvement of 1.05 lines in binocular group, compared to 1.35 lines	Although some benefit was observed with binocular group, it was not superior to patching

Contd...

Contd...

Title/Year	Purpose	Inclusion criteria	No. of patients	Follow-up	Results	Conclusion
ATS 19 2018	Effectiveness of binocular iPad game versus part time patching, for amblyopia in teenagers	• 13–17 years • 20/40–20/200 amblyopia	100	16 weeks	Mean improvement of 3.5 letters in binocular group versus 6.5 letters in patching group	Binocular iPad gaming was found inferior to patching, as a treatment for amblyopia in 13–17 years age group
ATS 20 2019	Binocular iPad treatment with glasses, versus glasses alone, in treatment of amblyopia	• 7–12 years of age • 20/40–20/200 amblyopia	138	4 weeks	Mean letter score improvement by 1.3 with binocular treatment (a new game-Dig rush iPad game was used), compared to 1.7 letters, with glasses alone	No additional benefit was demonstrated by dichoptic binocular game, in cases of residual amblyopia (7–12 years)

REFERENCES

1. Pediatric Eye Disease Investigator Group. A randomized trial of atropine vs. patching for treatment of moderate amblyopia in children. Arch Ophthalmol. 2002;120(3):268-78.
2. Repka MX, Wallace DK, Beck RW, Kraker RT, Birch EE, Cotter SA, et al. Two-year follow-up of a 6-month randomized trial of atropine vs patching for treatment of moder-ate amblyopia in children. Arch Opthalmol. 2005;123(2):149-57.
3. Holmes JM, Kraker RT, Beck RW, Birch EE, Cotter SA, Everett DF, et al. A randomized trial of prescribed patching regimens for treatment of severe amblyopia in children. Oph-thalmology. 2003;110(11):2075-87.
4. Repka MX, Beck RW, Holmes JM, Birch EE, Chandler DL, Cotter SA, et al. A Randomized Trial of Patching Regimens for Treatment of Moderate Amblyopia in Children. Arch Ophthalmol. 2003;121(5):603-11.
5. Holmes JM, Beck RW, Kraker RT, Astle WF, Birch EE, Cole SR, et al. Risk of amblyopia recurrence after cessation of treatment. J AAPOS. 2004;8(5):420-8.
6. Scheiman MM, Hertle RW, Beck RW, Edwards AR, Birch E, Cotter SA, et al. Randomized trial of treatment of amblyopia in children aged 7 to 17 years. Arch Ophthalmol. 2005;123(4):437-47.
7. Repka MX, Cotter SA, Beck RW, Kraker RT, Birch EE, Everett DF, et al. A randomised trial of atropine regimens for treatment of moderate amblyopia in children. Ophthalmology. 2004;111(11):2076-85.
8. Cotter SA; Pediatric Eye Disease Investigator Group, Edwards AR, Wallace DK, Beck RW, Arnold RW, Astle WF, et al. Treatment of anisometropic Amblyopia in children with refractive correction. Ophthalmology. 2006;113(6):895-903.
9. Wallace DK, Edwards AR, Cotter SA, Beck RW, Arnold RW, Astle WF, et al. A Randomized trial to evaluate two hours of daily patching for strabismic and anisometropic amblyopia in children. Ophthalmology. 2006;113(6):904-12.
10. Pediatric Eye Disease Investigator Group. A Randomized Trial of Near versus Distance Activities while Patching for Amblyopia in Children 3 to <7 years old. Ophthalmology. 2008;115(11):2071-8.
11. Wallace DK, Chandler DL, Beck RW, Arnold RW, Bacal DA, Birch EE, et al. Treatment of bilateral refractive amblyopia in children 3 to <10 years old. Am J Ophthalmol. 2007;144(4):487-96.
12. Pediatric Eye Disease Investigator Group. Pharmacologic plus optical penalization treatment for amblyopia: results of a randomized trial. Arch Ophthalmol. 2009;127(1):22-30.
13. Scheiman MM, Hertle RW, Kraker RT, Beck RW, Birch EE, Felius J, et al. Patching vs. atropine to treat amblyopia in children aged 7 to 12 years: a randomized trial. Arch Oph-thalmol. 2008;126(12):1634-42.
14. Repka MX, Kraker RT, Beck RW, Birch E, Cotter SA, Holmes JM, et al. Treatment of severe amblyopia with weekend atropine: results from 2 randomized clinical trials. J AAPOS. 2009;13(3):258-63.
15. Rutstein RP, Quinn GE, Lazar EL, Beck RW, Bonsall DJ, Cotter SA, et al. A randomized trial comparing Bangerter filters and patching for the treatment of moderate amblyopia in children. Ophthalmology. 2010;117(5):998-1004.
16. Wallace DK, Kraker RT, Beck RW, Cotter SA, Davis PL, Holmes JM, et al. A randomized trial to evaluate combined patching and atropine for residual amblyopia. Arch Ophthalmol. 2011;129(7):960-2.
17. Lyon DW, Hopkins K, Chu RH, Tamkins SM, Cotter SA, Melia BM, et al. Feasibility of a clinical trial of vision therapy for treatment of amblyopia. Optom Vis Sci. 2013;90(5):475-81.

18. Cotter SA, Foster NC, Holmes JM, Melia BM, Wallace DK, Repka MX, et al. Optical treatment of strabismic and combined strabismic-anisometropic amblyopia. Ophthalmology. 2012;119(1):150-8.
19. Repka MX, Kraker RT, Beck RW, Atkinson CS, Bacal DA, Bremer DL, et al. Pilot study of levodopa dosage as treatment for residual amblyopia in children 8 to younger than 18 years old. Arch Ophthalmol. 2010;128(9):1215-7.
20. Wallace DK, Lazar EL, Holmes JM, Repka MX, Cotter SA, Chen AM, et al. A randomized trial of increasing patching for amblyopia. Ophthalmology. 2013;120(11):2270-7.
21. Wallace DK, Lazar EL, Repka MX, Holmes JM, Kraker RT, Hoover DL, et al. A randomized trial of adding a plano lens to atropine for amblyopia. J AAPOS. 2015;19(1):42-8.
22. Repka MX, Kraker RT, Dean TW, Beck RW, Siatkowski RM, Holmes JM, et al. A randomized control trial of levodopa as treatment for residual amblyopia in older children. Ophthalmology. 2015;122(5):874-81.
23. Holmes JM, Manh VM, Lazar EL, Beck RW, Birch EE, Kraker RT, et al. A randomized trial of a binocular iPad game versus part-time patching in children 5 to 12 years of age with amblyopia. JAMA Ophthalmol. 2016;134(12):1391-1400.
24. Manh VM, Holmes JM, Lazar EL, Kraker RT, Wallace DK, Kulp MT, et al. A randomized trial of a binocular iPad game versus part-time patching in children 13 to 16 years of age with amblyopia. Am J Ophthalmol. 2018;186:104-15.
25. Holmes JM, Manny RE, Lazar EL, Birch EE, Kelly KR, Summers AI, et al. A Randomized Trial of Binocular Dig Rush Game Treatment for Amblyopia in children aged 7 to 12 years. Ophthalmology. 2019;126(3):456-66.

Clinical Trials in Neuro-ophthalmology

Anju Bhari, Swati Phuljhele

■ OPTIC NEURITIS AND MULTIPLE SCLEROSIS

Optic Neuritis Treatment Trial (ONTT)[1-3]

Purpose

1. To assess the beneficial and adverse effects of corticosteroid treatment for optic neuritis.
2. To determine the natural history of vision in patients who suffer from optic neuritis.
3. To identify risk factors for the development of multiple sclerosis in patients with optic neuritis.

Background

Optic neuritis is an inflammatory condition affecting the optic nerve, usually affecting young adults, especially females, between 18 and 45 years of age. In this disorder, closely linked to multiple sclerosis (MS), prognosis for visual recovery is generally good. However, return of visual function is almost never complete. Optic Neuritis Treatment Trial (ONTT) was the first major study that provided the information on the natural history, role of steroids in treatment of optic neuritis and risk of development of MS. Multiple sclerosis is a chronic, inflammatory, demyelinating disease of the central nervous system (CNS) that most commonly affects women, with an onset typically between 20 and 40 years of age. The association between optic neuritis and MS is well established. Optic neuritis may be the first manifestation of MS, or it may occur later in its course. A strong case can be made for "isolated" optic neuritis being a *forme fruste* of MS, based on similarities between the two in such epidemiologic factors as gender, age, geographic distributions, cerebrospinal fluid changes, histocompatibility data, magnetic resonance imaging (MRI) changes, and family history. The magnitude of the risk of MS after optic neuritis varies from region to region, it is more prevalent in western countries as compared to Asian region.

Description

The treatment phase of the study was called the Optic Neuritis Treatment Trial, whereas the long-term follow-up phase was called the Longitudinal Optic Neuritis Study (LONS). The study was conducted at 15 clinical centers in the United States. Resource centers included a data coordinating center and a visual field reading center.

Patients were randomized to one of the three following treatment groups at 15 clinical centers:
1. Oral prednisone (1 mg/kg/day) for 14 days
2. Intravenous methylprednisolone (250 mg every 6 hours) for 3 days, followed by oral prednisone (1 mg/kg/day) for 11 days
3. Oral placebo for 14 days

The oral prednisone and placebo groups were double masked, whereas the intravenous methylprednisolone group was single masked.

Baseline testing included blood tests to evaluate for syphilis and systemic lupus erythematosus, a chest X-ray to evaluate for sarcoidosis, and a brain MRI scan to evaluate for changes suggestive of multiple sclerosis.

Inclusion Criteria

The major eligibility criteria for enrolment included the following:
- Age range of 18–46 years
- Acute unilateral optic neuritis with visual symptoms for 8 days or less
- A relative afferent pupillary defect and a visual field defect in the affected eye
- No previous episodes of optic neuritis in the affected eye
- No previous corticosteroid treatment for optic neuritis or multiple sclerosis
- No systemic disease other than multiple sclerosis that might be the cause of the optic neuritis.

Study Measures

The rate of visual recovery and the long-term visual outcome were both assessed by measures of visual acuity, contrast sensitivity, color vision, and visual field at baseline, at seven follow-up visits during the first 6 months, and then yearly. A standardized neurologic examination with an assessment of multiple sclerosis status was made at baseline, after 6 months, and then yearly.

Results

The study has defined the value of baseline ancillary testing, the typical course of visual recovery with and without corticosteroid treatment, the risks and benefits of corticosteroid treatment, and the 5-year risk of the development of MS after optic neuritis. These results are briefly summarized here:

- Routine blood tests, chest X-ray, brain MRI, and lumbar puncture are of limited value for diagnosing optic neuritis in a patient with typical features of optic neuritis.

1-year results:

At 1-year follow-up there was no statistical difference in visual function among the groups. Visual acuity was 20/40 or better in 95% of the placebo group, 94% of the intravenous steroid group and 91% of the oral steroid group.

2-year results:

- At 2 year the risk of development of clinically defined multiple sclerosis (CDMS) was 8% of the patients treated with intravenous steroids had CDMS, 18% of the placebo group, 16% of the oral steroid group developed multiple sclerosis. However, by 3 years of follow-up, this treatment effect had subsided.
- Patients with oral regimen had a twofold greater rate of recurrent optic neuritis either in the fellow eye or in the affected eye (oral steroids 30% vs. intravenous steroid group 13% vs. placebo group 16%)

5-year results:

- Brain MRI is a powerful predictor of the early risk of MS after optic neuritis. The risk of development of CDMS at 5 years depends on number of demyelinating lesions on MRI. The risk is 16% with no lesions on MRI, 37% with one or two lesions and 51% if more than two lesions. Recurrences within 5 years of follow-up, the probability of a recurrence in either eye was almost 2-fold higher in the oral prednisone group than in either the placebo group or the intravenous group.
- The following features of the optic neuritis are associated with a low 5-year risk of MS: lack of pain, optic disc edema (particularly if severe), peripapillary hemorrhage, retinal exudates, and mild visual loss.
- Treatment with the intravenous followed by oral corticosteroid regimen provided a short-term reduction in the rate of development of multiple sclerosis, particularly in patients with brain MRI changes consistent with demyelination.

15-year results:

The cumulative probability of developing MS by 15 years after onset of optic neuritis was 50%.

- Overall, 72% of affected eyes had visual acuity of 20/20 or better.

Conclusion

- Chest X-ray, blood tests, and lumbar puncture are not necessary in evaluating patients with typical clinical features of acute optic neuritis (young adult with sudden visual loss, with progression of symptoms of 1 week or less accompanied by pain on eye movement, with visual improvement beginning within 1 month, with either a swollen or normal optic disc but no more than a minimal vitreous cellular reaction, and with no history of a systemic disease that might produce optic neuritis).

- Brain MRI should be considered to assess the risk of MS. At present, the decision to perform an MRI scan should be made on an individual patient basis.
- Treatment with oral prednisone in standard doses should be avoided, but treatment with intravenous methylprednisolone should be considered, particularly if brain MRI demonstrates multiple signal abnormalities consistent with MS or if a patient is one-eyed or needs to recover vision rapidly.

■ CLINICALLY ISOLATED SYNDROME (CIS) AND RELATED CLINICAL TRIALS

The term "clinically isolated syndrome (CIS)" has been used to describe a first neurologic episode that lasts at least 24 hours and is caused by inflammation/demyelination in one or more sites in the CNS. The episode can be monofocal or multifocal:
- *Monofocal episode*: The person experiences a single neurologic sign or symptom—for example, an attack of optic neuritis—that is caused by a single lesion.
- *Multifocal episode*: The person experiences more than one sign or symptom—for example, an attack of optic neuritis accompanied by weakness on one side—caused by lesions in more than one place.

Individuals who experience a CIS may or may not go on to develop multiple sclerosis. The challenge for the physician is to determine the likelihood that a person experiencing this type of demyelinating event is going to experience a second demyelinating event in the future, thereby meeting the criteria for a definite diagnosis of MS.
- *High Risk:* When the CIS is accompanied by MRI-detected brain lesions that are like those seen in MS, the person has a high-risk (60–80%) of a second neurologic event, and therefore a diagnosis of clinically definite multiple sclerosis (CDMS), within several years. *A diagnosis of CDMS requires the occurrence of at least two neurologic events consistent with demyelination that are separated both anatomically in the CNS and temporally.*
- *Lower Risk:* When the CIS is not accompanied by MRI-detected lesions, the person has a lower risk (20%) of developing MS over the same time period.

Four large-scale clinical trials have been conducted to determine whether early treatment following a CIS can delay the second clinical event, and therefore the diagnosis of CDMS:
1. The CHAMPS (Controlled High-Risk Subjects Avonex® MS Prevention Study) study
2. The ETOMS (Early Treatment of MS) study

3. The BENEFIT (Betaseron® in Newly Emerging MS for Initial Treatment) study
4. The PRECISE study.

Because treatment of MS is typically life-long, once started, determining when to start the patient with CIS on treatment is a critical clinical and economic decision. The results of these trials, and the FDA's approval of expanded labeling for Avonex, Betaseron, and Copaxone support the earliest possible treatment for MS with the use of disease-modifying therapies (DMTs), which many believe may suppress subsequent relapse and MRI lesion formation and delay the development of permanent clinical disabilities. Since ophthalmologists frequently encounter patients with optic neuritis, it is imperative to be aware of these trials.

Controlled High-risk Subjects Avonex Multiple Sclerosis Prevention Study (CHAMPS)[4]

Purpose

To determine whether weekly intramuscular injections of interferon beta-1a (IFN β-1a, Avonex) in patients with a first demyelinating event and with MRI evidence of prior subclinical demyelination in the brain reduced the incidence of clinically definite multiple sclerosis.

Background

Magnetic resonance imaging of the brain can identify lesions consistent with the occurrence of demyelination. The presence of such MRI-identified lesions in a patient with an isolated syndrome of the optic nerve (optic neuritis), spinal cord (incomplete transverse myelitis), or brain stem or cerebellum of recent onset is associated with a high-risk of CDMS. When the cause is demyelination, all three syndromes are presumed to have a common pathogenesis.

Interferon-beta has demonstrated benefits in the treatment of patients with established multiple sclerosis, including slowing the progression of physical disability, reducing the rate of clinical relapses, and reducing the development of brain lesions, as assessed by MRI, and brain atrophy. However, it is not known whether treatment of patients earlier in the course of multiple sclerosis is of value.

Description

Randomized, double-blind, placebo-controlled clinical trial of 383 patients conducted at 50 clinical centers in the United States and Canada from April 1996 until March 2000.

All patients received intravenous methylprednisolone 1 g/d followed by prednisone 1 mg/kg for 11 days. After this initial treatment with corticosteroids, 193 patients were randomly assigned to receive weekly intramuscular injections of 30 μg of IFN β-1a and 190 were assigned to receive weekly injections of placebo. To minimize the symptoms of the interferon-related influenza-like syndrome, patients were instructed to take 650 mg of acetaminophen before each injection and then every 6 hours after each injection for 24 hours during the first 6 months of treatment.

At the end of the first month (and again at the end of the second month, if the patient's condition was not considered to be stable or improving at month 1), each patient was examined by a treating and an examining neurologist, both of whom were unaware of the patient's treatment assignment. Subsequent examinations were scheduled at month 6 and every 6 months thereafter; additional examinations were performed within 7 days after a patient reported new visual or neurologic symptoms. The treating neurologist was responsible for asking the patient about adverse events and visual or neurologic symptoms, whereas the examining neurologist performed a structured neurologic examination without knowledge of the patient's history during or before the study.

The treatment period was planned to be 3 years. The trial was terminated in March 2000 at the recommendation of the data and safety monitoring committee after the single preplanned interim analysis of efficacy. This analysis revealed that treatment with IFN β-1a was significantly better than treatment with placebo and met the stopping guidelines.

Inclusion Criteria

Eligible subjects were patients between the ages of 18 and 50 who had a first isolated, well-defined acute neurologic event consistent with demyelination and involving the optic nerve (unilateral optic neuritis), spinal cord (incomplete transverse myelitis), or brain stem or cerebellum (brain-stem or cerebellar syndrome) that was confirmed on ophthalmologic or neurologic examination. Patients also had to have two or more clinically silent lesions of the brain that were at least 3 mm in diameter on MRI scans and were characteristic of multiple sclerosis (at least one lesion had to be periventricular or ovoid).

Study Measures

The primary prespecified end point was the development of clinically definite multiple sclerosis. Changes in findings on MRI of the brain served as a secondary prespecified end point.

Results

- During 3 years of follow-up, the cumulative probability of the development of CDMS was significantly lower in the IFN β-1a group than in the placebo group (rate ratio, 0.56; 95% confidence interval, 0.38 to 0.81; $p = 0.002$). At 3 years, the cumulative probability was 35% in the

IFN β-1a group and 50% in the placebo group. IFN β-1a reduced the rate of development of CDMS within 3 years by about half.
- The effect of treatment was similar among subgroups classified according to the type of initial event and the number of lesions on the T2-weighted MRI scan at screening.
- As compared with the patients in the placebo group, patients in the IFN β-1a group had a relative reduction in the volume of brain lesions ($p < 0.001$), fewer new or enlarging lesions ($p < 0.001$), and fewer gadolinium-enhancing lesions ($p < 0.001$) at 18 months.
- During the first 6 months, an influenza-like syndrome was reported by 54% of the patients in the IFN β-1a group and by 26% of the patients in the placebo group ($p < 0.001$). Depression was the only other adverse event whose incidence was at least 5 percentage points higher in the IFN β-1a group than in the placebo group.
- There has been controversy about the importance of performing MRI of the brain at the time of a first acute demyelinating event, particularly in patients who present with optic neuritis, since a clinical diagnosis of this syndrome generally can be established without ancillary testing. The results of this study provide justification for obtaining MRI scans of the brain at the time of a first event to determine whether there is further evidence of multiple sclerosis. This study's results indicate that treatment with IFN β-1a is beneficial in patients who are deemed to be at high-risk for CDMS because they have subclinical demyelinating lesions on MRI of the brain.

Conclusion

Initiating once-weekly treatment with intramuscular IFN β-1a at the time of a first demyelinating event is beneficial for patients with brain lesions on MRI that indicate a high-risk of CDMS.

Controlled High-risk Avonex Multiple Sclerosis Prevention Study in Ongoing Neurologic Surveillance Study (CHAMPIONS)[5,6]

Purpose
- To determine the long-term neurological outcome in patients treated with IFN β-1a from onset of a first clinical demyelinating event.
- To determine if immediate initiation of IFN β-1a therapy (the CHAMPS Avonex treatment group) confers long-term benefits compared to delayed initiation of therapy (the CHAMPS placebo group) on the rate of development of CDMS, annualized relapse rates, the development of permanent disability and MR measures of disease activity and progression.
- To determine predictors of long-term disease activity and disability in patients following a first clinical demyelinating event.

Description

It was an investigator-initiated, open-label extension study designed to address a number of issues unresolved by the CHAMPS Study.

All patients of the CHAMPS study were informed of the study results and offered participation in a safety extension study without knowledge of their treatment assignment during CHAMPS. CHAMPS patients at participating CHAMPIONS sites were enrolled in the study from February 2001 to March 2003. All patients were offered, but not required to take, IFN β-1a 30 μg intramuscular once weekly for up to 5 years (from CHAMPS randomization). Patients who received placebo in CHAMPS were considered the delayed treatment (DT) group, and patients who received IFN β-1a in CHAMPS were considered the immediate treatment (IT) group.

Study visits occurred every 6 months with additional urgent visits to evaluate relapses within 2 weeks of symptom onset. Because patients were enrolled in the CHAMPIONS Study at variable time points after randomization into CHAMPS, the study schedule was adjusted to allow for a uniform study visit 5 years following CHAMPS randomization. All patients were then placed on the same 6-month follow-up schedule. The last 5-year follow-up evaluation occurred in June 2003.

Inclusion Criteria

All patients who initially participated in the CHAMPS Study (and could be followed at one of the participating CHAMPIONS study sites) were eligible to participate in CHAMPIONS, regardless of outcome or treatment during/after CHAMPS, if they met the following criteria:
1. Completion of the 1-month follow-up visit in CHAMPS
2. Willingness to enroll in CHAMPIONS less than 5 years after CHAMPS enrolment
3. No evidence of systemic disease with significant organ dysfunction or potential mortality within 3 years of CHAMPIONS enrolment
4. No alternative neurologic diagnosis other than multiple sclerosis following enrolment in CHAMPS
5. No participation in another clinical trial of an investigational drug or device.

Study Measures

The primary outcome measure was the rate of development of CDMS.

The secondary outcome measures determined by the unblinded site neurologist at 5 years were:
- Number of confirmed relapses
- Disease course classification
- Neurologic disability as measured by the Expanded Disability Status Scale (EDSS; conducted during a period of neurologic stability defined as no relapses or corticosteroid treatments in the previous 2 months).

The secondary outcome measures determined by the central MRI reading center (blinded to previous/current treatment) at 5 years were:
- The number of new or enlarging T2 lesions
- Change in T2 lesion volume from CHAMPS baseline to 5 years
- The percentage of patients with Gd+ lesions at 5 years.

Results
- 64% (32/50) of CHAMPS study sites participated in CHAMPIONS. 53% (203/383) of patients enrolled in CHAMPIONS ($n = 100$, IT group; $n = 103$, DT group). Of these 203 patients, 28% (57/203) developed CDMS during CHAMPS, 6% (12/203) withdrew from the CHAMPS Study (but elected to return for CHAMPIONS), and 66% (134/203) completed the CHAMPS Study per protocol without CDMS.
- The 100 patients from the original CHAMPS IFN β-1a group received IFN β-1a immediately after onset of their first symptoms and thus are referred to as the "immediate treatment (IT)" group in CHAMPIONS. The 103 patients from the original CHAMPS placebo group initiated IFN β-1a at the time CDMS developed or after the CHAMPS closeout visit and thus are referred to as the "delayed treatment (DT)" group. The median time to initiation of IFN β-1a therapy in the DT group was 29 months.
- The cumulative probability of development of CDMS was significantly lower in the IT group compared with the DT group (5-year incidence 36 ± 9 vs. $49 \pm 10\%$; $p = 0.03$).
- Multivariate analysis suggested that the only factors independently associated with an increased rate of development of CDMS were randomization to the DT group and younger age at onset of neurologic symptoms. Few patients in either group developed major disability within 5 years.
- The majority of patients (72%) in CHAMPIONS had relapsing-stable disease. At 5 years, very few patients had developed significant neurologic disability, as measured by the EDSS.

Conclusion
These results support the use of IFN β-1a after a first clinical demyelinating event and indicate that there may be modest beneficial effects of immediate treatment compared with delayed initiation of treatment.

Early Treatment of Multiple Sclerosis Study (ETOMS)[7]

Purpose
To assess the effects of low-dose IFN β-1a (Rebif) on the occurrence of relapses in patients after first presentation with neurological events, who are at high-risk of conversion to CDMS.

Description

57 centers in 14 European countries took part in this double-blind placebo-controlled randomized study. Patients were enrolled between August 1995 and July 1997. Of the 375 patients screened, 309 were randomized into two groups.

Patients were randomly assigned either 22 µg IFN β-1a ($n = 154$) or placebo ($n = 155$) by subcutaneous injection once weekly for 2 years. The dose of Rebif used in the study was 1/6th of that generally used to treat relapsing remitting MS.

Neurological and clinical assessments were done every 6 months and brain MRI every 12 months.

Inclusion Criteria

Eligible patients aged 18–40 years, had a first episode of neurological dysfunction suggesting MS within the previous 3 months, and had strongly suggestive brain MRI findings.

Study Measures

The primary outcome measure was the conversion to CDMS as defined by the occurrence of a second exacerbation. Secondary outcome measures included change in the SNRS score, time to second exacerbation, and several MRI measures.

Results

241 (78%) of 308 randomized patients received study treatment for 2 years; 278 (90%) remained in the study until termination. 57 (85%) of 67 who stopped therapy did so after conversion to CDMS.

Fewer patients developed CDMS in the interferon group than in the placebo group [52/154 (34%) vs. 69/154 (45%); $p = 0.047$]. The time at which 30% of patients had converted to CDMS was 569 days in the interferon group and 252 in the placebo group ($p = 0.034$). The annual relapse rates were 0.33 and 0.43 ($p = 0.045$). The number of new T2-weighted MRI lesions and the increase in lesion burden were significantly lower with active treatment.

Conclusion

Interferon β-1a treatment at an early stage of MS had significant positive effects on clinical and MRI outcomes.

Prevention of Relapses and Disability by Interferon β-1a Subcutaneously in Multiple Sclerosis (PRISMS)[8]

Purpose

To evaluate the efficacy of subcutaneous interferon β-1a in relapsing/remitting multiple sclerosis.

Background

The efficacy of IFN β-1a in delaying the onset of CDMS was proved with previous studies however the route of administration and dosage use was different in different studies. The PRISM study was conceptualized to study the relapse rate, disability, and disease activity and burden of disease shown by MRI.

Methods

This was a double-blind placebo-controlled study where in 560 patients with expanded disability status scale (EDSS) scores of 0–5.0 were randomly given either 22 µg of IFN β-1a subcutaneously or 44 µg of IFN β-1a subcutaneously or placebo three times a week for 2 years.

Neurological examination was done every 3 months and MRI was done every 6 months. 205 patients had monthly MRI scans for first 9 months of treatment.

Results

The relapse rate was significantly lower in patients treated with interferon β-1a; mean number per patient was 1.82 for 22 µg group, 1.73 for 44 µg group and 2.56 for placebo group. Time to first relapse was prolonged by 3 and 5 months in the 22 µg and 44 µg group respectively, and the proportion of patients who were relapse free was increased significantly. Interferon β-1a delayed progression in disability and decreased accumulated disability. Interferon β-1a decreased accumulation of burden of disease and number of active lesions on MRI.

Conclusion

Subcutaneous IFN β-1a is an effective treatment of relapsing/remitting multiple sclerosis to decrease relapse rate, disability, MRI lesions and is well tolerated.

BEtaseron in Newly Emerging Multiple Sclerosis for Initial Treatment Study (BENEFIT)[9,10]

Purpose

To compare the effects of early and delayed treatment with interferon beta-1b (IFN β-1b, Betaseron) on time to CDMS and other disease outcomes, including disability progression.

Background

Several controlled studies provide evidence that treatment with interferon beta in patients with a first event suggestive of MS delays conversion to

CDMS. However, it has not been studied whether early initiation of treatment with IFN β prevents development of confirmed disability in MS.

Description

The initial phase was a placebo-controlled, double-blinded study. Patients with a first event suggestive of MS and a minimum of two clinically silent lesions in MRI were randomized to receive either IFN β-1b 250 μg ($n = 292$) or placebo ($n = 176$) subcutaneously every alternate day for 2 years, or until diagnosis of CDMS. Patients were then eligible to enter the follow-up phase with open-label IFN β-1b. In the current prospectively planned analysis 3 years after randomization (maximum 5), the effects of early IFN β-1b treatment were compared with those of delayed treatment initiated after diagnosis of CDMS or after 2 years on the study.

Study Measures

The primary outcomes were time to diagnosis of CDMS, time to confirmed expanded disability status scale (EDSS) progression, and score on a patient-reported functional assessment scale—the functional assessment of multiple sclerosis trial outcomes index (FAMS-TOI).

Results

Of the 468 patients originally randomized, 418 (89%) entered the follow-up phase; 392 (84%) completed 3 years' post-randomization follow-up.
- After 3 years, 99 (37%) patients in the early group developed CDMS compared with 85 (51%) patients in the delayed treatment group.
- Early treatment reduced the risk of CDMS by 41% (hazard ratio 0.59, 95% CI 0.44–0.80; $p = 0.0011$; absolute risk reduction 14%) compared with delayed treatment.
- Over 3 years, 42 (16%) patients in the early group and 40 (24%) in the delayed group had confirmed EDSS progression; early treatment reduced the risk for progression of disability by 40% compared with delayed treatment (0.60, 0.39–0.92; $p = 0.022$; absolute risk reduction 8%). The FAMS-TOI score was high and stable in both groups over the 3-year period ($p = 0.31$).
- 235 (80%) patients from the early treatment and 123 (70%) from the delayed treatment group completed the 5-year study. Early treatment reduced the risk of CDMS by 37% [hazard ratio (HR) 0.63, 95% CI 0.48–0.83; $p = 0.003$] compared with delayed treatment. The risk for confirmed disability progression was not significantly lower in the early treatment group (0.76, 0.52–1.11; $p = 0.177$). At 5 years, median FAMS-TOI scores were 125 in both groups. No significant differences in other disability-related outcomes were recorded.

Conclusion

Early initiation of treatment with IFN β-1b prevents the development of confirmed disability, supporting its use after the first manifestation of relapsing-remitting MS. Effects on the rate of conversion to CDMS and the favorable long-term safety and tolerability profile support early initiation of treatment with IFN β-1b, although a delay in treatment by up to 2 years did not affect long-term disability outcomes.

PreCISe study[11]

Purpose

To study the effect of glatiramer acetate (Copaxone) on conversion to CDMS in patients with CIS.

Background

Glatiramer acetate, approved for the treatment of relapsing-remitting MS, reduces relapses and disease activity and burden monitored by MRI. The efficacy of early treatment with glatiramer acetate in delaying onset of clinically definite multiple sclerosis was assessed in this study.

Description

Phase III, randomized, double-blind, placebo-controlled, international multicenter clinical trial undertaken in 80 sites in 16 countries. Patients were enrolled between January 2004 and January 2006.

481 patients presenting with a CIS with unifocal manifestation, and two or more T2-weighted brain lesions measuring 6 mm or more, were randomly assigned to receive either subcutaneous glatiramer acetate 20 mg per day ($n = 243$) or placebo ($n = 238$) for up to 36 months, unless they converted to CDMS. A preplanned interim analysis was done for data accumulated from 81% of the 3-year study exposure.

MRI evaluations were performed at screening, baseline, and every 3 months until conversion to CDMS. Evaluations included the total number of gadolinium-enhancing and T2 hyperintense lesions, counts of the number of new lesions, percentage brain volume change, and normalized brain volumes.

Inclusion Criteria

Subjects aged 18–45 years with a single focal demyelinating event accompanied by evidence of focal demyelination on brain MRI (MRI; ≥2 lesions on T2 MRI, each of which was ≥6 mm) enrolled within 90 days of the first episode were included.

Study Measures
The primary endpoint was time to CDMS, based on a second clinical attack.

Results
- Glatiramer acetate reduced the risk of developing CDMS by 45% compared with placebo (HR 0.55, 95% CI 0.40–0.77; $p = 0.0005$).
- The time for 25% of patients to convert to CDMS was prolonged by 115%, from 336 days for placebo to 722 days for glatiramer acetate.
- The proportion of patients with a second attack was also lower with Glatiramer acetate than placebo (42.9% vs. 24.7% for the Glatiramer acetate and placebo groups, respectively; $p < 0.0001$).
- Treatment with Glatiramer acetate also reduced MRI evidence of disease activity, including the number of new T2 lesions and the cumulative number of T2 and gadolinium-enhancing lesions.
- The most common adverse events in the glatiramer acetate group were injection-site reactions and immediate post-injection reactions.

Conclusion
Early treatment with glatiramer acetate is efficacious in delaying conversion to CDMS in patients presenting with CIS and brain lesions detected by MRI.

TRAUMATIC OPTIC NEUROPATHY

National Acute Spinal Cord Injury Study (NASCIS) 1990[12]

A multicenter, randomized, double blind control trial of methylprednisolone, naloxone or placebo in the treatment of acute spinal cord injury. It is based on results of this study the treatment for traumatic optic neuropathy was considered. Thus, this study gives us an indirect evidence for the treatment of traumatic optic neuropathy within 6 hours of presentation. However, later studies have found no beneficial use of oral steroids in patients with traumatic optic neuropathy.

Purpose
To compare the efficacy and safety of methylprednisolone, naloxone or placebo in the treatment of acute spinal cord injury.

Background
In National Acute Spinal Cord Injury Study 1, 1000 mg infusion of methylprednisolone sodium succinate was compared with a 100 mg dose of methylprednisolone given as a bolus and daily thereafter for 10 days.

No significant difference in motor and sensory outcomes was observed because the dose was below the theoretical therapeutic threshold.

Inclusion Criteria

Patients with spinal cord injury, diagnosed by a physician associated with the study, who presented within 12 hours and willing to give consent to participate in the study.

Exclusion Criteria

- Patients with involvement of nerve root or cauda equina only
- Gunshot wounds or life-threatening morbidity
- Pregnancy
- Narcotic addiction
- Age less than 13 years
- On maintenance steroids for other condition
- Already received >100 mg methylprednisolone or its equivalent or 1 mg naloxone
- Difficult to follow-up.

Methods

- Group 1: Methylprednisolone 30 mg/kg bolus, then 5.4 mg/kg/h for 23 hours ($n = 162$)
- Group 2: Naloxone 5.4 mg/kg bolus, then 4.5 mg/kg/h for 23 hours ($n = 154$)
- Group 3: Placebo ($n = 171$)

Bolus was given over 15 minutes, followed by a 45 minutes pause and a 23 hours maintenance infusion. Neurological function was assessed after drug administration at 6 weeks, 6 months and 1 year followed by a statistical analysis.

Results

- At 1 year, there was no significant improvement in neurological functions in 3 groups.
- Post-hoc analysis found statistically significant improvement on the motor score at 6 months and 1 year in subgroup of patients receiving steroids within 8 hours.

Conclusion

- The study failed to convincingly demonstrate the benefit of steroids in the management of acute spinal cord injury.
- Validity of statistical significance in post-hoc analysis of a subgroup is controversial.

International Optic Nerve Trauma Study (IONTS)[13]

Purpose

To compare visual outcome after traumatic optic neuropathy on treatment with corticosteroids or optic canal decompression surgery or observation.

Description

A comparative nonrandomized interventional study (1999).

Inclusion Criteria

Patients with unilateral or bilateral traumatic optic neuropathy with initial visual assessment within 3 days of injury and who received treatment within 7 days of injury and who were willing for 1 month of follow-up.

Method

Total 133 patients were included in the study. 127 with unilateral and 6 patients with bilateral traumatic optic neuropathy were included. Based on treatment received, patients with unilateral traumatic optic neuropathy were divided into three groups: (1) untreated ($n = 9$), (2) corticosteroid ($n = 85$), or (3) optic canal decompression surgery ($n = 33$).

Visual acuity was the main outcome assessed.

Results

Visual acuity increased by 3 or more lines in 52% of the steroid group, 32% of the surgery group and 57% of the untreated group. The baseline visual acuity was no light perception in more patients in surgery group. After adjustment of the baseline visual acuity, there was no significant difference in visual outcome of the three treatment groups.

Conclusion

No clear benefit was found on treatment with corticosteroids or optic canal decompression in traumatic optic neuropathy patients.

Corticosteroid Randomization after Significant Head Injury (CRASH) Trial[14]

Purpose

To evaluate efficacy and safety of steroids in patients with acute traumatic brain injury.

Background

Corticosteroids had been used to head injury for more than 30 years. Steroids were believed to improve the blood flow and reduce the risk of herniation by reducing the intracranial edema and pressure. This trial was done to confirm or refute the efficacy of steroids to reduce the risk of death in patients with head trauma.

Methods

It was a randomized control trial (2005). 10,008 patients presenting within 8 hours of head trauma, with Glasgow Coma Scale score of 14 or less were included in the study. They were given either placebo or megadose of intravenous methylprednisolone (2 g over an hour followed by 0.4 g/h for 48 hours).

Results

At 6 months, the risk of death was higher in the steroid group (25.7%) than in the placebo group (22.3%), as well as the risk of death and severe disability was also higher in steroid group (38.1%) than in the placebo group (36.3%).

Conclusion

Corticosteroids should not be used routinely in the treatment of head trauma.

Ischemic Optic Neuropathy Decompression Trial (IONDT)[15]

Purpose

- To assess the safety and efficacy of optic nerve decompression surgery versus careful follow-up
- To describe the natural history of nonarteritic anterior ischemic optic neuropathy (NAION) in untreated patients
- To assess changes in quality of life in NAION patients.

Background

The Ischemic Optic Neuropathy Decompression Trial was the first prospective, multicenter, randomized, controlled trial primarily designed to assess the safety and efficacy of optic nerve decompression surgery compared with "careful" follow-up in patients with NAION. The study began in October 1992 and completed data was made available in 1996.

Methods

A total of 420 patients were diagnosed with NAION. Of these 420 patients, 258 patients met the visual acuity requirement, and were randomized either to surgery or observation. The remaining 162 patients were followed for observing the natural history of the disease.

Inclusion Criteria

- Age 50 or older at randomization
- Duration of symptoms fewer than 14 days at baseline eligibility visit
- Best corrected visual acuity (BCVA) in the study eye between and including 20/64 and light perception
- Visual field defects consistent with optic neuropathy and ≤-3.0 dB
- Relative afferent pupillary defect
- Disc edema
- Willingness to give consent.

Exclusion Criteria

Medical

- Clinical evidence of temporal arteritis
- History of collagen vascular disease or other inflammatory disease
- Pain on eye movement
- History of optic neuritis
- History of multiple sclerosis
- Intolerance or allergy to inhalation anesthetics
- Myocardial infarction within the past 6 months
- Current anticoagulation therapy that cannot be discontinued for at least 2 weeks
- Abnormal Westergren sedimentation rate (>40 mm/h)
- Platelet count <160 × 10^3 mm^3 or hematocrit indicative of excessive surgical risk to the patient <35% for males, <30% for females.

Ophthalmologic

- Bilateral NAION (defined as previous NAION event in non-study eye within 14 days at onset of symptoms in study eye)
- Lens opacity, macular disease, retinopathy, or other eye disease limiting visual acuity
- Prior ophthalmic surgery, including cataract surgery within 3 months
- Vitreous hemorrhage, iritis, or cells in the vitreous
- Glaucoma or IOP greater than 30 mm Hg
- Any abnormality suggestive of non-ischemic etiology
- Use of any drugs known to affect the optic nerve or retina that cannot be discontinued.

General

- Inability or unwillingness of patient to comply with study requirements
- Unwillingness of physician to randomize the patient to treatment

Patients were randomized to optic nerve decompression group or careful follow-up group and followed for at least 2 years.

Primary Outcome

Change of at least three lines of visual acuity, measured using the New York Lighthouse charts (Lighthouse Low Vision Products, Long Island City, NY) at 6 months after randomization.

Secondary Outcomes

- Change of at least three lines of visual acuity at 1 year and at subsequent follow-up times after randomization
- Change in visual field as measured by automated Humphrey perimetry
- Occurrence of systemic and ophthalmic complications
- Change in quality of life
- Other morbidity or mortality.

Results

Results showed a lack of beneficial effect and a possible harmful effect of optic nerve decompression surgery on visual acuity in NAION patients and further recruitment was stopped.
- The gain in visual acuity of three lines or more at 6 months was 32.6% in the surgery group and 42.7% in the careful follow-up group.
- The risk of loss of three or more lines of vision was 23.9% in the surgery group and 12.4% in the careful follow-up group.

Conclusion

Optic nerve head decompression surgery is not recommended in NAION patients.

LEBER'S HEREDITARY OPTIC NEUROPATHY (LHON)

Rescue of Hereditary Optic Disease Outpatient Study (RHODOS)[16]

Purpose

To study the efficacy, safety, and tolerability of oral Idebenone in LHON.

Background

Leber's hereditary optic neuropathy is a mitochondrial genetic disease transmitted maternally, characterized by bilateral visual loss affecting young males. The primary mechanism of optic neuropathy in LHON is the mitochondrial mutation affecting complex I and thus electron transport chain. The treatment in such cases is mainly supportive in form of visual rehabilitation. Idedenone is a CoQ derivative that acts as an electron carrier in the electron transport chain. Idebenone also prevents lipid peroxidation of mitochondria, thus reducing the mitochondrial membrane damage. Rescue of Hereditary Optic Disease Outpatient Study (RHODOS) group investigated the efficacy, safety, and tolerability of oral idebenone in LHON.

Description
It was prospective, randomized, double-blind, placebo-controlled study where in 85 patients were enrolled inclusion criteria:
- Age between 14 and 64 years of age
- Positive m.3460G >A, m.11778G >A, or m.14484T >C mitochondrial DNA mutations
- Vision loss due to LHON within 5 years
- No drug abuse
- Neither pregnant or breastfeeding.

Patients were randomly assigned following a centralized randomization procedure to receive idebenone (Catena® 150 mg, Santhera Pharmaceuticals) 900 mg/day (300 mg three times a day during meals) or placebo for 24 weeks in a 2:1 ratio.

Primary Outcome
The primary endpoint was the best recovery of visual acuity between baseline and week 24 on ETDRS chart.

Secondary Outcome
- Change from baseline to Week 24 in BCVA
- Change in visual acuity of the best eye at baseline
- Change in visual acuity for both eyes in each patient.

Results
- In the placebo group BCVA changed by logMAR −0.071 (95% CI: −0.176 to 0.034), while the idebenone group changed by logMAR −0.135 (95% CI: −0.216 to −0.054)
- The differences between groups did not reach statistical significance at 24 weeks (logMAR −0.064; 95% CI: −0.184 to 0.055; $p = 0.291$)
- Trend toward improvement with idebenone was observed for the secondary end-points of change in best visual acuity (Idebenone: change in logMAR: −0.035; 95% CI: −0.126 to 0.055; Placebo: logMAR +0.085; 95% CI: −0.032 to 0.203; difference between groups: logMAR −0.120; 95% CI: −0.255, 0.014; $p = 0.078$)
- Excluding patients with the m.14484T >C mutation, which is known for its spontaneous recovery rate in visual acuity, led to a larger difference in the change of visual acuity between idebenone- and placebo-treated patients.

- The estimated mean difference among the patients with discordant visual acuities (difference of >0.2 logMAR) in best recovery in visual acuity between the idebenone and placebo group was logMAR = −0.285; 95% CI: −0.502 to −0.068; $p = 0.011$.

Conclusion

- Idebenone does not prevent the involvement of the second eye even if started early.
- However, affected individuals with discordant visual acuities (defined as a difference of >0.2 LogMAR between the two eyes), that means the patients with less duration of disease and are at highest risk for further visual loss in the least affected eye were more likely to benefit from the treatment with idebenone.
- In the follow-up study (RHODOS-OFU), the beneficial effect of 6 months of treatment with idebenone seemed to persist despite discontinuation of the active medication at the end of the trial.
- An important finding of the study was that the high dose of idebenone (900 mg/day) was found to be safe for clinical use and good compliance.

Clinical Trials in Neuro-ophthalmology

Table 1: Summary of different clinical trials in the field of neuro-ophthalmology.

Title	Purpose	No. of patients	Inclusion criteria	Outcome measure	Result/conclusion
ONTT (1991)	Effects of corticosteroid treatment for optic neuritis	454	First episode of acute unilateral optic neuritis with visual symptoms for 8 days or less in age range of 18 to 46 years	Rate of visual recovery and the long-term visual outcome	• High-dose, intravenous corticosteroids followed by oral corticosteroids accelerated visual recovery but provided no long-term benefit to vision • Oral prednisone alone did not improve the visual outcome and was associated with an increased rate of new attacks of optic neuritis
CHAMPS (1996)	Avonex (interferon beta-1a) in reducing the incidence of CDMS	383	Patients between the ages of 18 and 50 who had a first isolated, well-defined acute neurologic event consistent with demyelination	Development of CDMS	IFN β-1a at the time of a first demyelinating event is beneficial for patients with brain lesions on MRI that indicate a high-risk of CDMS
CHAMPIONS (2001) (further 5 year follow-up after CHAMPS)	Long-term neurological outcome in patients treated with IFN β-1a	203	Patients who initially participated in the CHAMPS Study	Rate of development of CDMS	Results support the use of IFN β-1a after a first clinical demyelinating event Modest beneficial effects of immediate treatment compared with delayed initiation of treatment
ETOMS (1995)	Effect of low-dose IFN β-1a (Rebif) on the relapses in patients after first presentation with neurological events	309	Patients 18–40 years, with first episode suggesting MS within the previous 3 months and strongly suggestive brain MRI	Conversion to CDMS	IFN β-1a treatment at an early stage of MS had significant positive effects on clinical and MRI outcomes

Contd...

Contd...

Title	Purpose	No. of patients	Inclusion criteria	Outcome measure	Result/conclusion
BENEFIT (2005)	Effect of early and delayed treatment with interferon beta-1b (IFN β-1b, Betaseron) on time to CDMS	392	Patients with a first event suggestive of MS and a minimum of two clinically silent lesions in MRI	Time to diagnosis of CDMS	Early treatment with IFN β-1b prevents the development of confirmed disability. Delay in treatment by up to 2 years did not affect long-term disability outcomes
PreCISe (2004)	Effect of glatiramer acetate (Copaxone) on conversion to CDMS	481	Patients with a single focal demyelinating event accompanied by evidence of focal demyelination on brain MRI enrolled within 90 days	Time to diagnosis of CDMS	Early treatment with glatiramer acetate is efficacious in delaying conversion to CDMS
PRISM	Efficacy of subcutaneous interferon beta-1a in relapsing/remitting multiple sclerosis	560	Patients with expanded disability status scale (EDSS) scores of 0–5.0	Time to first relapse	Subcutaneous interferon beta-1a is an effective treatment of relapsing/remitting Multiple Sclerosis to decrease relapse rate, disability, MRI lesions and is well-tolerated

(CDMS: clinically definite multiple sclerosis)

REFERENCES

1. Beck RW, Optic Neuritis Study Group. The Optic Neuritis Treatment Trial. Three-year follow-up results. Arch Ophthalmol. 1995;113:136-7.
2. Beck RW, Optic Neuritis Study Group. The Optic Neuritis Treatment Trial: Implications for clinical practice. Arch Ophthalmol. 1992;110:331-2.
3. Optic Neuritis Study Group. The five-year risk of multiple sclerosis after optic neuritis. Experience of the Optic Neuritis Treatment Trial. Neurology. 1997;49:1404-13.
4. Jacobs LD, Beck RW, Simon JH, Kinkel RP, Brownscheidle CM, Murray TJ, et al. Intramuscular interferon beta-1a therapy initiated during a first demyelinating event in multiple sclerosis. CHAMPS Study Group. N Engl J Med. 2000;343:898-904.
5. Kinkel RP, Kollman C, O'Connor P, Murray TJ, Simon J, Arnold D, et al. CHAMPIONS Study Group. IM interferon beta-1a delays definite multiple sclerosis 5 years after a first demyelinating event. Neurology. 2006;66:678-84.
6. Kinkel RP, Dontchev M, Kollman C, Skaramagas TT, O'Connor PW, Simon JH, et al. CHAMPIONS Investigators. Association between immediate initiation of intramuscular interferon beta-1a at the time of a clinically isolated syndrome and long-term outcomes: a 10-year follow-up of the Controlled High-Risk Avonex Multiple Sclerosis Prevention Study in Ongoing Neurological Surveillance. Arch Neurol. 2012;69:183-90.
7. Comi G, Filippi M, Barkhof F, Durelli L, Edan G, Fernández O, et al. Early Treatment of Multiple Sclerosis Study Group. Effect of early interferon treatment on conversion to definite multiple sclerosis: a randomised study. Lancet. 2001;357:1576-82.
8. PRISM study group. Randomized double-blind placebo-controlled study of interferon beta-1a in relapsing/remitting multiple sclerosis. PRISMS (Prevention of Relapses and disability by Interferon beta-1a subcutaneously in Multiple Sclerosis) Study group. Lancet. 1998;352(939):1498-504.
9. Kappos L, Freedman MS, Polman CH, Edan G, Hartung HP, Miller DH, et al. BENEFIT Study Group. Effect of early versus delayed interferon beta-1b treatment on disability after a first clinical event suggestive of multiple sclerosis: a 3-year follow-up analysis of the BENEFIT study. Lancet. 2007;370:389-97.
10. Kappos L, Freedman MS, Polman CH, Edan G, Hartung HP, Miller DH, et al. BENEFIT Study Group. Long-term effect of early treatment with interferon beta-1b after a first clinical event suggestive of multiple sclerosis: 5-year active treatment extension of the phase 3 BENEFIT trial. Lancet Neurol. 2009;8:987-97.
11. Comi G, Martinelli V, Rodegher M, Moiola L, Bajenaru O, Carra A, et al. PreCISe Study Group. Effect of glatiramer acetate on conversion to clinically definite multiple sclerosis in patients with clinically isolated syndrome (PreCISe study): a randomised, double-blind, placebo-controlled trial. Lancet. 2009;374:1503-11.
12. Bracken MB, Shepard MJ, Collins WF, Holford TR, Young W, Baskin DS, et al. A randomized, controlled trial of methylprednisolone or naloxone in the treatment of acute spinal cord injury. N Engl J Med. 1990;322:1405-11.
13. Levin LA, Beck RW, Joseph MP, Seiff S, Kraker R. The treatment of traumatic optic neuropathy: the international optic trauma study. Ophthalmology. 1999;106(7):1268-77.
14. CRASH trial collaborators. Final results of MRC CRASH, a randomized placebo control trial of intravenous corticosteroids in adults with head injury-outcome at 6 months. Lancet. 2005;365:1957-59.
15. The IONDT research group. The ischemic optic neuropathy decompression trial (IONDT): design and methods, Control Clin Trials. 1998;19(3):276-96.
16. Klopstock T, Yu-Wai-Man P, Dimitriadis K, Rouleau J, Heck S, Bailie M, et al. A randomized placebo controlled trial of idebenone in Leber's hereditary optic neuropathy. Brain. 2011;134(9):2677-86.

18 CHAPTER

Miscellaneous Clinical Trials: Collaborative Ocular Melanoma Study

Neha Goel, Vinod Kumar

■ COLLABORATIVE OCULAR MELANOMA STUDY (COMS)[1-6]

Purpose

1. To evaluate therapeutic interventions for patients who have choroidal melanoma, and to assess the potential life-preserving as well as sight-preserving role of radiation therapy.
2. To determine which of two standard treatments, enucleation or brachytherapy, is more likely to prolong survival of eligible patients with medium-sized choroidal melanoma.
3. To determine whether preoperative radiation prolongs life for patients whose eyes with large choroidal melanoma are enucleated.

Background

Choroidal melanoma is the most common primary eye cancer affecting adults. For more than 100 years, enucleation has been the standard treatment for choroidal melanoma. Before the COMS was initiated in 1986, interest in radiation therapy had increased because of the potential for saving the eye and perhaps some vision. However, the merits of radiation with respect to prolonging patient survival were unknown. The best data from nonrandomized studies suggested that there was no difference in length of remaining life between patients treated with radiation and those whose eyes were enucleated. Thus, it was appropriate and necessary to conduct a randomized, controlled clinical trial in which a large number of patients would be followed for many years in order to compare enucleation and radiation with respect to relative success in prolonging survival of choroidal melanoma patients.

Description

The COMS was a set of long-term, multicenter, randomized controlled trials conducted in 43 clinical centers located in major population areas of the United States and Canada. It consisted of two multicenter clinical trials designed to compare the outcome of therapies for large and medium choroidal melanomas and a third arm to assess the natural history of small choroidal melanomas. From November 1986 through July 1998, 8,712 patients with choroidal melanoma of all sizes were screened for eligibility for a COMS clinical trial.

In the trial for patients with tumors of medium size, enucleation and irradiation with an iodine-125 episcleral plaque were compared on the basis of length of remaining life. All randomized patients were followed for 5-15 years or until death. For patients randomly assigned to enucleation, the eye was removed following a standard procedure. For patients assigned to plaque irradiation, the margins of the tumor were located and the dimensions of the tumor were measured by the ophthalmic surgeon. A gold plaque with a plastic seed carrier that contained the proper dosage and configuration of radioactive iodine seeds was sutured to the outside (sclera) of the eye over the base of the tumor. This procedure made possible the delivery of a high dose of radiation to a very localized area (85 Gy to the tumor apex). The plaque typically was removed from the eye after 3-7 days. Enrolment was completed in this trial in July 1998 with 1,317 patients enrolled. Clinical follow-up of patients ended in July 2003.

In the COMS trial of preoperative radiation, patients with large tumors were randomized to enucleation alone or to enucleation preceded by 20 Gy of external beam radiation. The two randomly assigned groups of patients were followed for at least 5 years or until death and have been compared on the basis of length of remaining life and other outcomes. Enrolment in this trial was completed in December 1994, with 1,003 patients enrolled. Clinical follow-up of all patients in this trial ended in July 2000.

Accrual to a nonrandomized pilot study to assess the feasibility of a randomized trial for small tumors was halted in 1989. Additional follow-up of those 204 patients was carried out from 1994-1996.

Inclusion Criteria

Men and women eligible for the study had to be age 21 or older, have primary choroidal melanoma in only one eye, and have no evidence of metastatic disease. Accurate estimation of tumor thickness by echography also was required. Entrance criteria established at the beginning of the study defined large choroidal melanomas more than 8 mm in thickness and/or greater than 16 mm in longest base diameter. Medium choroidal tumors were 3.1-8 mm in thickness and no more than 16 mm in longest base diameter. Small choroidal melanomas were 1-3 mm in apical thickness and at least 5 mm in diameter.

Patients with coexisting disease that could compromise survival or those on immunosuppressive therapy were ineligible. Patients with medium-size melanoma near the optic nerve were excluded because it precluded application of the radioactive plaque. Also, patients with predominately ciliary body melanomas were not included.

Study Measures

The primary outcome was time to death from all-cause mortality. Secondary outcomes included metastasis-free survival, cancer-free survival, and years of useful vision. Information gathered and analyzed includes time to death from all causes, time to death from cancer (whether metastatic choroidal melanoma or not), diagnosis of other tumors, complications of radiation, and changes in visual acuity. A parallel study of quality of life for patients enrolled in the trial of radioactive plaque was initiated in January 1995.

Results

Nonrandomized Small Tumor Pilot Study[1,2]

The treatment and mortality results of the COMS nonrandomized small tumor pilot study were reported in 1997. From December 1986 to August 1989, 204 patients with small choroidal melanoma, defined as 1.0–3.0 mm in apical height and at least 5.0 mm in basal diameter, were enrolled in a prospective follow-up study. The median length of follow up was 92 months. Eight percent of patients were treated at the time of study enrolment and an additional 33% were treated during follow-up. Based on 27 deaths, the Kaplan-Meier estimate of 5-year all-cause mortality was 6.0% (95% confidence interval, 2.7–9.3%) and 8-year all-cause mortality was 14.9% (95% confidence interval, 9.6–20.2%). Mortality findings and analysis of predictors of growth have been published (COMS Reports Nos. 4 and 5).

The Randomized Trial of Pre-enucleation Radiation for Large Choroidal Melanoma[3,4]

- Initial mortality findings published in 1998 (COMS Report No. 10) showed that patients with large choroidal melanoma had similar survival rates regardless of whether they were treated with radiation prior to removal of the eye or had their eye removed without prior radiation therapy. 5-year survival rates were approximately 60% in both treatment arms.
- There were no significant differences in the two groups in terms of local orbital outcome, although there were fewer biopsy-confirmed tumor recurrences of the orbit in patients receiving pre-enucleation radiation (none for the radiation group vs. five in the nonradiation group; $p = 0.03$).
- The COMS large tumor trial found neither benefit nor harm from treating ocular melanoma patients with radiation before removal of the eye. However, patients who had pre-enucleation radiation had fewer local complications (COMS Report No. 11).

The Randomized Trial of I-125 Brachytherapy for Medium Choroidal Melanoma[5,6]

- Initial mortality findings published in 2001 (COMS Report No. 18) showed that survival rates for radiation therapy (I-125 brachytherapy)

and enucleation are about the same. The 5-year survival rate of patients who were treated with either radiation therapy or eye removal was 82%, considerably better than the 70% 5-year survival rate that had been projected when the study was designed in 1985.
- Compared to immediate loss of vision when the eye is removed, eyes treated with radiation steadily lost vision gradually, with 63% having visual acuity of 20/200 or worse by 3 years after treatment (COMS Report No. 16). The risk of vision loss was associated with a history of diabetes, thick tumors, tumors close to or beneath the macula, tumors with secondary retinal detachments, and tumors that were not dome-shaped.
- After the first 5 years following brachytherapy, the risk of treatment failure was 10.3%. Risk factors for treatment failure were greater tumor thickness, older age, and proximity of tumor to the foveal avascular zone.

CONCLUSION

The COMS was one of the largest and most challenging clinical trials ever conducted by the National Eye Institute. To date, its major findings are: (1) that pre-enucleation external-beam radiation to the orbit for large choroidal melanoma does not improve survival compared with enucleation alone; and (2) that there is no difference in 5-year survival of patients with medium-size choroidal melanoma treated with Iodine-125 brachytherapy or enucleation.

Table 1: Summary of Collaborative Ocular Melanoma Study (COMS).

Title	Purpose	No. of patients	Inclusion criteria	Follow-up	Result/conclusion
COMS small tumor 1989	Clinical characteristics and survival experience of small sized choroidal melanoma	204	Melanomas 1–3 mm in apical thickness and at least 5 mm in diameter	92 months (mean)	• Otherwise healthy patients who have small choroidal melanomas have a low risk of dying within 5 years (6%) • Small melanomas managed by observation—21% demonstrated growth by 2 years and 31% by 5 years
COMS medium tumor 1998	Brachytherapy vs. enucleation in medium sized choroidal melanoma	1,317	Tumor 3.1–8 mm in thickness and <16 mm in longest base diameter	5–15 years or till death	• Survival rates for both groups are similar (82%) • Compared to immediate loss of vision when the eye is removed, eyes treated with radiation steadily lost vision gradually
COMS large tumor 1994	Enucleation vs. enucleation preceded by radiotherapy in large melanomas	1,003	Melanomas >8 mm in thickness and/or > 16 mm in longest base diameter	5 years or till death	• Similar survival rates were seen in both groups (60%) • Fewer biopsy-confirmed tumor recurrences of the orbit in patients receiving pre-enucleation radiation

REFERENCES

1. Collaborative Ocular Melanoma Study Group. Mortality in patients with small choroidal melanoma. COMS Report No. 4. Arch Ophthalmol. 1997;115: 886-93.
2. Collaborative Ocular Melanoma Study Group. Factors predictive of growth and treatment of small choroidal melanoma. COMS Report No. 5. Arch Ophthalmol. 1997;115:1537-44.
3. Collaborative Ocular Melanoma Study Group. The Collaborative Ocular Melanoma Study (COMS) randomized trial of pre-enucleation radiation of large choroidal melanoma, II: Initial mortality findings. COMS Report No. 10. Am J Ophthalmol. 1998;125:779-96.
4. Collaborative Ocular Melanoma Study Group. The Collaborative Ocular Melanoma Study (COMS) randomized trial of pre-enucleation radiation of large choroidal melanoma, III: Local complications and observations following enucleation. COMS Report No. 11. Am J Ophthalmol. 1998;126:362-72.
5. Collaborative Ocular Melanoma Study Group. Collaborative Ocular Melanoma Study (COMS) randomized trial of I-125 brachytherapy for medium choroidal melanoma, I: Visual acuity after 3 years. COMS Report No. 16. Ophthalmology. 2001;108:348-66.
6. Collaborative Ocular Melanoma Study Group. The COMS randomized trial of Iodine 125 brachytherapy for choroidal melanoma, III: Initial mortality findings. COMS Report No. 18. Arch Ophthalmol. 2001;119:969-82.

CHAPTER 19
Clinical Trials in Ocular Complications of AIDS

Neha Goel, Vinod Kumar

■ LONGITUDINAL STUDY OF THE OCULAR COMPLICATIONS OF AIDS (LSOCA)[1]

Purpose

1. To monitor trends over time, in the incidence of cytomegalovirus (CMV) retinitis and other ocular complications of AIDS.
2. To determine the effect of highly active anti-retroviral therapy (HAART)-induced immune status on the risk of developing CMV retinitis and other ocular complications of AIDS.
3. To determine the characteristics (clinical, virologic, hematologic, and biochemical) of a population at high-risk for CMV retinitis and other ocular complications of AIDS.
4. To evaluate the effects of treatments for CMV retinitis and other ocular complications on visual function, quality of life, and survival.

Background

Ocular abnormalities in patients with AIDS were first reported in 1982. The most common finding is a noninfectious "HIV retinopathy," characterized by cotton wool spots, intraretinal hemorrhages, and/or microaneurysms. These changes occur in approximately 50% of patients with AIDS. HIV retinopathy alone is not typically associated with clinical loss of vision, but functional deficits in patients with AIDS without other ocular complications may be due to this phenomenon.

Cytomegalovirus retinitis has had the most clinical importance of all the associated complications of AIDS. It is commonly seen in late-stage AIDS, and even when treated it has the potential to cause substantial loss of vision. CMV retinitis is also the most costly AIDS-related opportunistic infection; the mean monthly cost of treatment has been estimated at $7,825. The incidence of CMV retinitis has varied with changes in the therapeutic and prophylactic strategies for AIDS and its complications. It has been on the decline in recent years related to the increased use of HAART.

Other ocular complications of AIDS such as ocular toxoplasmosis, herpes zoster retinitis, and pneumocystis choroidopathy occur less frequently than CMV retinitis and HIV retinopathy. Their frequency has also changed over the course of the AIDS epidemic.

Because the epidemiology of AIDS is rapidly evolving, with HIV becoming more like a chronic disease, new information is needed on the incidence and course of ocular complications. There is little information about the effect of HAART therapy over time on changes in immune status and the risk of ocular complications of AIDS. More information is also needed to determine who is at risk for developing ocular complications of AIDS, and how treatment is affecting their visual function, quality of life, and survival.

Description

LSOCA was a prospective observational study of patients with AIDS that began in September 1998 and was designed to document the incidence of ocular complications of AIDS in the era of HAART and their impact on vision. Patients with a prior diagnosis of AIDS according to the 1993 Center for Disease Control and Prevention (CDC) criteria were recruited from 19 clinical centers across the United States. Patients were enrolled with or without ocular complications and across a spectrum of immunologic functions (as determined by CD4+ T-cell count). Approximately 2,000 patients were to be enrolled in the study. Enrolment of patients with CMV retinitis at baseline was to be between 300 and 600 patients.

Follow-up visits for patients without ocular complications were scheduled every 6 months. Follow-up visits for patients with ocular complications at baseline or diagnosed during follow-up were every 3 months.

Cytomegalovirus retinitis was diagnosed by study-certified ophthalmologists with expertise in AIDS. *Newly diagnosed retinitis* was defined as CMV retinitis either diagnosed ≤45 days prior to study enrolment or diagnosed during follow-up (incident cases). *Previously diagnosed retinitis* was defined as CMV retinitis diagnosed >45 days prior to enrolment. *Retinitis progression* was defined as the movement of a border of a CMV lesion at least ½ standard disc diameter along a front ½ disc diameter in size or the occurrence of a new lesion ¼ disc area in size. Retinal detachments (RD) and immune recovery uveitis (IRU) were diagnosed clinically. *IRU* was defined as either the occurrence of new intraocular inflammation or an increase in intraocular inflammation (cells in the anterior chamber or vitreous) in an eye with CMV retinitis in the setting of immune recovery. *Immune recovery* was defined as an increase in CD4+ T cells from <100 cells/µL to a level ≥100 cells/µL, as this level is the one that is used to recommend discontinuation of the anti-CMV therapy. The incidence of IRU was calculated from the date that the CD4+ T cells rose to >100 cells/µL. For those participants with immune recovery at enrolment, the date the CD4+ T cells became >100 cells/µL was estimated, assuming a linear increase from the nadir CD4+ T cells to the enrolment CD4+ T cells with the increase beginning at the time HAART was started.

Inclusion Criteria

Males and females aged 13 years and older with diagnosis of AIDS were eligible.

Study Measures

- All participants gave a detailed medical history, including information on AIDS-related illnesses, nadir CD4+ T cell count (lowest count prior to enrolment), and antiretroviral therapy.
- A complete ophthalmologic examination was performed, including best-corrected visual acuity with logarithmic visual acuity charts, slit-lamp examination, and dilated indirect ophthalmoscopy. Standardized fundus photographs were obtained and forwarded to a centralized reading center for grading. In addition, contrast sensitivity and visual field (VF) examination was carried out.
- Laboratory testing included hematology, serum chemistry, CD4+ T cells, and collection of plasma and blood cells for banking. Analysis of banked specimens included HIV RNA levels (HIV load) and CMV DNA levels.

Results

Ocular Diagnoses at Enrolment[1]

As of March 31, 2003, 1632 participants with AIDS were enrolled.
- The cohort had a history of severe immune deficiency, as evidenced by a median nadir CD4+ T-cell count of 30 cells/μL. At enrolment, the median CD4+ T-cell count was 164 cells/μL. CD4+ T-cell counts were <50 in 24.1% but ≥100 in 63.6% and ≥200 in 43.0%.
- CMV retinitis was present in 22.1%, whereas other ocular opportunistic infections each were present in ≤0.6%. The incidence of CMV retinitis estimated from retrospective data was 5.60/100 person-years (PY). Of the 360 patients with CMV retinitis, 22.5% were newly diagnosed at enrolment, and the remainder had more long-standing CMV retinitis (median, 2.8 years).

Ocular Examination Results at Enrolment[2]

As of March 31, 2003, 1632 participants with AIDS were enrolled.
- The evidence of intraocular inflammation was substantially more common among patients with CMV retinitis or other major ocular complications than among those without, as were the complications of

infection and inflammation, including cataracts, pseudophakia, macular edema, and epiretinal membrane.
- Among patients with CMV retinitis, macular edema and epiretinal membrane formation were most common among patients with long-standing retinitis and immune recovery. Patients with newly diagnosed retinitis had eye examination findings similar to those reported in the pre-HAART era.
- Visual impairment (<20/40) in the better-seeing eye was present in 9.2% of patients with CMV retinitis, 41.4% of patients with other major ocular complications (primarily ocular opportunistic infections), and only 0.6% of patients with no major ocular complication ($p < 0.0001$).
- Although patients without major ocular complications generally had good visual acuity, approximately 9.8% of eyes and 6.6% of participants had contrast sensitivity loss sufficient to impair reading speed.

Risk Factors for Mortality[3]

1,583 patients with AIDS, of whom 374 had CMV retinitis (1998–2003), were analyzed. The overall mortality rate was 0.07 deaths/PY. In a multivariate analysis, the following baseline risk factors were associated with an increased mortality:
- Higher HIV viral load [relative risk (RR) = 4.6 for HIV viral load >100,000 copies/mL vs. <400 copies/mL; $p < 0.0001$]
- Lower CD4+ T-cell count at enrolment (RR = 3.8 for CD4+ T-cell count 0–49 cells/µL vs. ≥200 cells/µL; $p < 0.0001$)
- CMV viral load ≥ 400 copies/mL (RR = 1.9; $p = 0.002$)
- Lower hemoglobin (RR = 1.7 for hemoglobin < 10 g/dL; $p = 0.009$)
- A history of cryptococcal meningitis (RR = 1.7; $p = 0.02$)
- CMV retinitis (RR = 1.6; $p = 0.0002$)
- Karnofsky score ≤ 80 (RR = 1.4; $p = 0.008$)

Incidence of Cytomegalovirus Retinitis[4]

A total of 1,600 participants with AIDS but without CMV retinitis at enrolment who completed at least one follow-up visit were assessed.

The incidence rate of CMV retinitis in individuals with AIDS was 0.36/100 PY based upon 29 incident cases during 8,134 PY of follow-up.

The rate was higher for those with a CD4+ T-cell count at the immediately prior visit below 50 cells/µL (3.89/100 PY, $p < 0.01$), whereas only one individual with a CD4+ T-cell count of 50–99 cells/µL and two individuals with a CD4+ T-cell count of >100 cells/µL developed CMV retinitis. Having a CD4+ T-cell count below 50 cells/µL at the clinical visit prior to CMV retinitis evaluation was the single most important risk factor [HR: 136, 95% confidence interval (CI): 30–605, $p < 0.0001$) for developing retinitis.

Course of Cytomegalovirus Retinitis[5-7]

271 patients with AIDS and CMV retinitis were analyzed.

- *Retinitis progression*: The overall rate of retinitis progression was 0.10/PY; among those with CD4+ T-cell counts of <50/µL, it was 0.58/PY, compared to 0.02/PY among those with CD4+ T-cell counts of ≥200/µL ($p < 0.0001$). In the multivariate analysis, significant risk factors for retinitis progression included a low CD4+ T-cell count, positive CMV load, longer time for AIDS diagnosis, and low Karnofsky score.
- *Second (contralateral) eye involvement*: The overall rate of second eye involvement among patients with unilateral CMV retinitis was 0.07/PY; among those with CD4+ T-cell counts of <50/µL it was 0.34/PY, compared with 0.02/PY among those with CD4+ T-cell counts of ≥200/µL ($p < 0.0001$). The risk factors for contralateral eye involvement included low CD4+ T-cell count and detectable CMV load.
- *Retinal detachment*: The overall rate of RD was 0.06/PY; among those with CD4+ T-cell counts of <50/µL it was 0.30/PY, compared with 0.02/PY among those with CD4+ T-cell counts of ≥200/µL ($p < 0.0001$). The risk factors for RD included a low CD4+ T-cell count and a larger area of CMV retinitis.
- *5-year outcomes*:[7] 503 patients with AIDS and CMV retinitis were classified as having previously diagnosed CMV retinitis and immune recovery, previously diagnosed retinitis and immune compromise, and newly diagnosed CMV retinitis.
    - The overall mortality was 9.8 deaths/100 PY. Rates varied by group at enrolment from 3.0/100 PY for those with previously diagnosed retinitis and immune recovery to 26.1/100 PY for those with newly diagnosed retinitis.
    - The rate of retinitis progression was 7.0/100 PY and varied from 1.4/100 PY for those with previously diagnosed retinitis and immune recovery to 28.0/100 PY for those with newly diagnosed retinitis.
    - The rate of RD was 2.3/100 eye-years (EY) and varied from 1.2/100 EY for those with previously diagnosed retinitis and immune recovery to 4.9/100 EY for those with newly diagnosed retinitis.
    - The rate of IRU was 1.7/100 PY and varied from 1.3/100 PY for those with previously diagnosed retinitis and immune recovery at enrolment to 3.6/100 PY for those with newly diagnosed retinitis who subsequently experienced immune recovery.
    - The rates of visual loss to worse than 20/40 and to 20/200 or worse were 7.9/100 EY and 3.4/100 EY, respectively; they varied from 6.1/100 and 2.7/100 EY for those with previously diagnosed retinitis and immune recovery to 11.8/100 and 5.1/100 EY for those with newly diagnosed retinitis. Although the event rates tended to decline with time, in general, at no time did they reach zero.

Visual Acuity Loss in Cytomegalovirus Retinitis[8,9]

379 patients with AIDS and CMV retinitis (494 eyes) were evaluated for incidence, risk factors, and causes of visual acuity loss.
- The baseline frequencies of visual acuity loss to 20/50 or worse and to 20/200 or worse were 29% and 15%, respectively. Over a median follow-up period of 3.1 years, the incidences of visual acuity loss to 20/50 or worse, to 20/200 or worse, and of doubling of the visual angle were 0.10/EY, 0.06/EY, and 0.13/EY, respectively.
- Immune recovery was associated with a 42% reduction in vision loss to 20/50 or worse and with a 61% reduction in vision loss to 20/200 or worse after adjusting for confounding. Of the patients with immune recovery at baseline, 17% had IRU. In these patients, the incidence rate of 20/50 or worse vision was similar to that observed in patients without immune recovery (0.17/EY vs. 0.16/EY), but the incidence of 20/200 or worse vision was similar to that observed among patients with immune recovery (0.04/EY vs. 0.04/EY).
- Overall, involvement of the posterior pole with CMV retinitis (zone 1 retinitis) accounted for approximately one half of incident visual acuity loss of 20/50 or worse, 20/200 or worse, and of doubling of the visual angle. Cataract and retinitis-related RD were the second and third most common causes of vision loss, accounting for 22–33% and 13–20% of vision loss for the three outcomes, respectively. In subset analysis, cataract and cystoid macular edema (CME) accounted for approximately 50% of incident vision loss in the eyes of patients with long-standing CMV retinitis and immune recovery at baseline, but these complications accounted for <10% of incident vision loss in eyes of patients with newly diagnosed CMV retinitis at baseline. Of the eyes that had a vision-threatening complication of CMV retinitis, the eyes that developed RD had the highest risk of vision loss, with 100% of eyes developing visual impairment (20/50 or worse vision) and 42% of eyes developing legal blindness (20/200 or worse vision) at 12 months after diagnosis of the RD.

Visual Field Loss in Cytomegalovirus Retinitis[10]

A total of 476 patients with AIDS and CMV retinitis were assessed for VF loss.
- Over a median follow-up of 4 years (range, 0.5–9 years), the incidence rates of VF loss to 75% and 50% of normal were 0.22/EY (95% CI, 0.20–0.25) and 0.08/EY (95% CI, 0.06–0.10), respectively. The observed rates were six- to seven-fold less than the observed rates of VF loss in the era before HAART.
- Decreased CD4+ T-cell count, whether measured at enrolment or over follow-up time, was associated with increased rates of VF loss for all VF outcomes in a dose-dependent fashion. The risk factors for VF loss included lower CD4+ T-cell count, CMV lesion size > 25% of the total retinal area, and active CMV retinitis after controlling for potential confounding.

HAART use and immune recovery (CD4+ T-cell count > 100 cells/μL) were associated with reduced risk of VF loss in multiple regression models. Immune recovery was statistically significantly associated with a lower risk of VF loss to 75% of normal [relative risk (RR) = 0.63; 95% CI, 0.49–0.86; p = 0.003) and to 50% of normal (RR = 0.60; 95% CI, 0.44–0.82; p = 0.001) after controlling for demographic characteristics, HIV viral load, HAART use, CMV lesion location and size, and retinitis activity.

Noncytomegalovirus Ocular Opportunistic Infections in Patients with AIDS[11]

At enrolment, 37 non-CMV ocular opportunistic infections were diagnosed: 16 patients, herpetic retinitis; 11 patients, toxoplasmic retinitis; and 10 patients, choroiditis. During the follow-up period, the estimated incidences (and 95% CI) of these were: herpetic retinitis, 0.007/100 PY (95% CI 0.0004, 0.039); toxoplasmic retinitis, 0.007/100 PY (95% CI 0.004, 0.039); and choroiditis, 0.014/ 100 PY (95% CI 0.0025, 0.050). The mortality rates appeared higher among those patients with newly diagnosed or incident herpetic retinitis and choroiditis [rates = 21.7 deaths/100 PY (p = 0.02) and 12.8 deaths/100 PY (p = 0.04)], respectively, than those for patients with AIDS without an ocular opportunistic infection (4.1 deaths/100 PY); toxoplasmic retinitis did not appear to be associated with greater mortality (6.4/100 PY, p = 0.47). Eyes with newly diagnosed herpetic retinitis appeared to have a poor visual prognosis, with high rates of visual impairment (37.9/100 PY) and blindness (17.5/100 PY), whereas those outcomes in eyes with choroiditis appeared to be lower (2.3/100 and 0/100 PY, respectively).

Conclusion

- Although there is the possibility of oversampling patients with AIDS and ocular complications (as compared with a random sample), which would lead to increased estimates of prevalent and incident ocular morbidities, these data still suggest a substantial decline in the incidence of CMV retinitis from the pre-HAART era. Nevertheless, new cases of CMV retinitis continue to occur, and there is a population of patients with long-standing retinitis who will require management.[1]
- In the HAART era, CMV retinitis and other ocular opportunistic infections are associated with intraocular inflammation, structural ocular complications, and visual impairment. Patients with newly diagnosed CMV retinitis have eye examination findings similar to those seen in the pre-HAART era.[2]
- In the era of HAART, CMV disease as manifested by CMV retinitis and a detectable CMV viral load were associated with an increased risk for mortality, even after adjusting for demographic, treatment, immunologic, and HIV virologic factors.[3]

- Patients with AIDS, especially those with severely compromised immune systems, remain at risk for developing CMV retinitis in the HAART era, although the incidence rate is reduced from that observed in the pre-HAART era.[4]
- Compared with the rate of retinitis progression (approximately 3.0/PY) reported in the pre-HAART era, the rate of retinitis progression was reduced among patients in the HAART era, even among those with low CD4+ T-cell counts, who might be expected to behave most like patients from the pre-HAART era. However, these events also occurred among patients with high CD4+ T-cell counts and presumed immune recovery. Continued ophthalmologic follow-up of patients with immune recovery is recommended to detect early retinitis progression.[5]
- Compared with the rates reported in the pre-HAART era of second eye involvement (approximately 0.40/PY) and RD (approximately 0.50/PY), the rates of these events were reduced among patients in the HAART era. However, among patients with CD4+ T-cell counts of <50/µL, the rates were more similar to those from the pre-HAART era.[6]
- Despite the availability of HAART, patients with AIDS and CMV retinitis remain at increased risk for mortality, retinitis progression, complications of the retinitis, and visual loss over a 5-year period.[7]
- CMV retinitis is associated with a substantial risk of incident vision loss in the era of HAART. Those who have HAART-induced immune recovery have approximately 50% lower risk of visual acuity loss. Presence of IRU at baseline attenuated the protective effect of immune recovery for moderate vision loss but not for blindness. Zone 1 involvement and RD remain the most common causes of visual acuity loss among patients with CMV retinitis. Cataract and CME also are common causes of loss of visual acuity, primarily in those patients with HAART-induced immune recovery.[8,9]
- Cytomegalovirus retinitis was associated with a substantial risk of incident VF loss, but the incidence is approximately six-fold lower than that observed in the pre-HAART era. Those who have HAART-induced immune recovery have approximately 40% lower risk of VF loss for both outcomes after controlling for confounding.[10]
- Although uncommon, non-CMV ocular opportunistic infections may be associated with high rates of visual loss and/or mortality.[11]

FOSCARNET–GANCICLOVIR CYTOMEGALOVIRUS RETINITIS TRIAL (FGCRT)[12-14]

Purpose
- To evaluate the relative efficacy and safety of foscarnet and ganciclovir for the treatment of CMV retinitis in patients with AIDS.

- To compare the relative benefits of immediate treatment versus deferral of the treatment for patients with disease not involving the posterior pole.

Background

Cytomegalovirus retinitis is the most common intraocular infection in patients with AIDS and is estimated to affect 35–40% of patients with AIDS. Untreated CMV retinitis is a progressive disorder, the end result of which is total retinal destruction and blindness.

The first two drugs approved by the United States Food and Drug Administration (FDA) for the treatment of CMV retinitis were ganciclovir and foscarnet, respectively. Ganciclovir suppresses CMV infections, and relapse occurs in virtually all AIDS patients when ganciclovir is discontinued. Because of their similar hematologic (blood) toxicities, the simultaneous use of ganciclovir and zidovudine (AZT) is not recommended. Studies with the drug foscarnet indicate that remission of CMV retinitis occurs in 36–77% of patients and that relapse occurs in virtually all patients when the drug is discontinued. At the time of this trial, both ganciclovir and foscarnet were available only as intravenous formulations. Both drugs were given in a similar two-step fashion: an initial 2-week course of high-dose therapy (induction) to control the infection followed by long-term lower dose therapy to prevent relapse (maintenance).

The relative effectiveness of foscarnet compared with ganciclovir for the immediate control of CMV infections is unknown. Further, the long-term effects of foscarnet or ganciclovir on CMV retinitis, survival, and morbidity are unknown. There is also no definitive information on the relative effectiveness and safety of deferred versus immediate treatment for CMV retinitis confined to zones 2 and 3.

Description

FGCRT was a multicenter, randomized, controlled, unmasked, clinical trial. Enrolment in the trial began in March 1990 and was completed in October 1991. 240 patients with previously untreated CMV retinitis who enrolled in this trial were assigned randomly to treatment with either foscarnet or ganciclovir. In October 1991, the treatment protocol was suspended due to a greater mortality in the ganciclovir-assigned group.

Prior to randomization, patients were assigned to one of two strata based upon the location and the extent of retinitis in the more severely involved eye:
1. Patients with any retinitis in zone 1 (posterior pole) or patients with extensive retinitis involving 25% or more of zones 2 and 3 (peripheral retina)
2. Patients in whom retinitis is confined to <25% of zones 2 and 3 of the retina.

Half the patients in group 1 got immediate treatment with ganciclovir; the other half received immediate treatment with foscarnet. Patients in group 2 were treated with foscarnet or ganciclovir either immediately or treatment was deferred. Patients preferring to choose either immediate treatment or deferral (treatment preference design) were randomized only to foscarnet or ganciclovir for treatment of CMV retinitis. Patients in the deferral group were started on drug treatment when the retinitis became more immediately sight-threatening by virtue of either location (involvement of zone 1) or size (extent >25% of the retina).

Inclusion Criteria

Males and females eligible for the FGCRT must have been 13 years or older and have had AIDS (CDC definition) or laboratory confirmation of HIV infection and CMV retinitis. They could not have received previous treatment with an anti-CMV drug for their CMV retinitis. Furthermore, they must have had an absolute neutrophil count (ANC) ≥ 1,000 cells/mL and a serum creatinine ≤ 2.0 mg/dL in order to tolerate either drug.

Study Measures

Outcome measures included survival, retinitis progression, visual function (visual acuity and VF), drug side effects, and morbidity.

Results

- The efficacy of the two drugs in controlling the CMV retinitis as measured by the time to first progression was similar. The relative risk for progression of the retinitis was 0.97 (ganciclovir vs. foscarnet; $p = 0.833$), and the median time to first progression was 53 days in the foscarnet-assigned patients compared with 47 days in the ganciclovir-assigned patients ($p = 0.997$), as determined by a masked reading at a central fundus photograph reading center. By 120 days after randomization, progression was observed in 85% of patients in each treatment group.
- Visual acuity outcomes were similar for both groups; at 6 months after randomization, 88% of the foscarnet-assigned patients and 93% of the ganciclovir-assigned patients had a best-corrected visual acuity of 20/40 or better in the better eye ($p = 0.325$).
- VF scores were similar in the two groups; in all eyes affected with CMV retinitis, there was a mean 29°/month loss of VF in foscarnet-assigned patients compared with a 31°/month loss in ganciclovir-assigned patients ($p = 0.674$).
- On October 7, 1991, the trial's independent Policy and Data Monitoring Board recommended suspending the protocol because the data indicated that patients treated with foscarnet lived on average 4 months longer than those treated with ganciclovir. The median survival for those treated with

foscarnet was approximately 12 months, compared to 8 months for those treated with ganciclovir. The difference in survival could not be explained by variations in disease severity at the time the patients entered the study or by other chance factors. The difference in mortality between the foscarnet-treated patients and the ganciclovir-treated patients could also not be fully explained by differential antiretroviral use. However, the trial was not designed to study possible interactions between anti-CMV and anti-HIV treatments. Therefore, such an explanation cannot be ruled out.

- While a survival benefit for foscarnet was seen in most patients, in the group of patients who entered the study with a predicted creatinine clearance < 1.2 mL/min/kg, a survival benefit was seen for ganciclovir.

Conclusion

Although foscarnet was associated with a longer survival than ganciclovir, the two drugs appear equivalent in controlling CMV retinitis and preserving vision. Foscarnet may be the preferable initial treatment for CMV retinitis. A possible exception is the subgroup of patients with decreased renal function (predicted creatinine clearance < 1.2 mL/min/kg) who appeared to do better on ganciclovir.

Table 1: Summary of clinical trials AIDS in ophthalmology.

Title	Purpose	No. of patients	Inclusion criteria	Result/Conclusion
LSOCA 1998	Monitor incidence of CMV retinitis and other ocular complications of AIDS and effect of HAART on these	1,632	Patients ≥ 13 years with diagnosis of AIDS	• There is decline in the incidence of CMV retinitis from the pre-HAART era • In the HAART era, CMV retinitis is associated with intraocular inflammation • The rate of retinitis progression, second eye involvement, and RD was reduced among patients in the HAART era • CMV retinitis is associated with a substantial risk of vision loss and visual field loss even in the era of HAART thought it is reduced compared to the pre-HAART era
FGCRT 1990	Foscarnet versus ganciclovir for the treatment of CMV retinitis	240	Patients ≥ 13 years with AIDS or HIV infection and CMV retinitis	• Foscarnet was associated with a longer survival than ganciclovir • The two drugs appear equivalent in controlling CMV retinitis and preserving vision

(CMV: cytomegalovirus; HAART: highly active anti-retroviral therapy)

REFERENCES

1. Studies of the Ocular Complications of AIDS Research Group; Jabs DA, Natta MLV, Holbrook JT, Kempen JH, Meinert CL, et al. Longitudinal study of the ocular complications of AIDS: 1. Ocular diagnoses at enrollment. Ophthalmology. 2007;114:780-6.
2. Studies of the Ocular Complications of AIDS Research Group; Jabs DA, Natta MLV, Holbrook JT, Kempen JH, Meinert CL, et al.. Longitudinal study of the ocular complications of AIDS: 2. Ocular examination results at enrollment. Ophthalmology. 2007;114:787-93.
3. Studies of Ocular Complications of AIDS Research Group; Jabs DA, Holbrook JT, Natta MLV, Clark R, Jacobson MA, et al. Risk factors for mortality in patients with AIDS in the era of highly active antiretroviral therapy. Ophthalmology. 2005;112:771-9.
4. Studies of the Ocular Complications of AIDS Research Group. Incidence of cytomegalovirus retinitis in the era of highly active antiretroviral therapy. Am J Ophthalmol. 2012;153:1016-24.e5.
5. Studies of Ocular Complications of AIDS Research Group; Jabs DA, Natta MVL, Thorne JE, Weinberg DV, Meredith TA, et al. Course of cytomegalovirus retinitis in the era of highly active antiretroviral therapy: 1. Retinitis progression. Ophthalmology. 2004;111:2224-31.
6. Studies of Ocular Complications of AIDS Research Group; Jabs DA, Natta MVL, Thorne JE, Weinberg DV, Meredith TA, et al. Course of cytomegalovirus retinitis in the era of highly active antiretroviral therapy: 2. Second eye involvement and retinal detachment. Ophthalmology. 2004;111:2232-9.
7. Studies of Ocular Complications of AIDS Research Group; Jabs DA, Ahuja A, Natta MV, Lyon A, Srivastava S, et al. Course of cytomegalovirus retinitis in the era of highly active antiretroviral therapy: Five-year outcomes. Ophthalmology. 2010;117:2152-61.e2.
8. Studies of Ocular Complications of AIDS Research Group; Thorne JE, Jabs DA, Kempen JH, Holbrook JT, Nichols C, et al. Incidence of and risk factors for visual acuity loss among patients with AIDS and cytomegalovirus retinitis in the era of highly active antiretroviral therapy. Ophthalmology. 2006;113:1432-40.
9. Studies of Ocular Complications of AIDS Research Group; Thorne JE, Jabs DA, Kempen JH, Holbrook JT, Nichols C, et al. Causes of visual acuity loss among patients with AIDS and cytomegalovirus retinitis in the era of highly active antiretroviral therapy. Ophthalmology. 2006;113:1441-5.
10. Studies of Ocular Complications of AIDS Research Group; Thorne JE, Natta MLV, Jabs DA, Duncan JL, Srivastava SK. Visual field loss in patients with cytomegalovirus retinitis. Ophthalmology. 2011;118:895-901.
11. Studies of the Ocular Complications of AIDS (SOCA) Research Group; Gangaputra S, Drye L, Vaidya V, Thorne JE, Jabs DA, et al. Non-cytomegalovirus ocular opportunistic infections in patients with acquired immunodeficiency syndrome. Am J Ophthalmol. 2013;155:206-12.e5.
12. Studies of ocular complications of AIDS Foscarnet-Ganciclovir Cytomegalovirus Retinitis Trial: 1. Rationale, design, and methods. AIDS Clinical Trials Group (ACTG). Control Clin Trials. 1992;13:22-39.
13. Foscarnet-Ganciclovir Cytomegalovirus Retinitis Trial: 4. Visual outcomes. Studies of Ocular Complications of AIDS Research Group in collaboration with the AIDS Clinical Trials Group. Ophthalmology. 1994;101:1250-61.
14. Foscarnet-Ganciclovir Cytomegalovirus Retinitis Trial: 5. Clinical features of cytomegalovirus retinitis at diagnosis. Studies of ocular complications of AIDS Research Group in collaboration with the AIDS Clinical Trials Group. Am J Ophthalmol. 1997;124:141-57.

Index

Page numbers followed by *t* refer to table.

A

Acetonide 111
ACG *See* Angle closure glaucoma
Acute spinal cord injury, treatment of 385
Acyclovir 3
    prevention trial 3
Advanced glaucoma 37
    intervention study 36
Aflibercept 118, 174, 175
    group 174, 176
Age-related choroidal neovascularization 233
Age-related eye disease study 273, 276, 282
Age-related macular degeneration 109, 171, 186, 188, 194, 195, 202, 237, 249, 253, 257, 258, 273, 275
    clinical trials in 186, 207, 245*t*, 253, 273, 281*t*
    prevention trial, complication of 278, 282
    subfoveal neovascular 220
    treatment of 191
        trials 230
Ahmed glaucoma valve 49
Albuminuria 81
Allergen 132
Allograft reaction episodes 12
Amblyopia 328, 337
    clinical trials in 328
    treatment 359
        index 330
        study 328, 331-335, 338, 340, 342-344, 346, 347, 349, 350, 352-355, 357-360, 363*t*
    vision therapy for 349
Amblyopic eye 363*t*
Amikacin 296
Andhra Pradesh Eye Disease Study 59
Angioid streaks 188
Angle closure glaucoma 60, 64, 65*t*, 74
    diagnosis of 58
Antiangiogenic drugs 133, 135
Antiglaucoma medications 14, 45

Antihypertensive drug therapy, moderate 85
Anti-retroviral therapy, active 402, 412
Anti-vascular endothelial growth factor 109, 210, 309
    therapy 109, 120
    treatment 147
Applanation tonometry 62
Aravind Comprehensive Eye Survey 61
Argon laser
    trabeculoplasty 27
    treatment 39
Argon study 186, 188
Aspergillus species 6
Aspirin 97
Atenolol 83
Atropine 331, 339, 347
    eye drops 346
    protocol 329
Autorefraction 127
Avastin 227, 228, 310

B

Bacterial endophthalmitis 295
    management of 295
    postoperative 295
Bacterial keratitis 8
Baseline vision 119
BCVA *See* Best corrected visual acuity
Benzoporphyrin 190
Best-corrected visual acuity 31, 53, 101, 110, 127, 132, 141, 151, 183, 201, 202, 219, 224, 255, 271, 389
    score 194
Beta blocker betaxolol 27
Beta radiation epiretinal therapy 264
Bevacizumab 109, 118, 140, 146, 147, 174, 175, 227, 228, 230, 231, 237, 309
    group 139
    treatment 175
    use of 140
Bilateral refractive amblyopia 343
    treatment of 344

Biopsy 296
Blepharitis 4
Blood
    glucose 86
        control 83
        group B 199
    pressure 86
        control 85, 88, 89
        duration of 79
    samples 12
    tests 374
Brain, magnetic resonance imaging of 376
Branch retinal vein 165, 177
    occlusion 153, 183
Branch vein occlusion study 153
Brolucizumab 148, 243
BRVO *See* Branch retinal vein occlusion

C

Canaloplasty
    groups 44
    results of 43
Captopril 83
Cardiovascular disease, risk of 97
Cataract 145, 198, 276, 405
    extraction 42, 43, 84
    formation 146
    grading 59
    progression 170
    surgery 67, 105, 114, 115, 145, 325
Ceftazidime 296
Center for Disease Control and
    Prevention 403
Central corneal
    measurement 31
    scarring 10
    thickness 53, 166
Central foveal thickness 127, 151, 183, 220
Central keratometry 16
Central macula 122
Central macular thickness 127, 140, 146, 256
Central nervous system 372
Central retinal
    thickness 137, 151, 217, 219, 239
    vein occlusion 54, 156, 167, 171, 173, 178, 183
Central subfield macular thickness 166
Central vein occlusion study 156
Central-involved diabetic macular
    edema 121
    treatment for 120
Cerebrovascular accident 135, 136
CFT *See* Central foveal thickness
Chennai Glaucoma Study 63
Choriocapillaris 190
Choroidal melanoma 396, 398

Choroidal neovascularization 25, 202, 203*t*, 207, 210, 249, 253, 257, 258, 264, 279, 282
Chronic inflammation, cycle of 15
Clear lens extraction 45, 47
Clinically isolated syndrome 375
Clinically significant macular edema 88, 95, 101, 151
CMT *See* Central macular thickness
Collaborative initial glaucoma treatment
    study 29
Collaborative ocular melanoma study
    396, 400*t*
Color vision 93
Confirmed microbiologic growth 297
Conjunctival hemorrhage 141, 172, 217
Conjunctival sac 52
Conjunctivitis 4
Contact lenses 16, 324
Contralateral eye involvement 406
Contrast sensitivity testing 303
Cornea 40
    clinical trials in 1, 20*t*
    donor study 13
Corneal allograft 12
Corneal astigmatism 16
Corneal endothelial cell density 13
Corneal scarring 10
Corneal tissue 1
Corneal transplantation 12
    studies, collaborative 11
Corneal ulcers trial, steroid in 8
Corticosteroid 120, 131
    treatment 2
Cotton-wool spots 91
Creatinine clearance 86
CRT *See* Central retinal thickness
CRVO *See* Central retinal vein occlusion
Cryotherapy 301, 303, 304
    multicenter trial of 301
CSME *See* Clinically significant
    macular edema
Cycloplegic refraction 16
Cytomegalovirus 402, 403, 405-407, 409, 410, 412

D

De novo glaucoma procedure 51
Deferred panretinal photocoagulation 116
Dense macular hemorrhage 162
Denver developmental screening test 306
Dexamethasone 132, 144, 145, 146-148, 168, 175, 177-179
    dose of 169
    group 178
    implant 147

intravitreal implant 168
single-dose 177
Diabetes
complications of 80
type 2 85
control 88, 113
and complications trial 80
duration of 79
effect of 113
epidemiology of 88
interventions and complications, epidemiology of 82
macula in 132
related deaths 85
treatment of 80
Diabetes mellitus 134, 151
insulin-dependent 88
non-insulin-dependent 85
type 1 141, 142
type 2 79, 83, 96, 141, 142
Diabetic macular edema 101, 103, 127, 136, 137, 143, 144, 146, 147, 151
development of 107
focal photocoagulation for 111
management of 139, 198
mild 106
pharmacotherapy in 149*t*
study, center-involved 114
treatment for 108-110, 115, 134
vision-impairing 118
Diabetic retinopathy 78-80, 83, 86, 87*t*, 101, 103, 115, 127, 131, 153, 188
clinical research network 103
clinical trials in 78, 90, 103, 131
landmark trials in 101*t*
regression of 91
risk of 121
study 90, 101
vitrectomy study 98, 101
Diabetic vascular complications 85
Disc stereophotographs 39
Disease-modifying therapies 376
Diurnal intraocular pressure 69
DME *See* Diabetic macular edema
Docosahexaenoic acid 282
Donor cornea, characteristics of 14
Dorzolamide 34
DR *See* Diabetic retinopathy
DRS *See* Diabetic retinopathy study
DRVS *See* Diabetic retinopathy vitrectomy study
Dry eye 15
disease 15
symptoms 15

E

Early lens extraction 45, 47
Early manifest glaucoma trial 27, 73
Early proliferative retinopathy 96
Early treatment diabetic retinopathy 101
study 46, 93, 133, 159, 291, 300
chart 256, 263
vision test 328
Edema, ranibizumab for 132
Eicosapentaenoic acid 22, 276
EMGT *See* Early manifest glaucoma trial
Emotional stress 4
Endophthalmitis 106, 117, 122, 138, 254
vitrectomy study 295, 299, 300t
Endothelial damage 190
Endothelial function 16
Endothelial tight junction proteins 168
Epimacular brachytherapy 264
Epiretinal membrane 18, 405
Epithelial keratitis 4
ETDRS *See* Early treatment diabetic retinopathy study
European Glaucoma Prevention Study 32, 33
Expanded disability status scale 379, 382, 383
Extracapsular cataract extraction 299
Eye 30, 94, 99, 100, 120, 170, 188
affected 6
course of 35
indicated for 97
involvement, second 406
natural history for 160
nepafenac in 115
number of 117
pain 141, 172
photocoagulation for 92
progression of 108
refractory 147, 148
treatment-naive 176
untreated 188

F

Fasting plasma glucose 84
Fibrocellular tissue 200
Fibrovascular proliferations 99
Fibrovascular tissue 200
Filtering surgery 35
Financial stress 4
First trabeculectomy fail 36
Fleischer's ring 10
Fluocinolone acetonide 143
sustained-release 131
Fluorescein angiography 138, 159, 187, 188, 211, 225, 235
Fluorouracil filtering surgery study 40
Focal laser photocoagulation 190

Focal photocoagulation 106
Foscarnet-ganciclovir cytomegalovirus
    retinitis trial 409
Fovea 154, 158
    avascular zone 186
Foveal study 186, 188
Fuchs' dystrophy 13
Fundus fluorescein
    angiograms 155
    angiography 132, 159
Fundus photographs 103
Fungal corneal ulcers 5
Fusarium species 6

G

Ganciclovir 410
Glasgow coma scale score 388
Glasses 16
Glaucoma 14, 27, 42, 58, 62, 63, 169
    clinical trials in 27
    detection of 62
    epidemiological studies of 57, 74*l*
    filtering surgery 40
    landmark trials in 72*l*
    laser in 66
    laser trial 39
        follow-up study 38
    medication 49, 51
        number of 68
    neovascular 54, 92, 99
    prevalence of 57, 62, 63
    research foundation 73
    secondary 62
    surgery 14, 46, 144
        risk of future 66
    uncontrolled 176
Glaucomatous optic nerve 62
Glial dysfunction 147
Glycated hemoglobin 79
Glycemic control 82
    duration of 79
Goldmann perimetry 95, 303
Gonioscopy 62
Good vision, chances of 100
Good visual acuity 196
Graft rejection, risk of 14
Gram stain 297
Gram-negative organisms 298

H

Head injury trial 387
Health and vision, perception of 198
Hematology testing 132
Hemiretinal vein occlusion 162

Hemorrhage 200
    preretinal 164
    retinal 159, 164
    suprachoroidal 42
Hereditary optic disease outpatient study,
    rescue of 390, 391
Herpes simplex virus
    epithelial keratitis trial 3
    eye disease 4
Herpes simplex virus
    infection 3
    iridocyclitis 2
    management of 1
Herpes stromal keratitis 1, 2
Herpetic eye disease 1, 3
    management of 3
Horizon study 67
Hyperglycemia 84
    severe 81

I

Idiopathic neovascular membranes 202
Immune recovery uveitis 403
Implantable dexamethasone 168
Indocyanine green angiography 260
Infant aphakia treatment study 324, 325, 327*l*
Infectious endophthalmitis 163
Infectious keratitis 5
Inflammatory cells 168
Influence glaucoma 27
Insulin 83, 84
    injections 81
    therapy 83
Intensive blood glucose control 84
International Optic Nerve Trauma Study 387
International Retina Group 147
Interquartile range 140
Intraocular injections 134, 166, 168
Intraocular lens 295, 324, 327
    implantation 47
Intraocular pressure 42, 45, 51, 64, 65, 73, 92,
    104, 131, 158, 183
    elevation of 67
Intraocular ranibizumab 217
Intraocular steroids 135
Intraocular surgery 176
Intraoperative optical coherence
    tomography 17
Intraretinal edema 256
Intravitreal administration 171
Intravitreal aflibercept 118, 267, 271
    injection, safety of 175
Intravitreal bevacizumab 108, 131, 139, 146,
    234, 312
    monotherapy 312

Intravitreal corticosteroid injection 163
Intravitreal dexamethasone 146
Intravitreal injections 122, 131, 145, 162,
    171, 309
    safety of 167
Intravitreal lucentis, safety assessment of 221
Intravitreal ranibizumab 110, 111, 113, 116,
    117, 127, 271
Intravitreal steroids 109
Intravitreal triamcinolone 144, 164
    acetonide 127
Intravitreous bevacizumab 140
IOP *See* Intraocular pressure
Iridocyclitis 4
Iris neovascularization 183
Iritis 4
Ischemic central retinal vein occlusion,
    treatment of 54
Ischemic heart disease 79
Ischemic optic neuropathy decompression
    trial 388
IVR *See* Intravitreal ranibizumab
IVTA *See* Intravitreal triamcinolone
    acetonide

J

Jupiter study 69

K

Kaplan-Meier analysis 209
Keratitis 4
Keratoconus
    corneal scarring in 10
    evaluation of 9
    mild-to-moderate 10
Keratometry 326
Keratopathy 12
Kidney diseases 80
Krypton study 186, 188, 189

L

Landolt C chart 266
Laser 137
    monotherapy 137
    peripheral iridotomy 45
    photocoagulation 127, 137, 154, 175,
        186, 190, 202*t*
        role of 93
    therapy 139, 309
    trabeculoplasty failure 38
    treatment 39, 190
Laser-ranibizumab-triamcinolone study 109
Latanoprost 71
    monotherapy 71

Later perfluoropropane 284
Leber's hereditary optic neuropathy 390
Lens 40, 324
Lesion
    neovascular 188
    subgroup analyses of 196
    type of 186
Less severe retinopathy 96
Leukocyte
    movement 168
    recruitment 147
Lipid concentrations 86
Longitudinal optic neuritis study 373
Lower-extremity amputation 79
LP *See* Laser photocoagulation
Lucentis 134, 210
Lumbar puncture 374
Lymphocytotoxic antibodies 12

M

Macula 96
Macular edema 92, 95, 107, 118, 132, 134,
        136, 153, 157, 161, 163, 165, 168,
        179, 183, 255, 405
    development of 116
    duration of 169
    photocoagulation on 96
    treatment for 161, 165, 171
Macular grid laser photocoagulation 160
Macular laser 135
    photocoagulation 141
    procedures 136
Macular photocoagulation study 186
Macular program 58
Manifest refraction 10
Manual refraction 112
Mean binocular visual acuity 344
Menstrual periods 4
Mercury trial 71
Metamorphopsia score 291
Metformin 83, 84
Methylprednisolone 385, 386
Mild macular grid 127
Mitomycin C 42
MMG *See* Mild macular grid
Monoclonal antibody fragment 131
Monocular visual impairment 328
Monofocal episode 375
Multicenter cohort study 224
Multifocal episode 375
Multiple sclerosis 372, 374, 375, 381, 394
    study, early treatment of 380
    trial outcomes index, functional
        assessment of 383
Mycotic infections 7

Mycotic ulcer treatment trial 5, 7
Myocardial infarction 135
Myopia 63
    high 188
    pathologic 193, 194
Myopic choroidal neovascularization 194

N

Naloxone 385, 386
National Acute Spinal Cord Injury Study 385
National Eye Institute 5, 73, 90, 328
National Health Service 233
National Institute of Diabetes 80
National Institutes of Health 301
Neovascular age-related macular degeneration 207, 223, 225, 227, 243
    treatment of 225, 242
Neovascular complications, treatment of 162
Neovascular proliferation, active 100
Neovascularization, development of 153, 154, 156
Nephropathy 80
Netarsudil 71
    drop of 71
Neuronal cell death 147
Neuro-ophthalmology, clinical trials in 372, 393*t*
Neuropathy 80, 86
Neurosensory retina 190
Nocardia ulcers 9
Nonarteritic anterior ischemic optic neuropathy 388
Non-contact specular microscopy 326
Noncytomegalovirus ocular opportunistic infections 40
Nonfatal myocardial infarctions 136
Non-fusarium group 7
Noninfectious endophthalmitis 163
Non-nocardia ulcer 9
Nonocular safety 168
Nonproliferative diabetic retinopathy 90, 95, 127
Nonproliferative retinopathy, mild to moderate 81
Nonrandomized small tumor pilot study 398
Non-staphylococcus epidermidis 298
Normal tension glaucoma study, collaborative 34
NPDR *See* Nonproliferative diabetic retinopathy

O

OAG *See* Open-angle glaucoma
Occlusion therapy 328, 331
Ocular herpes simplex infection 4
Ocular histoplasmosis syndrome 198
Ocular hyperemia 141
Ocular hypertension 32, 69, 70, 73, 74, 169
    study 66
    treatment of 30, 52
Ocular hypotensive medication 32
Ocular inflammation 176
Ocular motility 326
Ocular neovascularization 208
Ocular treatment index 325
OHT *See* Ocular hypertension
Omega-3 long-chain polyunsaturated fatty acids 276
Open-angle glaucoma 27, 43, 52, 59, 63, 65, 70, 73, 74
    results of 64*t*
Open-label randomized controlled trial 319
Ophthalmic diseases, management of 17
Ophthalmology, clinical trials aids in 412*t*
Ophthalmoscopy, indirect 99
Optic disc 31, 32
Optic nerve
    evidence of 39
    typical 44
Optic neuritis 372
    treatment 373
    trial 372
Optical biometry 326
Optical coherence tomography 17, 105, 211, 217, 227, 255
Oral acyclovir, efficacy of 1
Oral voriconazole 7
Ozurdex 132

P

PACG *See* Primary angle closure glaucoma
Panretinal photocoagulation 90, 106, 116, 127, 135, 183
    treatment to 111
Parenting stress index 325
Pars plana vitrectomy 284, 290, 293, 296, 300
Patching protocol 329
PDR *See* Proliferative diabetic retinopathy
Pediatric eye disease 363*t*
    investigator group 328, 349
Pegaptanib 209
    sodium 208
Penetrating keratoplasty 3
Peribulbar triamcinolone acetonide 106
Peripheral diabetic retinopathy lesions 121
Peripheral retinal
    ablation 309
    vessels, development of 312
Peripheral vision, loss of 116
Phakic eyes 43

Pharmacotherapy 116
Photodynamic therapy 191, 202, 203t, 210, 253, 266, 271
   application of 190
Photokeratoscopy 16
Pigmentary glaucoma 29, 44
Placebo 386
   controlled clinical trial 376
Placental growth factor 171
Pneumatic retinopexy 290, 292
POAG See Primary open-angle glaucoma
Point-of-care glycated hemoglobin 113
Polymorphous dystrophy, posterior 13
Polypoidal choroidal vasculopathy 257, 261, 267, 271
   treatment of 266
Port delivery system 225
Prednisolone phosphate 1
Presumed ocular histoplasmosis 186, 202
Primary angle closure glaucoma 46, 58, 65, 66, 74
   treatment of 45, 47
Primary open-angle glaucoma 64, 74
Primary rhegmatogenous retinal detachment 290
   management of 290
Proliferative diabetic retinopathy 79, 90, 116, 127, 133
   development of high-risk 96
   severe 99
Proliferative retinopathy 90
Proteinuria, gross 79
PRP See Panretinal photocoagulation
Pseudoexfoliation 44
   glaucoma 29
Pseudophakia 405
Pseudophakic corneal edema 13
Pseudophakic eyes 147
Pulse oximetry 314

R

Radial keratotomy 16
   prospective evaluation of 16
Radiation therapy 264
Randomized clinical trial 261, 342, 348, 376
Randot preschool stereoacuity test 336
Ranibizumab 109, 110, 117, 118, 131, 134, 136, 165, 166, 177-179, 210, 212, 216, 225, 230, 253, 254, 260, 266, 271, 319, 320
   efficacy and safety of 216, 261
   efficacy of 136
   extension trial of 223
   injection 111, 134
   monotherapy 137, 138, 258, 260

   safety of 177, 178
   study of 219
   treatment 177
Refraction 57
Rehabilitative services 78
Renal disease, severe 99
Residual subretinal fluid 19
Restore lost vision 135
Retina 40
Retinal capillary perfusion 161
Retinal detachment 99, 106, 163, 198, 406
   clinical trials in 284, 293t
   management of 284
   rates of 299
Retinal disorders 103
Retinal glial cell 147
Retinal hemorrhages, extensive 91
Retinal ophthalmology 113
Retinal photographs 84
Retinal pigment epithelium 190
Retinal thickening 106, 107, 114, 148
   measurement of 114
Retinal vascular
   disease 158
   occlusions, clinical trials in 153, 180t
Retinal vein occlusion 153, 168, 175, 179
   comparative treatments for 174
   corticosteroid for 161
Retinitis 402, 403, 405-407, 409, 410
   previously diagnosed 403
   progression 403, 406
Retinopathy 176
   progression of 92
   severe 96
   stage of 92
Retinopathy of prematurity 301, 312, 319
   clinical trials in 301, 321t
   cryotherapy for 301
   effects of light reduction on 315
Retinopathy of prematurity study
   early treatment for 304
   high oxygen percentage in 314
   photographic screening for 316
Retinotomy 286
Rhegmatogenous retinal detachment 200, 201, 287, 293
Rhopressa 70
Rocket trial 70

S

Scanning laser ophthalmoscopy 32
Scleral buckling 287
Scleral flap 42
Selective laser trabeculoplasty 51
Severe vision loss, development of 91

Sham treatment 191
Silicone oil
    removal 286
    study 284
Silicone study 286
    classification system 286
    long-term outcome in 286
Slit-lamp
    biomicroscopy 62
    photograph 159
Smoking, history of 14
Snellen equivalent 138
Spectral-domain ocular coherence
        tomography 225
Staphylococcus
    aureus 297, 298
    epidermidis 298
    haemolyticus 298
    lugdunensis 298
Stereoscopic fundus evaluation 59
Steroid
    inflammatory action of 8
    related toxicities 163
    treatment 2
Stromal keratitis, development of 4
Subclinical diabetic macular edema
        study 108
Subfoveal lesions 188
Subfoveal recurrent 189
Submacular surgery 198, 201
    trials 198, 199, 204*t*
Subretinal fluid 254
Subretinal pigment epithelial fluid 256
Subtenon's injections 106
Sulfonylurea 83, 84
Sulfur hexafluoride 284
Sun exposure 4
Supplemental therapeutic oxygen 312
Systemic antibiotics 297
    role of 295
Systemic bevacizumab therapy 227

T

Teller acuity card procedure 306
Therapeutic keratoplasty 6, 7
Titmustest 336
Tonometry 326
Topical antibiotics 122
Topical antiglaucoma agents 31
Topical corticosteroids 2
Topical natamycin 8
Topical prednisolone phosphate 8
Topical steroids, receiving 2
Topical therapy 45
Topical trifluridine 4

Torpedo trial 255
Total macular volume 122
Trabeculectomy 42, 43, 45, 145
    group 43, 45
    study 42
Transient photosensitivity reactions 192
Transient visual disturbances 197
Traumatic optic neuropathy 385
Triamcinolone 109, 110, 111
Trifluridine prophylaxis 2

U

Ultrasonic corneal thickness 16
Urinalysis 132
Urine albumin 84

V

VA *See* Visual acuity 183
Vancomycin 296
Vascular endothelial growth factor 131, 183,
        207, 249, 253
    inhibition study 208
    trap-eye 238, 240
VEGF *See* Vascular endothelial growth factor
Vellore eye study 57
Verteporfin 190-193, 196, 210
    photodynamic therapy 190, 193,
            261, 271
    efficacy and safety of 260
    plus ranibizumab 257, 258
    therapy 193, 196, 197
        favor of 196
        use of 193
    treatment 193, 197
        group 195
Vision loss
    cause of 168
    from macular edema, risk for 154
    mild 119
    moderate 105, 195
    rate of 135
    severe 195
Vision related subscales 138
Vision specific quality 11
Visual activities 29
Visual acuity 29, 37, 41, 51, 57, 62, 84, 91, 99,
        100, 103, 120, 127, 133, 142,
        147, 159, 162, 164, 165, 188-190,
        192, 196, 199, 202, 208, 211, 215,
        221, 234, 254, 291, 327, 330, 331,
        333, 334, 339, 341, 346, 387
    course of 99
    improvement in 199, 350
    loss 191, 407
        risk of severe 201

masked assessment of 343
  measurements 164
    evaluation of 112
  monitoring 171
  reduced 172
  risk of 100
  spectacle-corrected 16
  stabilization 193
Visual benefit 144
Visual field 31, 93, 97, 404
  decrease of 38
  defects 389
  loss 27, 407
    advanced 28
  testing 303
Visual function 93
  preservation of 42
Visual impairment 138, 405
Visual improvement 119, 143, 170
Visual loss 35, 79, 92
Visual prognosis 298

Vitrectomy 97, 290, 295, 297
  early 98, 99
  evaluation of 105
  primary 287
Vitreomacular traction 105, 127
Vitreous hemorrhage 18, 99, 100, 113, 127, 158, 163, 164
  development of 154, 155
  experience 156
  severe 98, 99
Vitreous tap 296
Vogt's striae 10
Voriconazole 5, 6
Voyager study 52

X

Xenon technique 91

Z

Zidovudine 410

EU GSPR Authorised Reprsentative
Logos Europe, 9 rue Nicolas Poussin
1700, La Rochelle, France
Phone: +33 (0) 6 67 93 73 78
E-mail: contact@logoseurope.eu